W9-CDB-807

J. Michael Duncan, MD
6/2008

2008
YEAR BOOK OF
VASCULAR SURGERY®

The 2008 Year Book Series

Year Book of Anesthesiology and Pain Management™: Drs Chestnut, Abram, Black, Gravlee, Lee, Mathru, and Roizen

Year Book of Cardiology®: Drs Gersh, Cheitlin, Elliott, Graham, Sundt, and Waldo

Year Book of Critical Care Medicine®: Drs Dellinger, Parrillo, Balk, Bekes, Dorman, and Dries

Year Book of Dentistry®: Drs Olin, Belvedere, Davis, Henderson, Johnson, Ohrbach, Scott, Spencer, and Zakariasen

Year Book of Dermatology and Dermatologic Surgery™: Drs Thiers and Lang

Year Book of Diagnostic Radiology®: Drs Birdwell, Elster, Gardiner, Levy, Manaster, Oestreich, and Rosado de Christenson

Year Book of Emergency Medicine®: Drs Hamilton, Handly, Quintana, Werner, and Bruno

Year Book of Endocrinology®: Drs Mazzaferri, Bessesen, Clarke, Howard, Kennedy, Leahy, Meikle, Molitch, Rogol, and Schteingart

Year Book of Gastroenterology™: Drs Lichtenstein, Dempsey, Drebin, Jaffe, Katzka, Kochman, Makar, Morris, Osterman, Rombeau, and Shah

Year Book of Hand and Upper Limb Surgery®: Drs. Chang and Steinmann

Year Book of Medicine®: Drs Barkin, Berney, Frishman, Garrick, Loehrer, Phillips, and Khardori

Year Book of Neonatal and Perinatal Medicine®: Drs Fanaroff, Ehrenkranz, and Stevenson

Year Book of Neurology and Neurosurgery®: Drs Kim and Verma

Year Book of Obstetrics, Gynecology, and Women's Health®: Dr Shulman

Year Book of Oncology®: Drs Loehrer, Arceci, Glatstein, Gordon, Hanna, Morrow, and Thigpen

Year Book of Ophthalmology®: Drs Rapuano, Cohen, Eagle, Flanders, Hammersmith, Myers, Nelson, Penne, Sergott, Shields, Tipperman, and Vander

Year Book of Orthopedics®: Drs Morrey, Beauchamp, Huddleston, Peterson, Swiontkowski, and Trigg

Year Book of Otolaryngology-Head and Neck Surgery®: Drs Gapany, Keefe and Sindwani

Year Book of Pathology and Laboratory Medicine®: Drs Raab, Parwani, Bejarano, and Bissell

Year Book of Pediatrics®: Dr Stockman

Year Book of Plastic and Aesthetic Surgery™: Drs Miller, Bartlett, Garner, McKinney, Ruberg, Salisbury, and Smith

Year Book of Psychiatry and Applied Mental Health®: Drs Talbott, Ballenger, Buckley, Frances, Markowitz, and Sarles

Year Book of Pulmonary Disease®: Drs Phillips, Barker, Lewis, Maurer, Tanoue, and Willsie

Year Book of Sports Medicine®: Drs Shephard, Cantu, Feldman, Jankowski, McCrory, Nieman, Pierrynowski, Rowland, and Shrier

Year Book of Surgery®: Drs Copeland, Bland, Daly, Eberlein, Fahey, Jones, Mozingo, Pruett, and Seeger

Year Book of Urology®: Drs Andriole and Coplen

Year Book of Vascular Surgery®: Dr Moneta

2008

The Year Book of VASCULAR SURGERY®

Editor-in-Chief

Gregory L. Moneta, MD

Professor and Chief of Vascular Surgery, Oregon Health and Science University; and Chief of Vascular Surgery, Oregon Health and Science University Hospital and Portland VA Hospital, Portland, Oregon

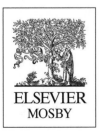

ELSEVIER
MOSBY

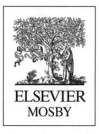

ELSEVIER
MOSBY

Vice President, Continuity: John A. Schrefer
Developmental Editor: Ruth Malwitz
Production Supervisor: Donna M. Adamson
Electronic Article Manager: Travis L. Ross
Illustrations and Permissions Coordinator: Dawn Vohsen

2008 EDITION

Printed in the United States of America
Composition by Thomas Technology Solutions, Inc.
Printing/binding by Sheridan Books, Inc

Editorial Office:
Elsevier
Suite 1800
1600 John F. Kennedy Blvd
Philadelphia, PA 19103-2899

International Standard Serial Number: 0749-4041
International Standard Book Number: 978-1-4160-5154-1

Contributors

David L. Cull, MD
Greenville Hospital System Professor of Clinical Surgery, University of South Carolina School of Medicine; Vice Chairman Surgical Research, Greenville Hospital System/University Medical Center, Greenville, South Carolina

Alan Dardik, MD, PhD
Assistant Professor of Surgery, Yale University School of Medicine; Attending Surgeon, VA Connecticut Healthcare System, West Haven, Connecticut

Mark A. Farber, MD
Associate Professor, Departments of Surgery and Radiology, and Medical Director, Endovascular Clinic, University of North Carolina School of Medicine, Chapel Hill, North Carolina

Nancy L. Harthun, MD
Associate Professor of Vascular and Endovascular Surgery, University of Virginia School of Medicine, Charlottesville, Virginia

Vikram S. Kashyap, MD, FACS
Staff, Departments of Vascular Surgery and Cell Biology, The Cleveland Clinic; Associate Professor, Division of Surgery, The Cleveland Clinic Lerner College of Medicine, Cleveland, Ohio

Brajesh K. Lal, MD
Associate Professor of Vascular Surgery and of Physiology, University of Medicine and Dentistry of New Jersey—New Jersey Medical School, Newark, New Jersey; Associate Professor of Biomedical Engineering, Stevens Institute of Technology, Hoboken, New Jersey

Table of Contents

Journals Represented

Journals represented in this YEAR BOOK are listed below.

American Journal of Cardiology
American Journal of Epidemiology
American Journal of Kidney Diseases
American Journal of Medicine
American Journal of Neuroradiology
American Journal of Physiology Heart and Circulation Physiology
American Journal of Physiology, Endocrinology and Metabolism
American Journal of Roentgenology
American Journal of Surgery
American Surgeon
Anesthesia and Analgesia
Annals of Internal Medicine
Annals of Surgery
Annals of Thoracic Surgery
Annals of Vascular Surgery
Archives of Surgery
Arthritis and Rheumatism
British Journal of Surgery
British Medical Journal
Chest
Circulation
Clinical Chemistry
Dermatologic Surgery
European Journal of Internal Medicine
European Journal of Vascular and Endovascular Surgery
Heart
Hypertension
International Journal of Cardiology
Journal of Computer Assisted Tomography
Journal of Neurology, Neurosurgery and Psychiatry
Journal of Neurosurgery
Journal of Surgical Research
Journal of Thoracic and Cardiovascular Surgery
Journal of Ultrasound in Medicine
Journal of Vascular Surgery
Journal of Vascular and Interventional Radiology: JVIR
Journal of the American College of Cardiology
Journal of the American College of Surgeons
Journal of the American Medical Association
Journal of the American Society of Nephrology
Kidney International
Lancet
Mayo Clinic Proceedings
Medicine
Neurology
New England Journal of Medicine
Radiology
Stroke
Surgery

Thrombosis Research
Vascular and Endovascular Surgery

STANDARD ABBREVIATIONS

The following terms are abbreviated in this edition: acquired immunodeficiency syndrome (AIDS), cardiopulmonary resuscitation (CPR), central nervous system (CNS), cerebrospinal fluid (CSF), computed tomography (CT), deoxyribonucleic acid (DNA), electrocardiography (ECG), health maintenance organization (HMO), human immunodeficiency virus (HIV), intensive care unit (ICU), intramuscular (IM), intravenous (IV), magnetic resonance (MR) imaging (MRI), ribonucleic acid (RNA), and ultrasound (US).

NOTE

The YEAR BOOK OF VASCULAR SURGERY® is a literature survey service providing abstracts of articles published in the professional literature. Every effort is made to assure the accuracy of the information presented in these pages. Neither the editors nor the publisher of the YEAR BOOK OF VASCULAR SURGERY® can be responsible for errors in the original materials. The editors' comments are their own opinions. Mention of specific products within this publication does not constitute endorsement.

To facilitate the use of the YEAR BOOK OF VASCULAR SURGERY® as a reference tool, all illustrations and tables included in this publication are now identified as they appear in the original article. This change is meant to help the reader recognize that any illustration or table appearing in the YEAR BOOK OF VASCULAR SURGERY® may be only one of many in the original article. For this reason, figure and table numbers will often appear to be out of sequence within the YEAR BOOK OF VASCULAR SURGERY®.

Introduction

Welcome to the 2008 YEAR BOOK OF VASCULAR SURGERY. I am sure those familiar with the YEAR BOOK will find this year's edition to be as informative and useful as previous editions. New readers are welcome and, hopefully, will come to appreciate the advantages of having a concise and comprehensive reference source where each article is carefully, but not always generously, critiqued by one of your peers.

In my 6 years as editor of the YEAR BOOK OF VASCULAR SURGERY I remember only one letter of complaint by someone who was disappointed with the YEAR BOOK OF VASCULAR SURGERY. That individual did not express disappointment with the content of the YEAR BOOK, but was unhappy his article had not been selected for inclusion in that year's edition. It was my decision not to include the article, and my prerogative as editor. I am ultimately responsible for what is included in the YEAR BOOK. Even my associate editors, who help tremendously with their enlightened comments, are asked to comment only upon articles I have selected for the YEAR BOOK. The YEAR BOOK OF VASCULAR SURGERY is a bit of a benevolent dictatorship in that regard. I do not ask Elsevier about my selections, and Elsevier never questions my selections for the YEAR BOOK or the commentaries of myself or my associate editors on those selections.

I review many hundreds of articles each year for possible selection in the YEAR BOOK. Sometimes, in retrospect, I have overlooked important articles. If any of you believe some article should be included in the YEAR BOOK, including your own work, send me a copy of the article, along with a letter explaining why the article is important. Such correspondence will be taken seriously. I still get to make the final decision. I would not edit the YEAR BOOK if I was told what to include or not include. However, while I insist on control of content and the final decision, I do not mind help with decisions.

Vascular surgeons are vascular specialists. We are technically talented, but also personally responsible for evaluating our patients, talking with their families, and the followup of our patients over time. This is crucial to maintaining vascular surgery as a viable specialty. One needs only to look at the current difficulties of our interventional radiology and cardiac surgical colleagues to understand this evolving medical paradigm. The goal is for the YEAR BOOK OF VASCULAR SURGERY to help vascular surgeons develop and maintain a broad knowledge base to ensure the continued vitality of our specialty. Knowledge, technical skill, a willingness to change, and dedication to long-term care of patients combine to make vascular surgery a thriving, and growing, specialty.

The YEAR BOOK is a team process. It is my pleasure to acknowledge the associate editors of the 2008 YEAR BOOK OF VASCULAR SURGERY and their contributions to the YEAR BOOK. These individuals are selected by me each year to participate in writing the comments that accompany each abstract. I appreciate their professionalism and willingness to give back to a profession that at times can seem so unforgiving and demanding.

My office staff works hard to transcribe the comments that accompany each abstract. Jenna Bowker, also in Portland, has for many years kept the whole YEAR BOOK process organized and running smoothly on my end. My principal contact at Elsevier is Ruth Malwitz. Both she and Elsevier are a pleasure to work with and are professional and savvy enough to keep me more or less on time and focused. I am sure there are times when both Ruth and Jenna feel they are roping the proverbial goat to keep this whole process going. I apologize for sometimes making their jobs a bit more difficult than they should be. This is probably Jenna's last year in helping with the YEAR BOOK. She is finishing nursing school and will be moving on in her career. Finally, my vascular surgical partners at Oregon Health and Science University (Gregory Landry, Timothy Liem, and Erica Mitchell) put up with the time required for me to put the YEAR BOOK together. It is good to have competent and understanding partners.

I hope everyone enjoys the YEAR BOOK. It is a great honor to be entrusted with the editorship of the YEAR BOOK, and no one learns more from each new edition than I do. As always, I welcome any comments on how the whole process can be improved.

Gregory L. Moneta, MD

1 Basic Considerations

Determinants of Arterial Wall Remodeling During Lipid-Lowering Therapy: Serial Intravascular Ultrasound Observations From the Reversal of Atherosclerosis With Aggressive Lipid Lowering Therapy (REVERSAL) Trial

Schoenhagen P, Tuzcu EM, Apperson-Hansen C, et al (Cleveland Clinic Found, Ohio)

Circulation 113:2826-2834, 2006

Background.—Coronary plaque progression and instability are associated with expansive remodeling of the arterial wall. However, the remodeling response during plaque-stabilizing therapy and its relationship to markers of lipid metabolism and inflammation are incompletely understood.

Methods and Results.—Serial intravascular ultrasound (IVUS) data from the Reversal of Atherosclerosis with Aggressive Lipid Lowering Therapy (REVERSAL) trial were obtained during 18 months of intensive versus moderate lipid-lowering therapy. In a subgroup of 210 patients, focal coronary lesions with mild luminal narrowing were identified. Lumen area, external elastic membrane (EEM) area, and plaque area were determined at the lesion and proximal reference sites at baseline and during follow-up. The remodeling ratio (RR) was calculated by dividing the lesion EEM area by the reference EEM area. The relationship between the change in remodeling, change in plaque area, lipid profile, and inflammatory markers was examined. At the lesion site, a progression in plaque area ($8.9\pm25.7\%$) and a decrease in the RR ($-3.0\pm11.2\%$) occurred during follow-up. In multivariable analyses, the percentage change in plaque area ($P<0.0001$), baseline RR ($P<0.0001$), baseline lesion lumen area (0.019), logarithmic value of the change in high-sensitivity C-reactive protein ($P=0.027$), and hypertension at baseline ($P=0.014$) showed a significant, direct relation with the RR at follow-up. Lesion location in the right coronary artery ($P=0.006$), percentage change in triglyceride levels ($P=0.049$), and age ($P=0.037$) demonstrated a significant, inverse relation with the RR at follow-up. Changes in LDL cholesterol, HDL cholesterol, and treatment group demonstrated no significant associations.

Conclusions.—Constrictive remodeling of the arterial wall was observed during plaque-stabilizing therapy with statin medications and appears related to their antiinflammatory effects.

▶ Plaque regression and stabilization appears to be accompanied by a reduction in vessel size. Correlation of these effects with C-reactive protein, but not serum levels of HDL or LDL cholesterol, suggests that drugs targeting arterial information may be more effective than just targeting measures of lipid metabolism. The anti-inflammatory effects of statins may turn out to be more important than their cholesterol-lowering effects.

G. L. Moneta, MD

Genetic polymorphisms of the platelet receptors P2Y$_{12}$, P2Y$_1$ and GP IIIa and response to aspirin and clopidogrel
Lev EI, Patel RT, Guthikonda S, et al (Baylor College of Medicine)
Thromb Res 119:355-360, 2007

Introduction.—There is wide variability in the responses of individual patients to aspirin and clopidogrel. Polymorphisms of several platelet receptors have been related to increased platelet aggregation. Therefore, we aimed to evaluate whether these polymorphisms are related to altered response to aspirin or clopidogrel.

Materials and Methods.—Patients ($n=120$) undergoing percutaneous coronary intervention who received aspirin for ≥ 1 week but not clopidogrel were included. Blood samples were drawn at baseline and 20–24h after a 300-mg clopidogrel dose. Aspirin insensitivity was defined as 5 µM ADP-induced aggregation $\geq 70\%$ and 0.5 mg/mL arachidonic acid-induced aggregation $\geq 20\%$. Clopidogrel insensitivity was defined as baseline minus post-treatment aggregation $\leq 10\%$ in response to 5 and 20 µM ADP. PlA polymorphism of glycoprotein IIIa, T744C polymorphism of the P2Y$_{12}$ gene and the 1622A>G polymorphism of the P2Y$_1$ gene were genotyped by polymerase chain reaction.

Results.—There were no differences in polymorphism frequencies between drug-insensitive vs. drug-sensitive patients. There were also no significant differences in response to aspirin (assessed by arachidonic acid-induced aggregation) or to clopidogrel (assessed by ADP-induced aggregation or activation markers) when patients were grouped according to genotype. The only trend observed was lower reduction in PAC-1 binding following clopidogrel in PlA$_2$ carriers ($P=0.065$).

Conclusions.—We did not find an association between polymorphisms in the platelet receptors GP IIIa, P2Y$_{12}$ or P2Y$_1$ and response to aspirin or clopidogrel in cardiac patients. These findings suggest that the variability in response to anti-platelet drugs is multi-factorial and is not caused only by single gene mutations.

▶ This study reaches somewhat different conclusions than others on this subject because it did not find an association between polymorphism of the platelet receptor (*A1/A2* gene) and aspirin insensitivity. Others[1] have found such a correlation. The authors studied slightly different patients and used slightly different assays than previous studies. This may be part of the explanation for their findings. It is also possible that various drug interactions, platelet turnover, drug absorption, and individual metabolism may also affect aspirin and clopidogrel sensitivity.

G. L. Moneta, MD

Reference

1. Szczeklik A, Undas A, Sanak M, Frolow M, Wegrzyn W. Relationship between bleeding time, aspirin and the P1A1/A2 polymorphism of platelet glycoprotein IIIa. *Br J Haematol.* 2000;110:965-967.

TCF7L2 Polymorphisms and Progression to Diabetes in the Diabetes Prevention Program

Florez JC, for the Diabetes Prevention Program Research Group (George Washington Univ, Rockville, Md)
N Engl J Med 355:241-250, 2006

Background.—Common polymorphisms of the transcription factor 7-like 2 gene (*TCF7L2*) have recently been associated with type 2 diabetes. We examined whether the two most strongly associated variants (rs12255372 and rs7903146) predict the progression to diabetes in persons with impaired glucose tolerance who were enrolled in the Diabetes Prevention Program, in which lifestyle intervention or treatment with metformin was compared with placebo.

Methods.—We genotyped these variants in 3548 participants and performed Cox regression analysis using genotype, intervention, and their interactions as predictors. We assessed the effect of genotype on measures of insulin secretion and insulin sensitivity at baseline and at one year.

Results.—Over an average period of three years, participants with the risk-conferring TT genotype at rs7903146 were more likely to have progression from impaired glucose tolerance to diabetes than were CC homozygotes (hazard ratio, 1.55; 95 percent confidence interval, 1.20 to 2.01; P<0.001). The effect of genotype was stronger in the placebo group (hazard ratio, 1.81; 95 percent confidence interval, 1.21 to 2.70; P=0.004) than in the metformin and lifestyle-intervention groups (hazard ratios, 1.62 and 1.15, respectively; P for the interaction between genotype and intervention not significant). The TT genotype was associated with decreased insulin secretion but not increased insulin resistance at baseline. Similar results were obtained for rs12255372.

Conclusions.—Common variants in *TCF7L2* seem to be associated with an increased risk of diabetes among persons with impaired glucose tolerance. The risk-conferring genotypes in *TCF7L2* are associated with impaired beta-cell function but not with insulin resistance.

▶ This important study adds to the understanding of progression from impaired glucose tolerance to diabetes. These authors found that variants of a transcription factor gene were associated with decreased insulin secretion. Understanding the molecular basis of a common chronic illness may lead to improved pharmacotherapy or targeting a particular treatment to a genetically defined patient group.

G. L. Moneta, MD

Treatment of Periodontitis and Endothelial Function
Tonetti MS, D'Aiuto F, Nibali L, et al (Univ of Connecticut, Farmington; Univ College London)
N Engl J Med 356:911-920, 2007

Background.—Systemic inflammation may impair vascular function, and epidemiologic data suggest a possible link between periodontitis and cardiovascular disease.

Methods.—We randomly assigned 120 patients with severe periodontitis to community-based periodontal care (59 patients) or intensive periodontal treatment (61). Endothelial function, as assessed by measurement of the diameter of the brachial artery during flow (flow-mediated dilatation), and inflammatory biomarkers and markers of coagulation and endothelial activation were evaluated before treatment and 1, 7, 30, 60, and 180 days after treatment.

Results.—Twenty-four hours after treatment, flow-mediated dilatation was significantly lower in the intensive-treatment group than in the control-treatment group (absolute difference, 1.4%; 95% confidence interval [CI], 0.5 to 2.3; P=0.002), and levels of C-reactive protein, interleukin-6, and the endothelial-activation markers soluble E-selectin and von Willebrand factor were significantly higher (P<0.05 for all comparisons). However, flow-mediated dilatation was greater and the plasma levels of soluble E-selectin were lower in the intensive-treatment group than in the control-treatment group 60 days after therapy (absolute difference in flow-mediated dilatation, 0.9%; 95% CI, 0.1 to 1.7; P=0.02) and 180 days after therapy (difference, 2.0%; 95% CI, 1.2 to 2.8; P<0.001). The degree of improvement was associated with improvement in measures of periodontal disease (r=0.29 by Spearman rank correlation, P=0.003). There were no serious adverse effects in either of the two groups, and no cardiovascular events occurred.

Conclusions.—Intensive periodontal treatment resulted in acute, short-term systemic inflammation and endothelial dysfunction. However, 6 months after therapy, the benefits in oral health were associated with improvement in endothelial function.

▶ The severity of periodontitis present in subjects of this study is likely present in no more than 0.5% to 1% of the adult U.S. population. Atherosclerosis is obviously considerably more common. It would be interesting to see if future studies can demonstrate improvement in endothelial function with periodontal treatment in patients with lesser degrees of periodontitis.

G. L. Moneta, MD

Chlamydia pneumoniae in foci of "early" calcification of the tunica media in arteriosclerotic arteries: an incidental presence?

Bobryshev YV, Lord RSA, Tran D (St Vincent's Hosp, Sydney, Australia; Univ of New South Wales, Sydney, Australia)
Am J Physiol Heart Circ Physiol 290:H1510-H1519, 2006

Only a few previous works investigated the involvement of *Chlamydia pneumoniae* (*Chlamydophila pneumoniae*) in arterial calcification. The present study investigated a possible association between *C. pneumoniae* and medial calcification. Carotid artery segments obtained by endarterectomy from 60 patients were examined by PCR and immunohistochemistry to identify the presence of *C. pneumoniae*. Arterial specimens showing double-positive ($n = 17$), double-negative ($n = 22$), and single-positive results ($n = 21$) were further analyzed by a combination of histology, immunohistochemistry, and electron microscopy. Medial calcification occurred in 10 of 17 (58.8%) *C. pneumoniae* double-positive arterial specimens, but no medial calcification was observed in any of 22 *C. pneumoniae* double-negative arterial specimens. Electron microscopy indicated *C. pneumoniae* in smooth muscle cells (SMCs) in foci of medial calcification. Medial SMCs showing damage to the cytoplasm and basement membrane contained the structures with the appearance of elementary, reticulate, and aberrant bodies of *C. pneumoniae*. The presence of *C. pneumoniae* in SMCs was confirmed by electron-microscopic immunocytochemistry. In the extracellular matrix, calcification was observed in *C. pneumoniae* aberrant bodies that exited the SMCs. The findings offer a new hypothesis of arterial calcification: they suggest that *C. pneumoniae* infection of medial SMCs may be associated with the pathophysiological events of arteriosclerotic calcification of the tunica media.

▶ There are two distinct forms of vascular calcification: intimal calcification, which occurs in the context of atherosclerosis, and medial calcification, which can occur without atherosclerosis. A variety of different mechanisms may contribute to vascular calcification. The present study suggests that the medial form of vascular calcification may be initiated by the infection of medial smooth muscle cells by *C pneumoniae*. Whether *C pneumoniae* is required for eventual narrowing of the arterial lumen or degeneration of the arterial wall is still unknown.

G. L. Moneta, MD

Plasma Sphingomyelin and Subclinical Artherosclerosis: Findings from the Multi-Ethnic Study of Atherosclerosis

Nelson JC, Jiang X-C, Tabas I, et al (Univ of Washington, Seattle; State Univ of New York, Brooklyn; Columbia Univ, New York)
Am J Epidemiol 163:903-912, 2006

Plasma sphingomyelin has been shown to be an independent risk factor for coronary heart disease, but the relation of plasma sphingomyelin to earlier, subclinical atherosclerotic disease has not been reported. The authors examined the association between plasma sphingomyelin and three measures of subclinical cardiovascular disease (carotid intimal-medial wall thickness, ankle-arm blood pressure index, and Agatston coronary artery calcium score) among 6,814 middle-aged, asymptomatic adults in the Multi-Ethnic Study of Atherosclerosis, which was initiated in 2000. The sphingomyelin level was positively correlated with lipids and the Framingham risk score ($p < 0.01$ for both), and the mean level was higher in women than men (50 (standard deviation (SD), 16) vs. 45 (SD, 15) mg/dl) ($p < 0.01$) and higher in never versus current smokers (49 (SD, 16) vs. 45 (SD, 17) mg/dl) ($p < 0.01$). Women with sphingomyelin levels of 60 or more mg/dl had more severe subclinical disease by all three measures than did the referent group with sphingomyelin levels of 39 or less mg/dl, although associations were not significant after multivariate adjustment for standard cardiovascular disease risk factors. Men with sphingomyelin levels of 60 or more mg/dl versus those with sphingomyelin levels of 39 or less mg/dl had higher calcium scores (135 vs. 99 Agatston units) ($p = 0.01$). These observations are consistent with the hypothesis that plasma sphingomyelin is in the biologic pathway that mediates the risk for subclinical disease attributable to standard cardiovascular disease risk factors.

▶ Sphingomyelin accumulates in atheromas in animal models and in human atheroma. Much sphingomyelin found in arteries arises from the synthesis within the arterial tissue.[1] However, synthesis of sphingomyelin within arterial tissue appears slow compared to the total amount accumulated, suggesting plasma levels of sphingomyelin may also contribute to accumulation of sphingomyelin within arterial tissue. The unadjusted data from this study provides some support that plasma sphingomyelin is a component of a pathway that mediates risk for subclinical disease attributable to traditional cardiovascular risk factors.

G. L. Moneta, MD

Reference

1. Zilversmit DB, McCandless EL, Jordan PH, Henley WS, Ackerman RF. The synthesis of phospholipids in human atheromatous lesions. *Circulation.* 1961;23: 370-375.

Differential effects of aging on limb blood flow in humans

Donato AJ, Uberoi A, Wray DW, et al (Univ of California, San Diego, La Jolla)
Am J Physiol Heart Circ Physiol 290:H272-H278, 2006

Aging appears to attenuate leg blood flow during exercise; in contrast, such data are scant and do not support this contention in the arm. Therefore, to determine whether aging has differing effects on blood flow in the arm and leg, eight young (22 ± 6 yr) and six old (71 ± 15 yr) subjects separately performed dynamic knee extensor [0, 3, 6, 9 W; 20, 40, 60% maximal work rate (WR_{max}] and handgrip exercise (3, 6, 9 kg at 0.5 Hz; 20, 40, 60% WR_{max}). Arterial diameter, blood velocity (Doppler ultrasound), and arterial blood pressure (radial tonometry) were measured simultaneously at each of the submaximal workloads. Quadriceps muscle mass was smaller in the old (1.6 ± 0.1 kg) than the young (2.1 ± 0.2 kg). When normalized for this difference in muscle mass, resting seated blood flow was similar in young and old subjects (young, 115 ± 28; old, 114 ± 39 ml · kg^{-1} · min^{-1}). During exercise, blood flow and vascular conductance were attenuated in the old whether expressed in absolute terms for a given absolute workload or more appropriately expressed as blood flow per unit muscle mass at a given relative exercise intensity (young, 1,523 ± 329; old, 1,340 ± 157 ml · kg^{-1} · min^{-1} at 40% WR_{max}). In contrast, aging did not affect forearm muscle mass or attenuate rest or exercise blood flow or vascular conductance in the arm. In conclusion, aging induces limb-specific alterations in exercise blood flow regulation. These alterations result in reductions in leg blood flow during exercise but do not impact forearm blood flow.

▶ Vascular surgeons understand the increased propensity of atherosclerosis to localize to the legs compared to the arms. This study demonstrates that, in the same subjects, arm blood flow does not change with age, whereas leg blood flow and vascular conductance decrease with age, even when normalized to diminished muscle mass with aging. The mechanism for this association and its relationship to disease remains elusive.

G. L. Moneta, MD

Gene transfer of extracellular superoxide dismutase protects against vascular dysfunction with aging

Brown KA, Chu Y, Lund DD, et al (Univ of Iowa Roy J and Lucille A Carver College of Medicine, Iowa City; Veterans Med Ctr, Iowa City, Iowa)
Am J Physiol Heart Circ Physiol 290:H2600-H2605, 2006

Aging is an independent risk factor for cardiovascular disease, but mechanisms leading to vascular dysfunction have not been fully elucidated. Recent studies suggest that oxidative stress may increase in blood vessels during aging. Levels of superoxide are influenced by the activity of SODs. The goal of this study was to examine the effect of extracellular superoxide dismutase (ECSOD) on superoxide levels and vascular function in an animal model of

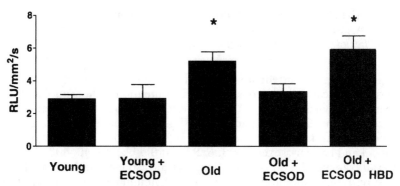

FIGURE 7.—Superoxide levels in aorta from Fischer 344 rats. Superoxide levels in young (untreated; n = 9), rats treated with AdECSOD (n = 5), and old (untreated; n = 6) rats treated with AdESCOD (n = 16) or AdECSODΔHBD (n = 6). Values are means ± SE. *P < 0.05 vs. young, young + ECSOD, and old + ECSOD. RLU, relative light units. *Abbreviations*: AdESCOD, adenovirus expressing human extracellular superoxide dismutase; HBD, heparin-binding domain. (Reprinted with permission from Brown KA, Chu Y, Lund DD. Gene transfer of extracellular superoxide dismutase protects against vascular dysfunction with aging. *Am J Physiol Heart Circ Physiol.* 2006;290:H2600-H2605.)

aging. Aortas from young (4–8 mo old) and old (29–31 mo old) Fischer 344 rats were examined in vitro. Relaxation of aorta to ACh was impaired in old rats compared with young rats; e.g., 3 µM ACh produced 57 ± 4% (mean ± SE) and 84 ± 2% relaxation in old and young rats, respectively (P < 0.0001). Three days after gene transfer of adenovirus expressing human ECSOD (AdECSOD), the response to ACh was not affected in young rats but was improved in old rats. There was no difference in relaxation to the endothelium-independent dilator sodium nitroprusside between young, aged, and AdECSOD-treated old rats. Superoxide levels (lucigenin-enhanced chemiluminescence) were significantly increased in aged rats compared with young rats. After gene transfer of ECSOD to aged rats, superoxide levels in aorta were similar in old and young rats. Gene transfer of an ECSOD with the heparin-binding domain deleted had no effect on vascular function or superoxide levels in old rats. These results suggest that 1) vascular dysfunction associated with aging is mediated in part by increased levels of superoxide, 2) gene transfer of ECSOD reduces vascular superoxide and dysfunction in old rats, and 3) beneficial effects of ECSOD in old rats require the heparin-binding domain of ECSOD (Fig 7).

▶ Endothelial dysfunction of aging is thought to involve nitric oxide (NO) and subsequent interaction of NO with reactive oxygen species (ROS). Using an established model of aging, these investigators show that vessel reactivity changes with aging and these changes associated with aging are mediated by ROS and superoxide. Gene transfer with superoxide dismutase inhibits these changes, suggesting new approaches to therapy in aged human vascular patients.

G. L. Moneta, MD

Effect of Very High-Intensity Statin Therapy on Regression of Coronary Atherosclerosis: The ASTEROID Trial

Nissen SE, for the ASTEROID Investigators (Cleveland Clinic Lerner School of Medicine, Ohio; et al)

JAMA 295:1556-1565, 2006

Context.—Prior intravascular ultrasound (IVUS) trials have demonstrated slowing or halting of atherosclerosis progression with statin therapy but have not shown convincing evidence of regression using percent atheroma volume (PAV), the most rigorous IVUS measure of disease progression and regression.

Objective.—To assess whether very intensive statin therapy could regress coronary atherosclerosis as determined by IVUS imaging.

Design and Setting.—Prospective, open-label blinded end-points trial (A Study to Evaluate the Effect of Rosuvastatin on Intravascular Ultrasound-Derived Coronary Atheroma Burden [ASTEROID]) was performed at 53 community and tertiary care centers in the United States, Canada, Europe, and Australia. A motorized IVUS pullback was used to assess coronary atheroma burden at baseline and after 24 months of treatment. Each pair of baseline and follow-up IVUS assessments was analyzed in a blinded fashion.

Patients.—Between November 2002 and October 2003, 507 patients had a baseline IVUS examination and received at least 1 dose of study drug. After 24 months, 349 patients had evaluable serial IVUS examinations.

Intervention.—All patients received intensive statin therapy with rosuvastatin, 40 mg/d.

Main Outcome Measures.—Two primary efficacy parameters were prespecified: the change in PAV and the change in nominal atheroma volume in the 10-mm subsegment with the greatest disease severity at baseline. A secondary efficacy variable, change in normalized total atheroma volume for the entire artery, was also prespecified.

Results.—The mean (SD) baseline low-density lipoprotein cholesterol (LDL-C) level of 130.4 (34.3) mg/dL declined to 60.8 (20.0) mg/dL, a mean reduction of 53.2% (P<.001). Mean (SD) high-density lipoprotein cholesterol (HDL-C) level at baseline was 43.1 (11.1) mg/dL, increasing to 49.0 (12.6) mg/dL, an increase of 14.7% (P<.001). The mean (SD) change in PAV for the entire vessel was −0.98% (3.15%), with a median of −0.79% (97.5% CI, −1.21% to −0.53%) (P<.001 vs baseline). The mean (SD) change in atheroma volume in the most diseased 10-mm subsegment was −6.1 (10.1) mm^3, with a median of −5.6 mm^3 (97.5% CI, −6.8 to −4.0 mm^3) (P<.001 vs baseline). Change in total atheroma volume showed a 6.8% median reduction; with a mean (SD) reduction of −14.7 (25.7) mm^3, with a median of −12.5 mm^3 (95% CI, −15.1 to −10.5 mm^3) (P<.001 vs baseline). Adverse events were infrequent and similar to other statin trials.

Conclusions.—Very high-intensity statin therapy using rosuvastatin 40 mg/d achieved an average LDL-C of 60.8 mg/dL and increased HDL-C by 14.7%, resulting in significant regression of atherosclerosis for all 3 prespecified IVUS measures of disease burden. Treatment to LDL-C levels below currently accepted guidelines, when accompanied by significant HDL-C increases, can regress atherosclerosis in coronary disease patients. Further studies are needed to determine the effect of the observed changes on clinical outcome.

▶ The study demonstrates convincing regression of atherosclerosis in the coronary circulation with high-dose statin therapy. The study has some limitations because there were no placebo controls and 22 patients were withdrawn because of ischemic events. Those patients may represent actual progression of atherosclerosis under the treatment protocol. Nevertheless, in the patients evaluated, coronary atherosclerosis was reduced with high-dose statin therapy employed in this study. There were minimal complications and intolerance associated with the drug. It does seem clear that high-dose statin therapy is indicated in patients with significant coronary disease. Regression of plaques may someday be routine clinical reality.

G. L. Moneta, MD

Statin Use and Sex-Specific Stroke Outcome in Patients With Vascular Disease
Bushnell CD, Griffin J, Newby LK, et al (Duke Univ, Durham, NC; Auckland City Hosp, New Zealand; Natl Health and Med Research Council Clinical Trials Centre, Camperdown, New South Wales, Australia; et al)
Stroke 37:1427-1431, 2006

Background and Purpose.—Although statins reduce the risk of stroke in patients with coronary heart disease, possible differing effects of statins on stroke outcomes based on sex remain uncertain. We investigated the relationships between statin use and sex-specific stroke incidence, severity, and mortality.

Methods.—Data from 3 trials of oral glycoprotein IIb/IIIa inhibitors (first and second Sibrafiban versus aspirin to Yield Maximum Protection from ischemic Heart events postacute cOroNary sYndromes [SYMPHONY] and Blockade of the glycoprotein IIb/IIIa Receptor to Avoid Vascular Occlusion [BRAVO]) were pooled and stroke outcomes compared among 8191 baseline statin users versus 14,752 nonusers. Time-to-event data were modeled with proportional hazards regression. Stroke severity was assessed retrospectively with the Canadian Neurological Scale (CNS) based on records with scoreable neurological examinations.

Results.—A total of 217 subjects had strokes (0.95%). Statin users had a lower risk of stroke in unadjusted (hazard ratio [HR], 0.69; 95% CI, 0.51 to 0.92) and risk-adjusted models (HR, 0.72; 95% CI, 0.53 to 0.97). There was no difference in stroke mortality with statin use ($P=0.8$). CNS scores could be assigned to 106 of the subjects, with no difference in severity among statin users and nonusers (median CNS=10.5 in users versus CNS=9.75 in nonusers; $P=0.14$). Women had more severe strokes than men (median CNS=10.5 in men versus 9.5 in women; Poisson regression $P=0.035$).

Women had more severe strokes after adjustment for statin use ($P=0.03$) and the combination of statin use, atrial fibrillation, and age ($P=0.03$).

Conclusions.—In patients included in these clinical trials of oral glycoprotein IIb/IIIa inhibitors, statin use is associated with a reduced risk of stroke but not severity or mortality. Women had more severe strokes than men, a difference that was not explained by baseline characteristics or statin use.

▶ The basis for this study were 217 stroke subjects, culled from a pooled sample of over 22,000 patients with vascular disease enrolled in secondary prevention trials. Statin use was associated with a modest reduction in stroke risk, but had no effect on stroke severity or mortality. This unplanned post hoc analysis suffers from inadequate statistical power. If its findings are corroborated by larger prospective trials, we may find that statins prevent strokes by stabilizing plaque but do not offer a neuroprotective effect.

G. L. Moneta, MD

Statin Use and Functional Decline in Patients With and Without Peripheral Arterial Disease

Giri J, McDermott MM, Greenland P, et al (Massachusetts Gen Hosp, Boston: Northwestern Univ, Chicago; Natl Inst on Aging, Bethesda, Md; et al)
J Am Coll Cardiol 47:998-1004, 2006

Objectives.—We determined whether statin use (vs. non-use) is associated with less annual decline in lower-extremity functioning in patients with and without lower-extremity peripheral arterial disease (PAD) over three-year follow-up.

Background.—It is unclear whether statin use is associated with less functional decline in patients with PAD.

Methods.—Participants included 332 men and women with an ankle brachial index (ABI) <0.90 and 212 with ABI 0.90 to 1.50. Functional outcomes included 6-min walk distance and usual and rapid-pace 4-m walking velocity. A summary performance score combined performance in walking speed, standing balance, and time for five repeated chair rises into an ordinal score ranging from 0 to 12 (12 = best).

Results.—Adjusting for age, race, gender, comorbidities, education, health insurance, total cholesterol/high-density lipoprotein level, body mass index, pack-years of smoking, leg symptoms, immediately previous year functioning, statin use/non-use, ABI, and change in ABI, the PAD participants using statins had less annual decline in usual-pace walking velocity (0.002 vs. −0.024 m/s/year, p = 0.013), rapid-pace walking velocity (−0.006 vs. −0.042 m/s/year, p = 0.006), 6-min walk performance (−34.5 vs. −57.9 feet/year, p = 0.088), and the summary performance score (−0.152 vs. −0.376, p = 0.067) compared with non-users. These associations were attenuated slightly by additional adjustment for high-sensitivity C-reactive protein levels. Among non-PAD participants, there were no significant associations between statin use and functional decline.

Conclusions.—The PAD patients on statins have less annual decline in lower-extremity performance than PAD patients who are not taking statins.

▶ Statins are the cure-all! In patients with PAD, statin use ameliorated the decline in walking distance and velocity. Despite a well-done prospective study, the mechanism of statins' pleotrophic effect on lower extremity function remains unclear.

G. L. Moneta, MD

Family History of Diabetes Is a Major Determinant of Endothelial Function

Goldfine AB, Beckman JA, Betensky RA, et al (Joslin Diabetes Ctr, Boston; Brigham and Women's Hosp, Boston; Harvard School of Public Health, Boston)
J Am Coll Cardiol 47:2456-2461, 2006

Objectives.—We evaluated whether endothelial dysfunction was present in nondiabetic persons with a family history (FH) of diabetes and assessed its relationship with insulin resistance and atherosclerosis risk factors.

Background.—Atherosclerosis is frequently present when type 2 diabetes (T2D) is first diagnosed. Endothelial dysfunction contributes to atherogenesis.

Methods.—Oral glucose tolerance and brachial artery flow-mediated, endothelium-dependent vasodilation (EDV) were assessed in 38 nondiabetic subjects; offspring of two parents with T2D (FH+) or with no first-degree relative with diabetes (FH−).

Results.—Although fasting glucose was higher in FH+ than FH− (5.3 ± 0.1 mmol/l vs. 4.9 ± 0.1 mmol/l, p < 0.03), glycemic burden assessed as 2-h or area-under-the-curve glucose after glucose load or glycosylated hemoglobin (HbA1c), and measures of insulin sensitivity or inflammation did not differ. Brachial artery flow-mediated EDV was reduced in FH+ (7.1 ± 0.9% vs. 11.7 ± 1.6%, p < 0.02), with no difference in nitroglycerin-induced endothelium-independent vasodilatation. In the combined cohort, only FH+ (r^2 = 0.12, p < 0.02) and HbA1c (r^2 = 0.14, p < 0.02) correlated with EDV. Insulin resistance, assessed by tertile of homeostasis model assessment of insulin resistance (HOMA-IR), was associated with impaired endothelium-dependent vasodilatation in FH− (p < 0.03, analysis of variance), but not in FH+, as even the most insulin-sensitive FH− offspring had diminished endothelial function. In multiple regression analysis, including established cardiac risk factors, blood pressure and lipids, HbA1c, and HOMA-IR, FH remained a significant determinant of EDV (p = 0.04).

Conclusions.—Bioavailability of nitric oxide is lower in persons with a strong FH of T2D. Glycemic burden, even in the nondiabetic range, can contribute to endothelial dysfunction. Abnormalities of endothelial function may contribute to atherosclerosis before development of overt diabetes.

▶ If one accepts brachial artery flow-mediated determination of endothelial function represents global nitric oxide bioavailability, this paper has significant implications. Atherogenesis is prompted by endothelial dysfunction, which may precede overt diabetes in offspring of diabetic parents. Taking a family history has never been more important.

G. L. Moneta, MD

The vascular endothelial cell mediates insulin transport into skeletal muscle

Wang H, Liu Z, Li G, et al (Univ of Virginia Health System, Charlottesville)
Am J Physiol Endocrinol Metab 291:E323-E332, 2006

The pathways by which insulin exits the vasculature to muscle interstitium have not been characterized. In the present study, we infused FITC-labeled insulin to trace morphologically (using confocal immunohistochemical methods) insulin transport into rat skeletal muscle. We biopsied rectus muscle at 0, 10, 30, and 60 min after beginning a continuous ($10 \text{ mU} \cdot \text{min}^{-1}$) $\cdot \text{kg}^{-1}$), intravenous FITC-insulin infusion (with euglycemia maintained). The FITC-insulin distribution was compared with that of insulin receptors (IR), IGF-I receptors (IGF-IR), and caveolin-1 (a protein marker for caveolae) in skeletal muscle vasculature. We observed that muscle endothelium stained strongly for FITC-insulin within 10 min, and this persisted to 60 min. Endothelium stained more strongly for FITC-insulin than any other cellular elements in muscle. IR, IGF-IR, and caveolin-1 were also detected immunohistochemically in muscle endothelial cells. We further compared their intracellular distribution with that of FITC-insulin in cultured bovine aortic endothelial cells (bAECs). Considerable colocalization of IR or IGF-IR with FITC-insulin was noted. There was some but less overlap of IR or IGF-IR or FITC-insulin with caveolin-1. Immunoprecipitation of IR coprecipitated caveolin-1, and conversely the precipitation of caveolin-1 brought down IR. Furthermore, insulin increased the tyrosine phosphorylation of caveolin-1, and filipin (which inhibits caveolae formation) blocked insulin uptake. Finally, the ability of insulin, IGF-I, and IGF-I-blocking antibody to diminish insulin transport across bAECs grown on transwell plates suggested that IGF-IR, in addition to IR, can also mediate transendothelial insulin transit. We conclude that in vivo endothelial cells rapidly take up and concentrate insulin relative to plasma and muscle interstitium and that IGF-IR, like IR, may mediate insulin transit through endothelial cells in a process involving caveolae.

▶ Despite the expansive title, this study is limited to morphological analysis and the tracing of insulin, and receptors in rat muscle and cell culture. The confocal images are well done and tell a story of rapid insulin entry into skeletal muscle. Differential insulin transport from the bloodstream to its sites of action may explain insulin resistance in humans, but this remains poorly characterized.

G. L. Moneta, MD

The potassium channel opener levcromakalim causes expansive remodelling of experimental vein grafts
Wales L, Gosling M, Taylor GW, et al (Imperial College, London; Royal Free & Univ College Med School, London)
J Vasc Surg 44:159-165, 2006

Background.—Maintenance of luminal area is essential for the optimal performance of venous bypass grafts. However, injury and response to the arterial circulation evoke vascular remodelling that favors intimal hyperplasia, with luminal encroachment and inward remodelling. Potassium channel-opening drugs reduce tissue workload and peripheral vascular resistance and through these mechanisms could favor outward or expansive remodelling of vein grafts. We tested the hypothesis that levcromakalim, a potassium channel opener, would enhance expansive remodelling in vein grafts.

Methods.—A randomized, double-blind, placebo-controlled trial was conducted in 33 rats with vena cava-to-aorta bypass grafts. Drugs were administered via osmotic pump for 7 days after surgery. Half the cohort had bromodeoxyuridine (BrdU) infused at day 6. Morphometric analysis was conducted of pressure perfusion-fixed grafts harvested at 1 week and 4 weeks.

Results.—At 1 week, lumen area was similar in both groups (1.82 ± 0.39 mm^2 placebo vs 1.85 ± 0.36 mm^2 levcromakalim), although medial cell density and BrdU staining were significantly increased in the placebo group. At 4 weeks, lumen area was unchanged in the placebo group (1.88 ± 0.51 mm^2) but had increased to 2.32 ± 0.46 mm^2 in the levcromakalim group ($P = .039$ vs 1 week), with a very significant reduction in the intimal area (levcromakalim, 0.06 ± 0.02 mm^2 vs placebo, 0.33 ± 0.17 mm^2; $P = .001$).

Conclusions.—Early, short-term treatment with levcromakalim favors expansive remodelling of experimental vein grafts to mimic the effect of external stenting. This expansive remodelling was associated with a reduction in medial cell proliferation at 1 week.

Clinical relevance.—Critical limb ischemia can be treated by bypass surgery or angioplasty, but inward remodelling with restenosis is a common problem. There has been little previous experimental work to identify treatments associated with expansive remodelling, which would increase the chances of vessel patency. Here, in a randomized trial, we show that short-term treatment with a potassium channel opener (a class of drug that can be used to treat hypertension) results in strong, expansive remodelling, which increases the lumen area and graft size of experimental vein grafts by >25%.

▶ This study describes a novel approach to create larger vein graft lumen area by treatment with an antihypertensive drug. Intravenous treatment for 7 days resulted in larger vein grafts by 28 days. Although the relevance of rat studies to humans is often questioned, this is a different approach than the failed E2F-decoy human trial and may be worthy of trials in different models.

G. L. Moneta, MD

Controlled release of small interfering RNA targeting midkine attenuates intimal hyperplasia in vein grafts

Banno H, Takei Y, Muramatsu T, et al (Nagoya Univ, Japan; Aichi Gakuin Univ, Japan)
J Vasc Surg 44:633-641, 2006

Objective.—Intimal hyperplasia is a major obstacle to patency after vein grafting. Despite of a diverse array of trials to prevent it, a satisfactory therapeutic strategy for clinical use has not been established. However, sufficient inhibition of early stages of intimal hyperplasia may prevent this long-term progressive disease. Midkine (MK) is a heparin-binding growth factor that was originally discovered as the product of a retinoic acid-responsive gene. We previously demonstrated that MK-deficient mice exhibit a striking reduction of neointima formation in a restenosis model, which is reversed on systemic MK administration. In this study, we evaluated a strategy of using small interfering RNA (siRNA) targeting MK as a therapy for vein graft failure.

Methods.—We first made a highly effective siRNA to rabbit MK. Jugular vein-to-carotid artery interposition vein grafts, which are applied to a low flow condition, were made in Japanese white rabbits. Small interfering RNA mixed with atelocollagen was administered to the external wall of grafted veins. Cy3-conjugated stabilized siRNA was used to confirm its stability and successful transfer into the vein graft wall. Neointimal hyperplasia was evaluated 4 weeks after the operation. The proliferation index and leukocyte infiltration were determined.

Results.—MK expression was induced and reached the maximum level 7 days after operation. Fluorescence of Cy3-labeled siRNA could be detected in the graft wall even 7 days after operation. Knockdown of the gradually increasing expression was achieved by perivascular application of siRNA using atelocollagen. The intima-media ratio and the intima thickness at 28 days after grafting were both reduced >90% by this treatment compared with controls. This phenomenon was preceded by significant reductions of inflammatory cell recruitment to the vessel walls and subsequent cell proliferation in MK siRNA-treated grafts.

Conclusions.—These results suggest that midkine is a candidate molecular target for preventing vein graft failure. Furthermore, for clinical applications of siRNA, a single intraoperative atelocollagen-based nonviral delivery method could be a reliable approach to achieve maximal function of siRNA in vivo. This strategy may be a useful and practical form of gene therapy against human vein graft failure.

▶ This Japanese group demonstrates the use of a novel technology, siRNA, to inhibit rabbit vein graft neointimal hyperplasia. Although midkine is yet another of many targets that may eventually prove to be relevant, the use of siRNA is interesting even though the doses are quite high. The demonstration of adventitial application is also of interest to surgeons.

G. L. Moneta, MD

Transforming growth factor-β1 antisense treatment of rat vein grafts reduces the accumulation of collagen and increases the accumulation of h-caldesmon

Wolff RA, Malinowski RL, Heaton NS, et al (William S Middleton Mem Veterans Hosp, Madison, Wisc; Univ of Wisconsin, Madison)
J Vasc Surg 43:1028-1036, 2006

Background.—The main cause of occlusion and vein graft failure after peripheral and coronary arterial reconstruction is intimal hyperplasia. Transforming growth factor β-1 (TGF-β1) is a pleiotropic cytokine known to have powerful effects on cell growth, apoptosis, cell differentiation, and extracellular matrix synthesis.

Methods.—To investigate the role of TGF-β1 in intimal hyperplasia, we used adenovirus to deliver to superficial epigastric vein messenger RNA (mRNA) antisense to TGF-β1 (Ad-AST) or the sequence encoding the bioactive form of TGF-β1 (Ad-BAT). Infection with "empty" virus was used as a control (Ad-CMVpLpA). The treated vein was then used for an interposition graft into rat femoral artery. Grafts were harvested at 1, 2, 4, and 12 weeks and formalin-fixed for histologic studies or placed in liquid nitrogen for mRNA studies.

Results.—Ad-AST treatment resulted in an overall reduction of TGF-β1 expression ($P = .001$), and Ad-BAT treatment resulted in an overall increase in TGF-β1 expression ($P = .007$). Histologic analysis showed Ad-AST caused reduced collagen build up in the neointima at 12 weeks ($P = .0001$). Immunohistochemical staining for h-caldesmon at 12 weeks indicated Ad-AST increased smooth muscle cells throughout the vessel wall compared with Ad-CMVpLpA ($P = .0024$) or Ad-BAT ($P = .04$). Ad-AST also resulted in reduced CD68-positive cells in the media/adventitia ($P = .005$ vs Ad-CMVpLpA, $P = .01$ vs Ad-BAT). To further understand how Ad-AST was influencing the build up of collagen, we performed quantitative polymerase chain reaction on complimentary DNA (cDNA) from homogenates of the vein grafts. Tissue inhibitor of matrix metalloproteinase-1 (TIMP-1) was increased at 1 week by Ad-BAT ($P = .048$ vs Ad-CMVpLpA) and decreased by Ad-AST at all time points ($P \le .038$). The mRNA for collagen-1 α-1 was decreased by Ad-AST at 2, 4, and 12 weeks ($P \le .05$) and increased by Ad-BAT at 1 week ($P = .01$).

Conclusions.—TGF-β1 antisense treatment of vein grafts prevents the accumulation of collagen in the neointima in part by (1) changing the proportions of the cell types populating the vein graft wall, (2) reducing the mRNA for TIMPs, and (3) reducing the amount of collagen mRNA. With the Ad-AST and Ad-BAT treatments, we have been able to tip the maturation of the vein graft toward positive remodeling (artery-like phenotype) or toward negative remodeling (fibroproliferation and stenosis), respectively.

▶ Using complementary strategies to inhibit (antisense technology) or stimulate (CMV = cytomegalovirus) promoter driven expression) protein synthesis, this paper links TGF-β to collagen synthesis in rat vein grafts. The claim that vessel phenotype is altered is not well documented. However, it is not clear whether increasing the collagen content in vein grafts would be good (increased strength) or bad (increased stiffness).

G. L. Moneta, MD

VEGF Inhibits PDGF-Stimulated Calcium Signaling Independent of Phospholipase C and Protein Kinase C

Chandra A, Angle N (Univ of California, San Diego)
J Surg Res 131:302-309, 2006

Introduction.—Despite advances in both open and endovascular techniques for treatment of arterial occlusive disease, restenosis because of neointimal hyperplasia continues to be a major cause of graft failure and restenosis. This phenomenon has been attributed to vascular smooth muscle cell (VSMC) activation by several potent mitogens including platelet derived growth factor (PDGF) and vascular endothelial growth factor (VEGF) released at the site of injury. PDGF is known to stimulate calcium influx in VSMC that has been shown to be critical for VSMC migration and proliferation. We have previously shown that VEGF inhibits PDGF-stimulated VSMC proliferation. The objective of this set of experiments was to investigate whether VEGF modulated PDGF-stimulated Ca^{2+} influx in VSMC.

Materials and methods.—Primary cultured human aortic SMC were grown to subconfluency and assigned to the following groups: no stimulation, stimulation with PDGF-BB (20 ng/ml), stimulation with VEGF165 (40 ng/ml), or a combination of PDGF-BB + VEGF165. Ca^{2+} influx was measured using a Fura-2 fluorescence assay. The intracellular Ca^{2+} fraction was assayed with the Fura-2 assay by using Ca^{2+}-free media. Phospholipase $C\gamma_1$ ($PLC\gamma_1$), protein kinase C (PKC), and Akt phosphorylation was assessed with standard immunoblotting techniques at 1, 5, and 10 min time points. Ca^{2+}-calmodulin kinase II (CaMKII) activity was extrapolated from the phosphorylation of Phospholamban B (PLB), a well-known protein substrate, at 1, 5, and 10 min time points.

Results.—PDGF stimulation resulted in a 328 ± 9 nm total calcium influx in VSMC. The combination of VEGF + PDGF resulted in a 273 ± 21 nm total calcium influx, an amount significantly less than with PDGF alone ($P <$

0.04). PDGF stimulation resulted in a 72 ± 35 nm intracellular calcium release. The addition of VEGF to PDGF resulted in an intracellular calcium release of only 15 ± 11 nm, a significant decrease compared to PDGF alone ($P < 0.01$). The phosphorylation of $PLC\gamma_1$, PKC, and Akt was equivalent at 1, 5, and 10 min between the PDGF and the PDGF + VEGF treatment groups. There was an increase in CaMKII activity at 1 and 5 min time points in both the PDGF and PDGF + VEGF treatment groups suggesting that extracellular calcium influx is sufficient for CaMKII activation.

Conclusion.—VEGF inhibits PDGF-stimulated total calcium influx and, in particular, PDGF-stimulated intracellular calcium release in VSMC. The equivalent phosphorylation of $PLC\gamma1$, PKC, and Akt suggests that the inhibitory mechanism by VEGF on calcium influx occurs downstream of these proximal mediators. The inhibition of intracellular calcium release did not inhibit CaMKII activity. VEGF may play an important role in modulating PDGF induced VSMC proliferation by specifically inhibiting intracellular calcium release in response to PDGF.

▶ This paper provides another example of the complex interplay between growth factors and how in vitro culture conditions are a poor mimic of the in vivo environment. The relevance of these short-term phenomena to longer term changes leading to neointimal hyperplasia is not clear.

G. L. Moneta, MD

Slower Onset of Low Shear Stress Leads to Less Neointimal Thickening in Experimental Vein Grafts

Baldwin ZK, Chandiwal A, Huang W, et al (Univ of Chicago)
Ann Vasc Surg 20:106-113, 2006

Vein grafts respond to low flow and shear stress (τ_w) by generating thicker walls and smaller lumens through the processes of neointimal hyperplasia and remodeling. Clinically, however, vein grafts with obviously low τ_w, such as those distal to high-grade proximal obstructions, are not infrequently found to be widely patent and pliable. One possible explanation for this phenomenon may be that vein grafts remodel more favorably in response to changes in shear that occur gradually over time compared to abruptly. This hypothesis was tested in an experimental animal model in this report. Two separate models of experimental vein graft failure were created, causing either immediate exposure to ultralow τ_w (<1 dyne/cm^2) or delayed exposure to ultralow τ_w. Under general anesthesia and using a sterile technique, the right external jugular (EJ) veins of 28 New Zealand white rabbits were surgically exposed and isolated. An end-to-side distal EJ/common carotid artery anastomosis was created, resulting in a widely patent arteriovenous fistula. For the immediate exposure group ($n = 5$), the EJ was suture-ligated just proximal to the thoracic inlet, distal to a small 10-50 μm venous tributary. This created a reversed vein segment immediately and abruptly exposed to high wall tension (2.0 ± 0.3 × 10^4 dyne/cm) and ultralow τ_w (0.15 ± 0.08

dyne/cm^2). For the delayed exposure group (n = 22), the EJ was ligated over a 0.035 guidewire, leaving a small aperture to sustain some measure of blood flow and τ_w. This predictably resulted in slightly less wall tension (1.4 ± 0.2 × 10^4 dyne/cm) and higher τ_w (0.68 ± 0.21 dyne/cm^2) than the immediate exposure group. During the first week, the small outflow aperture in the delayed exposure grafts thrombosed, eventually exposing them to the same low level of τ_w as the immediate exposure grafts. Thus, the only difference in the two models was that delayed exposure grafts enjoyed a slower decline in τ_w than immediate exposure grafts. Fourteen rabbits in the delayed exposure group were harvested over the first 7 days to define the patency curve of the restricted outflow channel. As expected, the small aperture had thrombosed in all animals by 7 days. The remaining 14 grafts were harvested after 4 weeks, and 13/14 remained patent. Examination of the hemodynamic parameters at the time of death confirmed that wall tension and τ_w had equalized (wall tension 0.9 ± 0.1 vs. 1.1 ± 0.1 × 10^4 dyne/cm, τ_w 0.45 ± 0.12 vs. 0.30 ± 0.08 dyne/cm^2). Histological examination revealed less neointimal hyperplasia in the delayed exposure group compared to the immediate exposure group (wall thickness 266 ± 16 vs. 180 ± 24 µm, p = 0.025) as well as a slightly greater luminal diameter (0.30 ± 0.02 vs. 0.40 ± 0.02 cm, p = 0.038). The results of this experiment suggest that slow exposure to reduced τ_w results in more favorable remodeling (less thickening) than abrupt exposure. This finding may explain the occasional clinical observation of a widely patent vein graft even in the face of proximal arterial obstruction and very low flow; the change in τ_w presumably occurred slowly mitigating the remodeling response.

▶ This intriguing paper shows that gradually diminished flow through a vein graft allows the vein graft to successfully adapt to the low flow conditions, compared to increased amounts of neointimal hyperplasia when the flow is reduced quickly. The relevance of this finding in young rabbits with normal veins to elderly human patients is not clear.

G. L. Moneta, MD

Tumor necrosis factor-α and the early vein graft

Jiang Z, Shukla A, Miller BL, et al (Univ of Florida, Gainesville; Malcom Randall VA Med Ctr, Gainesville, Fla)
J Vasc Surg 45:169-176, 2007

Background.—Tumor necrosis factor-α (TNF-α) has been implicated in the blood vessel wall response to hemodynamic forces. We hypothesized that TNF-α activity drives neointimal hyperplasia (NIH) during vein graft arterialization and that anti-TNF-α therapy would inhibit NIH.

Methods.—Rabbits underwent bilateral vein grafting using jugular vein. All distal branches except the occipital artery were unilaterally ligated to create distinct flow environments between the bilateral grafts. Vein grafts were harvested sequentially up to 28 days for TNF-α messenger RNA (mRNA) quantitation. In separate experiments, animals received short-term or long-term dosing with pegylated soluble TNF-α type I receptor (PEG sTNF-RI) or vehicle. After 14 to 28 days, grafts were analyzed for morphometry, proliferation, apoptosis, and PEG sTNF-RI distribution.

Results.—Quantitative mRNA assay (TaqMan) revealed shear-dependent ($P < .001$) and time-dependent ($P < .001$) TNF-α expression. TNF-α induction was maximal at day 1 and gradually decreased over time, but was persistently elevated even 4 weeks later ($P < .001$). Low shear (associated with increased NIH) resulted in significantly higher TNF-α mRNA expression ($P = .03$). PEG sTNF-RI was found in high concentrations in the serum and localized to NIH. The high-flow and low-flow vein grafts from treated animals demonstrated similar volumes of NIH compared with controls. PEG-sTNF-RI had only modest impact on vascular wall cell turnover, as reflected by terminal deoxynucleotide transferase-mediated deoxy uridine triphosphate nick-end labeling ($P = .064$) and anti-Ki-67 ($P = .12$) assays.

Conclusions.—Placement of a vein into the arterial circulation acutely upregulates TNF-α; this expression level correlates with the degree of subsequent NIH. Pharmacologic interruption of this signaling pathway has no significant impact on NIH or wall cellular proliferation/apoptosis, suggesting that early vein graft adaptations can proceed via TNF-α-independent mechanisms.

▶ Placement of a vein, accustomed to low pressure and shear, into the arterial circulation results in short-term activation of TNF-α and other inflammatory pathways. Uncoupling the flow and pressure, so the vein is exposed to lower flow in the arterial circulation, results in increased TNF-α mRNA expression, but TNF-α is not linked to ultimate neointimal thickening.

G. L. Moneta, MD

Temporal gradients in shear, but not spatial gradients, stimulate ERK1/2 activation in human endothelial cells
White CR, Stevens HY, Haidekker M, et al (La Jolla Bioengineering Inst, Calif; Loma Linda Univ, Calif; Univ of California, San Diego, La Jolla)
Am J Physiol Heart Circ Physiol 289:H2350-H2355, 2005

We have previously demonstrated temporal gradients in shear stress stimulate endothelial cell proliferation, whereas spatial gradients do not. In the present study, the extracellular signal-regulated kinases 1 and 2 (ERK1/2) pathway was investigated as a possible mediator for the promitogenic effect of temporal gradients. The sudden expansion flow chamber (SEFC) model was used to differentiate the effect of temporal gradients in shear from that of spatial gradients on ERK1/2 activation in human umbilical vein endothelial cells (HUVEC). ERK1/2 activation in the SEFC was not significantly different from control when HUVEC were exposed to spatial gradients alone. When a single temporal impulse was superimposed on spatial gradients, ERK1/2 activation was stimulated 330% (relative to spatial alone) within the region of spatial gradients. Inhibition of the ERK1/2 pathway with U-0126 abolished all effects of temporal gradients. To further separate temporal and spatial gradients, a conventional parallel plate flow chamber was utilized. Acute exposure to oscillations in flow at a frequency of 1 Hz stimulated ERK1/2 activation $620 \pm 88\%$ relative to control, whereas a single impulse of flow increased ERK1/2 activation $166 \pm 19\%$. Flow without the temporal component did not significantly activate ERK1/2. These results suggest that the ERK1/2 pathway directly mediates the promitogenic effects of temporal gradients in shear stress.

▶ This paper relates activation of the endothelial mitogen-activated protein kinase (MAPK) system to temporal gradients in shear stress. Identification of this mechanism is still many steps from pharmacological approaches to inhibiting atherosclerosis and neointimal hyperplasia, not only from the long distance between in vitro models to in vivo applications, but also because of the ubiquitous activation of MAPK by many intracellular processes.

G. L. Moneta, MD

Matrix Metalloproteinase-8 and -9 Are Increased at the Site of Abdominal Aortic Aneurysm Rupture
Wilson WRW, Anderton M, Schwalbe EC, et al (Univ of Leicester, England; St George's Hosp Med School, London)
Circulation 113:438-445, 2006

Background.—Abdominal aortic aneurysm (AAA) expansion is characterized by extracellular matrix degradation and widespread inflammation. In contrast, the processes that characterize AAA rupture are not well understood. The aim of this study was to investigate the proteolytic and cellular activity of ruptured AAA, focusing on matrix metalloproteinases (MMPs) and their inhibitors (TIMPs).

Method and Results.—Anterior aneurysm wall biopsies were taken from 55 nonruptured and 21 ruptured AAAs. A further biopsy from the site of rupture was taken from 12 of the ruptured AAAs. MMP-1, -2, -3, -8, -9, and -13, as well as TIMP-1 and -2, were quantified in each biopsy with ELISA. A comparison of anterior aneurysm biopsies showed no difference in MMP or TIMP concentrations between nonruptured and ruptured AAA. In a comparison of ruptured AAA biopsies, MMP-8 and -9 levels were significantly elevated in the 12 rupture site biopsies compared with their 12 paired anterior wall biopsies, whereas other MMPs and TIMPs showed no difference (MMP-8, $P<0.001$; MMP-9, $P=0.01$). MMP-8 and -9 expression was mediated by native mesenchymal cells and was independent of the inflammatory infiltrate.

Conclusions.—A localized increase in MMP-8 and -9, mediated by native mesenchymal cells, presents a potential pathway for collagen breakdown and AAA rupture.

▶ The paper suggests a final common pathway in breakdown in extracellular matrix in AAA rupture. The corollary, of course, is that inhibition of MMP-8 or MMP-9 activity could potentially decrease the risk of aneurysm rupture. Perhaps, someday, patients with aortic aneurysms unsuitable for repair could be treated with inhibitors of MMP-9 or MMP-8 in an attempt to stabilize the aneurysm and prevent death from rupture.

G. L. Moneta, MD

Hypertension Accelerated Experimental Abdominal Aortic Aneurysm Through Upregulation of Nuclear Factor κB and Ets
Shiraya S, Miwa K, Aoki M, et al (Osaka Univ, Suita, Japan; Tottori Univ, Yonago, Japan)
Hypertension 48:628-636, 2006

In this study, we focused on the effect of hypertension on the transcription factors nuclear factor κB (NFκB) and ets in the mechanisms of abdominal aortic aneurysm (AAA), and we investigated how hypertension affects the progression of AAA. AAA was produced by elastase perfusion in hypertensive rats and normotensive rats. The size of AAA rapidly increased in hypertensive rats as compared with normotensive rats. Western blot analysis demonstrated that the expression of matrix metalloproteinase (MMP)-2, -3 , -9, and -12, as well as intercellular adhesion molecule, was increased in hypertensive AAA rats, accompanied by upregulation of NFκB and ets. Moreover, in situ zymography showed that the activity of MMPs was increased in the aorta of a hypertensive AAA model as compared with that in a normotensive AAA model. Interestingly, transfection of chimeric decoy oligodeoxynucleotide (ODN) resulted in significant inhibition of aortic dilatation both in normotensive and hypertensive rats at 4 weeks after transfection. Destruction of elastic fibers was also significantly inhibited by transfection of chimeric decoy ODN in both hypertensive rats and normotensive rats. The expression of MMP-2, -3, -9, and -12, as well as intercellular adhesion molecule, was significantly attenuated by the chimeric decoy ODN, accompanied by inhibition of the migration of macrophages. Also, the effect of chimeric decoy ODN was confirmed in an organ culture. The present study demonstrated that hypertension accelerated the progression of experimental AAA through upregulation of NFκB and ets. Inhibition of NFκB and ets could be a novel therapeutic strategy to treat AAA in hypertensive patients (Fig 1).

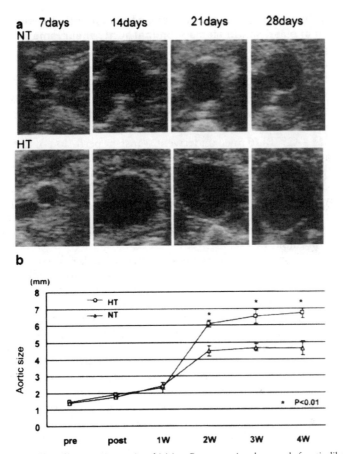

FIGURE 1.—Effect of hypertension on size of AAA. a, Representative ultrasound of aortic dilatation. b, Time course of aortic size after elastase perfusion as assessed by ultrasound. Pre indicates before elastase infusion; Post, after elastase infusion. N = 15 per group. *Abbreviations*: HT, hypertensive AAA model; NT, normotensive AAA model. (Courtesy of Shiraya S, Miwa K, Aoki M, et al. Hypertension accelerated experimental abdominal aortic aneurysm through upregulation of nuclear factor κB and Ets. *Hypertension.* 2006;48:628-636.)

▶ The study indicates hypertension accelerates progression of abdominal aortic aneurysm in an experimental rat model. Inhibition of NFκB and ets may someday be used as a method of decreasing aneurysm expansion in both normotensive and hypertensive patients. Potential drug therapy for aneurysms is slowly moving to target specific agents.[1]

G. L. Moneta, MD

Reference

1. Wilson WR, Anderton M, Schwalbe EC, et al. Matrix metalloproteinase-8 and -9 are increased at the site of abdominal aortic aneurysm rupture. *Circulation.* 2006;113:438-445.

Temporal changes in mouse aortic wall gene expression during the development of elastase-induced abdominal aortic aneurysms

Van Vickle-Chavez SJ, Tung WS, Absi TS, et al (Washington Univ, St Louis)
J Vasc Surg 43:1010-1020, 2006

Objective.—To characterize temporal changes in mouse aortic wall gene expression associated with the development of experimental abdominal aortic aneurysms.

Methods.—C57BL/6 mice underwent transient perfusion of the abdominal aorta with either elastase (n = 61) or heat-inactivated elastase as a control (n = 68). Triplicate samples of radiolabeled aortic wall complementary DNA were prepared at intervals of 0, 3, 7, 10, and 14 days, followed by hybridization to nylon microarrays (1181 genes). Autoradiographic intensity data were normalized by conversion to z scores, and differences in gene expression were defined by two-tailed z tests at a significance threshold of $P < .01$.

Results.—Elastase perfusion caused a progressive increase in aortic diameter up to 14 days accompanied by transmural inflammation and destructive remodeling of the elastic media. No aneurysms occurred in the control group. Compared with healthy aorta, 336 genes exhibited significant alterations during at least 1 interval after elastase perfusion (135 at more than 1 interval and 14 at all intervals), with pronounced increases for interleukin 6, cyclin E2, interleukin 1β, osteopontin, CD14/lipopolysaccharide receptor, P-selectin glycoprotein ligand 1, and gelatinase B/matrix metalloproteinase 9 (all >20-fold on day 3). Sixty-two genes exhibited synchronous alterations in the elastase and control groups, thus suggesting a nonspecific response. By direct comparisons between the elastase and control groups, there were 384 genes with significant differences in expression for at least 1 interval after aortic perfusion, including 234 with differential upregulation (eg, p44MAPK/ERK1, osteopontin, heat shock protein 84, hypoxia-inducible factor 1alpha, apolipoprotein E, monocyte chemotactic protein 3, MIG (monokine induced by gamma interferon), and interleukin 2 receptor γ and 163 with differential downregulation (eg, prothrombin, granzyme B, ataxia telangiectasia mutated, and interleukin-converting enzyme).

Conclusions.—Development of elastase-induced abdominal aortic aneurysms in mice is accompanied by altered aortic wall expression of genes associated with acute and chronic inflammation, matrix degradation, and vascular tissue remodeling. Knowledge of these alterations will facilitate further studies on the functional molecular mechanisms that underlie aneurysmal degeneration.

▶ A well-recognized animal model for aortic aneurysms served as the basis for DNA microarray techniques. Nearly 400 genes (out of 1,181 genes) had significantly different levels of expression compared to controls. As opposed to studies examining one gene and/or protein, this study reveals the complex nature of genetic changes involving cytokines, adhesion proteins, and much more during a disease state. We hear a symphony rather than a solo.

G. L. Moneta, MD

Deletion of p47^{phox}Attenuates Angiotensin II–Induced Abdominal Aortic Aneurysm Formation in Apolipoprotein E–Deficient Mice

Thomas M, Gavrila D, McCormick ML, et al (Univ of Iowa, Iowa City; VA Med Ctr, Iowa City; Univ of Kentucky, Lexington; et al)
Circulation 114:404-413, 2006

Background.—Angiotensin II (Ang II) contributes to vascular pathology in part by stimulating NADPH oxidase activity, leading to increased formation of superoxide (O_2^-). We reported that O_2^- levels, NADPH oxidase activity, and expression of the p47^{phox} subunit of NADPH oxidase are increased in human abdominal aortic aneurysms (AAAs). Here, we tested the hypothesis that deletion of p47^{phox} will attenuate oxidative stress and AAA formation in Ang II-infused apoE$^{-/-}$ mice.

Method and Results.—Male apoE$^{-/-}$ and apoE$^{-/-}$ p47$^{phox-/-}$ mice received saline or Ang II (1000 ng · kg^{-1} · min^{-1}) infusion for 28 days, after which abdominal aortic weight and maximal diameter were determined. Aortic tissues and blood were examined for parameters of aneurysmal disease and oxidative stress. Ang II infusion induced AAAs in 90% of apoE$^{-/-}$ versus 16% of apo$^{-/-}$ p47$^{phox-/-}$ mice ($P<0.05$). Abdominal aortic weight (14.1 ± 3.2 versus 35.6 ± 9.0 mg), maximal aortic diameter (1.5 ± 0.2 versus 2.4 ± 0.4

A

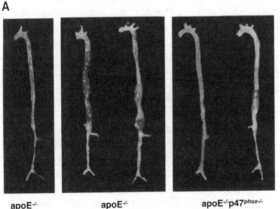

apoE$^{-/-}$ (NS infusion)	apoE$^{-/-}$ (ang II infusion)	apoE$^{-/-}$p47$^{phox-/-}$ (ang II infusion)

FIGURE 2A.—Representative photographs showing macroscopic features of aneurysms induced by Ang II. No animals infused with NS developed aneurysms (left specimen). Infusion of Ang II in apo E$^{-/-}$ animals led to the development of AAA and less frequently thoracic aortic aneurysms (middle specimens). The incidence of both types of aneurysms was markedly decreased by inactivation of the p47^{phox} gene (right specimens). *Abbreviation*: NS, normal saline. (Courtesy of Thomas M, Gavrila D, McCormick ML, et al. Deletion of p47^{phox} attenuates angiotensin II–induced abdominal aortic aneurysm formation in apolipoprotein E–deficient mice. *Circulation.* 2006;114:404-413.)

mm), aortic NADPH oxidase activity, and parameters of oxidative stress were reduced in apoE$^{-/-}$ p47$^{phox-/-}$ mice compared with apoE$^{-/-}$ mice ($P < 0.05$). In addition, aortic macrophage infiltration and matrix metalloproteinase-2 activity were reduced in apoE$^{phox-/-}$ mice compared with apoE$^{-/-}$ mice. Deletion of p47^{phox} attenuated the pressor response to Ang II; however, co-infusion of phenylephrine with Ang II, which restored the Ang II pressor response, did not alter the protective effects of p47^{phox} deletion on AAA formation (Fig 2A).

Conclusions.—Deletion of p47^{phox} attenuates Ang II-induced AAA formation in apoE$^{-/-}$ mice, suggesting that NADPH oxidase plays a critical role in AAA formation in this model.

▶ Another type of murine aneurysm model serves as the basis for this study. Double knockouts (apoE and p47^{phox} deficient) had less aneurysm formation, suggesting that NADPH oxidase plays a critical role in aneurysm formation. Understanding the mechanisms of aneurysm formation may lead to new therapies targeting NADPH oxidase.

G. L. Moneta, MD

Oral Administration of Diferuloylmethane (Curcumin) Suppresses Proinflammatory Cytokines and Destructive Connective Tissue Remodeling in Experimental Abdominal Aortic Aneurysms

Parodi FE, Mao D, Ennis TL, et al (Washington Univ, St Louis)
Ann Vasc Surg 20:360-368, 2006

Chronic transmural inflammation and proteolytic destruction of medial elastin are key mechanisms in the development of abdominal aortic aneurysms (AAAs). Diferuloylmethane (curcumin) is a major component of the food additive tumeric, which has been shown to have anti-inflammatory properties. To determine if ingestion of curcumin influences aneurysmal degeneration, C57Bl/6 mice underwent transient elastase perfusion of the abdominal aorta to induce the development of AAAs, followed by daily oral gavage with 100 mg/kg curcumin ($n = 36$) or water alone ($n = 31$). By 14 days, mice in the control group developed a mean increase in aortic diameter of $162.8 \pm 4.6\%$ along with a dense mononuclear inflammation and destruction of medial elastin. By comparison, the mean increase in aortic diameter in the curcumin-treated group was only $133.2 \pm 5.2\%$ ($p < 0.0001$). Although aortic wall inflammation was similar between the groups, the structural integrity of medial elastin was significantly greater in curcumin-treated mice. Curcumin-treated mice also exhibited relative decreases in aortic tissue activator protein-1 and nuclear factor κB DNA binding activities and significantly lower aortic tissue concentrations of interleukin-1β (IL-1β), IL-6, monocyte chemoattractant protein-1, and matrix metalloproteinase-9 (all $p < 0.05$). These data demonstrate for the first time that oral administration of curcumin can suppress the development of experimental AAAs, along with structural preservation of medial elastin fibers and reduced aortic wall expression of several cytokines, chemokines, and proteinases known to mediate aneurysmal degeneration. The possibility that dietary ingestion of curcumin may have a beneficial effect in degenerative aortic aneurysms warrants further consideration.

▶ A component of the food additive turmeric was found to suppress aneurysm formation in mice. Despite impressive decreases in cytokine production, curcumin treatment led to a modest 18% decrease in aortic dilatation after elastase perfusion. If these observations in mice were confirmed in humans, therapy would be straightforward. We could prescribe Indian food!

G. L. Moneta, MD

Regression of abdominal aortic aneurysm by inhibition of c-Jun N-terminal kinase
Yoshimura K, Aoki H, Ikeda Y, et al (Yamaguchi Univ, Ube, Japan; ETH Hönggerberg, Zurich, Switzerland)
Nature Med 11:1330-1338, 2005

Abdominal aortic aneurysm (AAA) is a common disease among elderly people that, when surgical treatment is inapplicable, results in progressive expansion and rupture of the aorta with high mortality. Although nonsurgical treatment for AAA is much awaited, few options are available because its molecular pathogenesis remains elusive. Here, we identify JNK as a proximal signaling molecule in the pathogenesis of AAA. Human AAA tissue showed a high level of phosphorylated JNK. We show that JNK programs a gene expression pattern in different cell types that cooperatively enhances the degradation of the extracellular matrix while suppressing biosynthetic enzymes of the extracellular matrix. Selective inhibition of JNK *in vivo* not only prevented the development of AAA but also caused regression of established AAA in two mouse models. Thus, JNK promotes abnormal extracellular matrix metabolism in the tissue of AAA and may represent a therapeutic target.

▶ This well-written manuscript describes a number of elegant experiments. Inhibition of JNK (stress-activated protein kinase) caused regression of abdominal aortic aneurysm (AAA) in mice. Instead of tissue destruction via matrix metalloproteinases, inhibition of JNK led to tissue repair with production of elastin and collagen. This compelling scientific study is the first showing regression of AAA that I am aware of.

G. L. Moneta, MD

How Critical Is Fibrous Cap Thickness to Carotid Plaque Stability? A Flow-Plaque Interaction Model

Li Z-Y, Howarth SPS, Tang T, et al (Univ of Cambridge and Addenbrooke's Hosp, England)
Stroke 37:1195-1199, 2006

Background and Purpose.—Acute cerebral ischemic events are associated with rupture of vulnerable carotid atheroma and subsequent thrombosis. Factors such as luminal stenosis and fibrous cap thickness have been thought to be important risk factors for plaque rupture. We used a flow-structure interaction model to simulate the interaction between blood flow and atheromatous plaque to evaluate the effect of the degree of luminal stenosis and fibrous cap thickness on plaque vulnerability.

Methods.—A coupled nonlinear time-dependent model with a flow-plaque interaction simulation was used to perform flow and stress/strain analysis in a stenotic carotid artery model. The stress distribution within the plaque and the flow conditions within the vessel were calculated for every case when varying the fibrous cap thickness from 0.1 to 2 mm and the degree of luminal stenosis from 10% to 95%. A rupture stress of 300 kPa was chosen to indicate a high risk of plaque rupture. A 1-sample t test was used to compare plaque stresses with the rupture stress.

Results.—High stress concentrations were found in the plaques in arteries with >70% degree of stenosis. Plaque stresses in arteries with 30% to 70% stenosis increased exponentially as fibrous cap thickness decreased. A decrease of fibrous cap thickness from 0.4 to 0.2 mm resulted in an increase of plaque stress from 141 to 409 kPa in a 40% degree stenotic artery.

Conclusions.—There is an increase in plaque stress in arteries with a thin fibrous cap. The presence of a moderate carotid stenosis (30% to 70%) with a thin fibrous cap indicates a high risk for plaque rupture. Patients in the future may be risk stratified by measuring both fibrous cap thickness and luminal stenosis.

▶ This is another bit of information which may eventually help differentiate high-risk from low-risk carotid plaque. The overall goal is to eventually decrease the number of patients required to treat to have an impact on stroke incidence of patients with asymptomatic carotid stenosis. As data and technology improve, plaque composition, immunologic factors, and fibrous cap thickening may all play a role in determining which patients with asymptomatic carotid stenosis are most likely to benefit from intervention.

G. L. Moneta, MD

Pregnancy-Associated Plasma Protein-A Is Markedly Expressed by Monocyte-Macrophage Cells in Vulnerable and Ruptured Carotid Atherosclerotic Plaques: A Link Between Inflammation and Cerebrovascular Events

Sangiorgi G, Mauriello A, Bonanno E, et al (Istituto Policlinico San Donato, Milan, Italy; Univ of Rome Tor Vergata; Mayo Clinic and Found, Rochester, Minn; et al)
J Am Coll Cardiol 47:2201-2211, 2006

Objectives.—The study aim was to evaluate serologic expression of pregnancy-associated protein-A (PAPP-A) in patients affected by cerebrovascular accidents and to correlate it with histopathologic carotid plaque complexity.

Background.—Little is known about PAPP-A expression in carotid atherosclerotic disease and whether this protein represents a marker of plaque vulnerability also in carotid district.

Methods.—Seventy-two carotid plaques from patients submitted to surgical endarterectomy (19 who suffered a major stroke, 24 transient ischemic attack, and 29 asymptomatic) were evaluated. Serologic PAPP-A levels were determined by enzyme-linked immunoadsorbent assay. Plaques were divided in three groups based on histology: 1) stable (n = 38); 2) vulnerable (n = 13); 3) ruptured with thrombus (n = 14). Immunohistochemical staining for PAPP-A, smooth muscle cells, macrophages, and T-lymphocytes was performed in all cases. Real-time polymerase chain reaction assessed local PAPP-A production, and double immunofluorescence confocal microscopy (ICM) characterized cell type expressing PAPP-A.

Results.—Pregnancy-associated protein-A (serologic values were 4.02 ± 0.18 mIU/l in Group 1, 7.43 ± 0.97 mIU/l in Group 2, and 6.97 ± 0.75 mIU/l in Group 3 [1 vs. 3, p = 0.01; 1 vs. 2, p = 0.004; 2 vs. 3, p = 0.71, respectively]). Pregnancy-associated protein-A (expression showed a mean score value of 0.62 ± 0.06 for stable plaques, 2.54 ± 0.14 for vulnerable plaques, and 2.71 ± 0.12 for ruptured plaques [1 vs. 2, p = 0.001; 1 vs. 3, p = 0.001; 2 vs. 3, p = 0.37, respectively]). Real-time polymerase chain reaction demonstrated local messenger ribonucleic acid PAPP-A production, and double ICM confirmed monocyte/macrophage expression of PAPP-A in Groups 2 and 3 but not Group 1.

Conclusions.—This study suggests that PAPP-A is a marker of carotid plaque destabilization and rupture. Further studies are necessary to determine if PAPP-A can represents a new target for stratifying the risk of cerebrovascular events.

▶ It appears that PAPP-A is another potential marker of carotid plaque destabilization. We are slowly moving toward identifying which plaques are most dangerous. What is truly needed, however, is the identification of the asymptomatic plaque most likely to result in a neurologic symptom. The next step should be to determine if PAPP-A values can predict which initially asymptomatic plaques will eventually be associated with neurologic symptoms.

G. L. Moneta, MD

Role of platelet-derived growth factor and transforming growth factor β_1 the in the regulation of metalloproteinase expressions
Borrelli V, di Marzo L, Sapienza P, et al (Univ of Rome "La Sapienza")
Surgery 140:454-463, 2006

Background.—We investigated the role and influence of platelet derived growth factor (PDGF) and transforming growth factor β_1 (TGF) in the pathologic mechanism at the basis of plaque instability regulating the expression of matrix metalloproteinases (MMPs).

Methods.—Plaques obtained from 70 patients who underwent carotid endarterectomy were classified histologically as stable or unstable. Serum levels of PDGF and TGF were measured pre- and postoperatively. The serum activities of MMP-2 and MMP-9 were also analyzed. Human umbilical artery smooth muscle cells (HUASMCs) were stimulated in vitro with PDGF at various concentrations (20 and 50 ng/mL) and TGF (2 and 5 ng/mL) in a serum-free medium. The release of MMPs in the conditioned medium was assessed by enzyme-linked immunosorbent assay. Release of the MMPs was confirmed by Western blot analysis; their activity and expression were determined by zymography and reverse transcription-polymerase chain reaction. Specific inhibition tests were performed on HUASMCs to evaluate the role of these growth factors.

Results.—Forty-two (60%) patients had an unstable carotid plaque and 28 (40%) a stable plaque. Preoperatively, patients affected with unstable carotid plaques had higher PDGF and lower TGF plasma levels than patients with stable carotid plaques ($P < .001$); the levels returned to normal at 1 and 30 days postoperatively, compared with 20 non-operated healthy volunteers. Release, activity, protein level, and expression of MMPs in PDGF-stimulated HUASMCs were greater than in the controls ($P < .001$), whereas these values in the TGF-stimulated HUASMCs were lower ($P < .001$). The addition of monoclonal anti-PDGF antibodies decreased the release, activity, protein level, and expression of MMPs, whereas the addition of monoclonal anti-TGF antibodies increased the release, activity, protein level and expression of MMPs ($P < .001$).

Conclusions.—TGF seems to be an important stabilizing factor and prevents plaque rupture through the decrease of MMPs.

▶ Identifying molecular markers using human specimens has the great potential of unlocking mechanisms of disease that are clinically relevant. In this paper, the authors correlate the stability of carotid plaque with plasma levels of MMPs, PDGF, and TGF. Rather than identifying the vulnerable plaque, the marked changes in these plasma markers with eventual normalization indicate a preoperative stress state that returns to normal. Perhaps further study will eventually lead to a preoperative plasma marker for plaque instability.

G. L. Moneta, MD

An engineered vascular endothelial growth factor-activating transcription factor induces therapeutic angiogenesis in ApoE knockout mice with hindlimb ischemia

Xie D, Li Y, Reed EA, et al (Duke Univ, Durham, NC; Durham VA Med Ctr, NC)
J Vasc Surg 44:166-175, 2006

Objective.—Angiogenesis is the growth and proliferation of blood vessels from existing vascular structures, and therapeutic angiogenesis seeks to promote blood vessel growth to improve tissue perfusion. Vascular endothelial growth factor (VEGF) is a prototypic angiogenic agent that exists in vivo in multiple isoforms, and studies with VEGF to date had used single isoform therapy with disappointing results. We tested plasmid and adenoviral vectors encoding a zinc-finger DNA-binding transcription factor (ZFP-32E) that was designed to increase the expression of all major VEGF isoforms in a preclinical model of peripheral arterial obstructive disease (PAOD) in hypercholesterolemic (ApoE knock-out) mice.

Methods.—Unilateral femoral artery ligation/excision was performed in 117 mice. At 7 days postoperatively, the ischemic tibialis anterior (TA) and gastrocnemius (GAS) muscles received either ZFP-32E treatment (125 µg of plasmid, 2.5×10^{11}) viral particle units [vpu] of adenovirus; some mice received a second plasmid injection 3 days later) or no-ZFP treatment (125 µg of β-galactosidase [β-gal], a plasmid-lacking insert, or an equal dose of adenoviral encoding β-gal; some mice received a second plasmid injection 3 days later). Group 1 mice (n = 31) were euthanized 3 days later, and VEGF messenger RNA (mRNA) and protein levels were measured. Group 2 mice (n = 38) were euthanized 7 days later, and measures of capillary density, cell proliferation, and apoptosis were quantified. Group 3 mice (n = 48) were euthanized 28 days later, and changes in lower limb blood flow perfusion were measured.

Results.—In group 1, VEGF mRNA and protein levels were significantly higher in those with ZFP-32E treatment vs β-gal. In group 2, capillary density and proliferating cells were significantly greater and apoptosis was significantly lower in those with ZFP-32E treatment vs β-gal. Finally, in group 3, changes in the perfusion ratio (ischemic/nonischemic limb) at 21 days after injection were significantly greater in those with ZFP-32E treatment vs no-ZFP treatment.

Conclusion.—The ability of this engineered zinc-finger VEGF-activating transcription factor to induce therapeutic angiogenesis in hypercholesterolemic mice suggests this approach warrants investigation as a novel approach to treat PAOD.

▶ The holy grail for medical treatment of ischemia is inducing angiogenesis. Using a novel transcription factor that activates vascular endothelial growth factor (VEGF), these investigators observed increases in VEGF and vascular density. This led to increased perfusion by 8% to 12%. Previous angiogenesis clinical trials have been disappointing, and this therapeutic approach still has many hurdles before successful application in humans.

G. L. Moneta, MD

Reconstitution of CD39 in liposomes amplifies nucleoside triphosphate diphosphohydrolase activity and restores thromboregulatory properties
Haller CA, Cui W, Wen J, et al (Emory Univ, Atlanta, Ga; Harvard Med School; Georgia Inst of Technology, Atlanta)
J Vasc Surg 43:816-823, 2006

Background.—CD39 (nucleoside triphosphate diphosphohydrolase [NTPDase-1]) expressed on the luminal surface of endothelial cells rapidly metabolizes extracellular adenosine triphosphate (ATP) and adenosine diphosphate (ADP) to adenosine monophosphate (AMP), and abrogates platelet reactivity. Optimization of CD39 enzymatic activity appears dependent upon the expression of both transmembrane domains within plasma membranes. Thus, motivation exists to examine therapeutic antiplatelet formulations that consist of liposomal CD39.

Methods.—Full-length human CD39 was produced by using a yeast expression system, purified, and reconstituted within lipid vesicles. The catalytic efficiency (kcat/Km) of CD39-mediated phosphohydrolysis of ADP and ATP was determined both for detergent-solubilized and protein-reconstituted CD39 within lipid membranes. The capacity of CD39-containing lipid vesicles to inhibit platelet activation induced by ADP, collagen, or thrombin was determined in vitro by platelet aggregometry. A murine model of thromboplastin-induced thromboembolism was used to determine the effectiveness of intravenous liposomal CD39 in limiting platelet consumption and mortality.

Results.—Reconstitution of human CD39 in lipid vesicles was associated with a decrease in Km of nearly an order of magnitude over the detergent-solubilized form. There was a concomitant increase in both ADPase and ATPase catalytic efficiencies (kcat/Km ADPase: sol CD39: 2.7×10^6 vs liposomal CD39: 1.4×10^7) min/M; kcat/Km ATPase: sol CD39: 7.2×10^6 vs liposomal CD39: 2.0×10^7 min/M). Furthermore, CD39 lipid vesicles effectively inhibited platelet aggregation when activated by ADP, collagen, or thrombin, and also promoted platelet disaggregation (60.4% ± 6.1%). Treatment with CD39 lipid vesicles preserved platelet counts after thromboplastin injection (pretreatment, 906.8 ± 42.9 platelets/μm^3; empty vesicles, 278.6 ± 34.8 platelets/μm^3; CD39 vesicles, 563.6 ± 42.2 platelets/μm^3; n =

10 mice/test group; $P < .0001$). In parallel survival studies, liposomal CD39 reduced mortality from 73% to 33% ($P \leq .05$; n = 12 mice/experimental test group, n = 15 mice/control test group).

Conclusions.—Incorporation of solubilized CD39 into a lipid bilayer restores enzyme activity and optimizes thromboregulatory potential. Treatment with CD39 in liposomal formulations decreased mortality in a murine model of thromboplastin-induced thromboembolism by limiting intravascular platelet aggregation and thrombosis.

▶ The authors use liposomal CD39 as an alternative and novel antiplatelet agent. Because CD39 inhibits platelet function by several mechanisms, this powerful agent may find clinical utility and additional safety beyond currently used agents.

G. L. Moneta, MD

Pulsed High-Intensity Focused Ultrasound Enhances Thrombolysis in an in Vitro Model

Frenkel V, Oberoi J, Stone MJ, et al (NIH, Bethesda, Md; Case Western Reserve Univ, Cleveland, Ohio)
Radiology 239:86-93, 2006

Purpose.—To evaluate the use of pulsed high-intensity focused ultrasound exposures to improve tissue plasminogen activator (tPA)-mediated thrombolysis in an in vitro model.

Materials and Methods.—All experimental work was compliant with institutional guidelines and HIPAA. Clots were formed by placing 1 mL of human blood in closed-off sections of pediatric Penrose tubes. Four experimental groups were evaluated: control (nontreated) clots, clots treated with pulsed high-intensity focused ultrasound only, clots treated with tPA only, and clots treated with pulsed high-intensity focused ultrasound plus tPA. The focused ultrasound exposures (real or sham) were followed by incubations of the clots in tPA with saline or in saline only. Thrombolysis was measured as the relative reduction in the mass of the clot. D-Dimer assays also were performed. Two additional experiments were performed and yielded dose-response curves for two exposure parameters: number of pulses per raster point and total acoustic power. Radiation force-induced displacements caused by focused ultrasound exposures were simulated in the clots. A Tukey-Kramer honestly significant difference test was performed for comparisons between all pairs of experimental groups.

Results.—The clots treated with focused ultrasound alone did not show significant increases in thrombolysis compared with the control clots. The clots treated with focused ultrasound plus tPA showed a 50% ([30.2/20.1]/20.1) increase in the degree of thrombolysis compared with the clots treated with tPA only ($P < .001$), further corroborating the D-dimer assay results ($P < .001$). Additional experiments revealed how increasing both the number of pulses per raster point and the total acoustic power yielded corresponding

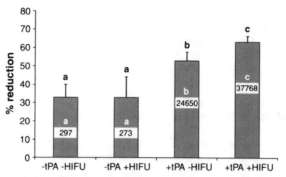

FIGURE 4.—Graph shows results of the standard pulsed high-intensity focused ultrasound (*HIFU*) experiments. The degree of thrombolysis in clots treated with focused ultrasound plus tPA was significantly greater than the degree of thrombolysis in clots treated with tPA only. In both these groups, the degree of thrombolysis was significantly greater than that in the control (untreated) clots and the clots treated with focused ultrasound exposures only. Differing lowercase letters between mean levels of thrombolysis indicate a significant difference of at least $P = .05$. Bars represent group means with standard deviations. D-Dimer values for the four experimental groups appear inside the bars and directly reflect the results of thrombolysis. (Courtesy of Frenkel V, Oberoi J, Stone MJ, et al. Pulsed high-intensity focused ultrasound enhances thrombolysis in an in vitro model. *Radiology.* 2006;239:86-93.)

increases in the thrombolysis rate. In the latter experiment, simulations performed at a range of power settings revealed a direct correlation between increased displacement and observed thrombolysis rate.

Conclusion.—The rate of tPA-mediated thrombolysis can be enhanced by using pulsed high-intensity focused ultrasound exposure in vitro (Fig 4).

▶ The use of a combination of thrombolytic drugs and focused US exposure has potential benefits with possible quicker resolution of thrombus and lower doses of thrombolytic agents. These are changes that could result in decreased bleeding risks and decreased treatment times. Presumably, US enhances thrombolysis through mechanical cavitation effects. A great deal of work will be required to evaluate the effective doses of both US and the thrombolytic agents in various clinical situations (venous thrombi, arterial thrombi, new versus old thrombi, etc). Work such as this presented here establishes the feasibility of dose ranging studies for thrombolytic agents and US for dissolving clots. Such work is crucial to future in vivo evaluation of a combination of US and thrombolytic agents.

G. L. Moneta, MD

Downregulation of desmuslin in primary vein incompetence

Yin H, Zhang X, Wang J, et al (First Affiliated Hosp, Guangzhou, People's Republic of China; Third Affiliated Hosp, Guangzhou, People's Republic of China; Sun Yat-sen Univ, Guangzhou, People's Republic of China)
J Vasc Surg 43:372-378, 2006

Objective.—Primary vein incompetence is one of the most common diseases of the peripheral veins, but its pathogenesis is unknown. These veins present obvious congenital defects, and examination of gene expression profiles of the incompetent vein specimens may provide important clues. The aim of this study was to screen for genes affecting the primary vein incompetence phenotype and test the differential expression of certain genes.

Methods.—We compared gene expression profiles of valvular areas from incompetent and normal great saphenous veins at the saphenofemoral junctions by fluorescent differential display reverse-transcription polymerase chain reaction (FDD RT-PCR). Differentially expressed complimentary DNAs (cDNAs) were confirmed by Northern blotting and semi-quantitative RT-PCR. Similarity of the cDNAs sequences to GenBank sequences was determined. Gene expression status was then determined by Western blot analysis and immunohistochemical techniques.

Results.—There were >30 differentially expressed cDNA bands. Sequence analysis revealed that a cDNA fragment obviously downregulated in incompetent great saphenous vein was a portion of the messenger RNA (mRNA) encoding desmuslin, a newly discovered intermittent filament protein. Northern blotting and semi-quantitative RT-PCR analysis revealed a similar mRNA expression profile of the desmuslin gene in other samples. Western blotting and immunohistochemical techniques localized the desmuslin protein mainly in the cytoplasm of venous smooth muscle cells. The amount of desmuslin was greatly decreased in the smooth muscle cells of incompetent veins.

Conclusions.—The expression of many genes is altered in primary vein incompetence. Up- or downregulation of these genes may be involved in the pathogenesis of this disease. Desmuslin expression is downregulated in the abnormal veins. Its effect on the integrity of smooth muscle cells might be related to malformation of the vein wall. Further studies are needed to investigate other differentially expressed cDNAs and the exact role of desmuslin in this disease.

Clinical Relevance.—Primary vein incompetence is a frequent and refractory disease of the peripheral veins. Exploring its pathogenesis may enhance our comprehension and management of this disease. We used reliable techniques to detect disease-related genes and confirmed downregulation of desmuslin in abnormal veins. Alteration of these genes might be used as disease markers or gene therapy targets.

▶ The authors describe downregulation of the intermediate filament protein demuslin in the veins of patients with reflux. It is not clear whether this downregulation is simply an association or whether this is mechanistic in the pathophysiology of the disease. However, this study attempts to close the gap between venous and arterial basic science.

G. L. Moneta, MD

Influence of gene polymorphisms in ulcer healing process after superficial venous surgery
Gemmati D, Tognazzo S, Catozzi L, et al (Univ of Ferrara, Italy)
J Vasc Surg 44:554-562, 2006

Objective.—Role of superficial venous surgery in reducing the time it takes for ulcers to heal is still controversial, although all studies confirm a significant reduction in ulcer recurrences. Recently, the *HFE-C282Y* and *FXIII-V34L* gene variants demonstrated a role in the risk of venous ulceration in primary chronic venous disorder (CVD) and in modulating lesion size in chronic venous ulcer (CVU), respectively. This study was conducted to investigate the role of *HFE-C282Y* and *FXIII* (*V34L* and *P564L*) gene variants in ulcer healing time after superficial venous surgery, by assessing the outcome of a cohort of homogeneous CVU patients.

Methods.—The study selected 91 patients affected by primary CVU (CEAP C6, Ep, Asp, Pr), with the exclusion of any other comorbidity factor involved in delayed healing process, who underwent surgery. We assessed the ulcer area and the healing time. Patients were genotyped by polymerase chain reaction for *FXIII* (*V34L* and *P564L*) and for *HFE-C282Y* substitutions.

Results.—Globally, CVU cases had a postoperative mean healing time of 8.5 ± 5.7 weeks. For the subset of cases above and below the median value (M = 8.0 weeks), *FXIII-V34L* genotype distribution significantly differed ($P < .0001$). In addition, Kaplan-Meier analysis yielded specific healing time profiles for the different *FXIII-V34L* classes of genotype ($P = .00001$), with an increased risk of delayed healing for the *FXIII-VV* genotype (hazard ra-

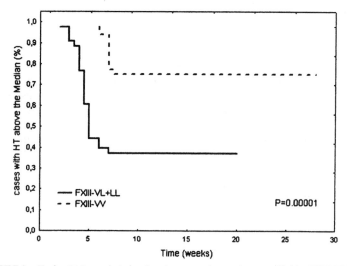

FIGURE 3.—Kaplan-Meier analysis for chronic venous ulcer patients stratified by *FXIII-V34L* genotypes (log-rank test, $P = .00001$). (Reprinted by permission of the publisher from Gemmati D, Tognazzo S, Catozzi L, et al. Influence of gene polymorphisms in ulcer healing process after superficial venous surgery. *J Vasc Surg.* 2006;44:554-562. Copyright 2006, Elsevier.)

tio, 4.14; 95% confidence interval, 2.1 to 8.2; $P = .00005$). Although *FXIII-P54L* genotype distributions did not differ, homozygous *564LL* cases ($P = .005$) and double carriers for both *FXIII* variants ($P < .0001$), had a significantly reduced healing time vs wild types. No differences in healing time were observed between carriers and noncarriers of the *HFE-C282Y* variant, whereas when these cases were stratified by *FXIII-V34L* genotypes, the *L34* carriers had a significantly shorter healing time, irrespective of the *HFE* genotype.

Conclusion.—The *FXIII-34L* variant was significantly associated with shorter healing time after superficial venous surgery, suggesting a role in the healing and tissue regeneration phases. Conversely, *HFE-C282Y*, despite its role in ulcer establishment, did not affect the postoperative healing time. In perspective, the identification of patients with a poor prognosis may give clinicians the opportunity to modify management and to target tailored therapies in the view of a new and alternative concept of treatment based on pharmacogenomics (Fig 3).

▶ These investigators carefully treated patients with venous ulcers and peered down to the molecular level to try to identify genetic reasons for poor healing. Their investigative efforts are to be applauded. The authors conclude that genotyping could identify patients that have poorer prognosis in venous ulcer healing and, thus, lead to modification of their management. In the context of this study with excellent venous surgery and wound care, I am not sure I see how.

G. L. Moneta, MD

Venous Ulcer Fibroblasts Respond to Basic Fibroblast Growth Factor at the Cell Cycle Protein Level

Seidman C, Raffetto JD, Overman KC, et al (Eugene Surgical Associates Peacehealth, Ore; Boston Med Ctr; Boston Univ; et al)
Ann Vasc Surg 20:376-380, 2006

Fibroblasts cultured from venous ulcers demonstrate phenotypic characteristics of cellular senescence including slow growth, altered morphology, upregulation of fibronectin, and increased senescence-associated β-galactosidase activity. In senescent cells, arrest of cell replication is related to overexpression of p21 and underexpression of phosphorylated tumor-suppressor protein retinoblastoma (ppRb). The regulatory mechanisms for cell proliferation in venous ulcer fibroblasts are unknown. In this study, venous ulcer fibroblasts are examined for cell cycle protein expression and modulation by basic fibroblast growth factor (bFGF). Fibroblasts were isolated from the venous ulcer of the distal lower extremity (fb-D) of patients with chronic venous insufficiency. A control biopsy was obtained from the proximal ipsilateral thigh (fb-P). Paired cultures were plated at 100,000 cells/plate and the cells synchronized. After 24 hr, one culture set was treated with bFGF (20 ng/mL) and the other was kept in culture medium only (untreated). All cultures, treated and untreated, were lysed following 24 hr of incubation, and the lysate was used to perform immunoblot analysis for p21, ppRb, and cyclin D1. Immunoblot samples were standardized to protein content. In all patients analyzed ($n = 4$), at basal levels (untreated) fb-D demonstrated significant overexpression of p21 versus fb-P ($p = 0.016$). Treatment with bFGF resulted in significant downregulation of p21 levels for fb-D ($p = 0.008$) and fb-P ($p = 0.037$) compared to untreated fibroblasts. ppRb was underexpressed in fb-D versus fb-P ($p = 0.069$). Treatment with bFGF increased ppRb significantly in fb-D ($p = 0.030$) and in fb-P ($p = 0.027$) compared to untreated fibroblasts. No differences were observed in cyclin D1 with respect to basal levels in fb-P versus fb-D or in treated versus untreated groups. Venous ulcer fibroblasts show phenotypic similarity to senescent cells, with overexpression of p21 as well as down regulation of phosphorylated pRb. The aberrations seen in the cell cycle proteins in fb-D are similar to those seen in senescent cells; however, bFGF can modulate important cell cycle regulatory proteins, promoting a proliferative environment in fb-D that is not possible in a senescent cell. The role of bFGF may be useful in the clinical treatment of venous ulcer pathology.

▶ In this study comparing fibroblasts from venous ulcers to similar cells from the proximal ipsilateral leg in 4 patients, the authors analyze the pathways of cellular senescence. The cell cycle proteins in fibroblasts from ulcers resembled the profile of senescent cells, and, importantly, could be altered by bFGF in culture. Whether this method is clinically applicable will require a larger clinical study of fibroblast responses in patients with active ulcers.

G. L. Moneta, MD

2   Coronary Disease

Optimal Medical Therapy with or without PCI for Stable Coronary Disease
Boden WE, for the COURAGE Trial Research Group (Buffalo Gen Hosp, NY; et al)
N Engl J Med 356:1-14, 2007

Background.—In patients with stable coronary artery disease, it remains unclear whether an initial management strategy of percutaneous coronary intervention (PCI) with intensive pharmacologic therapy and lifestyle intervention (optimal medical therapy) is superior to optimal medical therapy alone in reducing the risk of cardiovascular events.

Methods.—We conducted a randomized trial involving 2287 patients who had objective evidence of myocardial ischemia and significant coronary artery disease at 50 U.S. and Canadian centers. Between 1999 and 2004, we assigned 1149 patients to undergo PCI with optimal medical therapy (PCI group) and 1138 to receive optimal medical therapy alone (medical-therapy group). The primary outcome was death from any cause and nonfatal myocardial infarction during a follow-up period of 2.5 to 7.0 years (median, 4.6).

Results.—There were 211 primary events in the PCI group and 202 events in the medical-therapy group. The 4.6-year cumulative primary-event rates were 19.0% in the PCI group and 18.5% in the medical-therapy group (hazard ratio for the PCI group, 1.05; 95% confidence interval [CI], 0.87 to 1.27; P=0.62). There were no significant differences between the PCI group and the medical-therapy group in the composite of death, myocardial infarction, and stroke (20.0% vs. 19.5%; hazard ratio, 1.05; 95% CI, 0.87 to 1.27; P=0.62); hospitalization for acute coronary syndrome (12.4% vs. 11.8%; hazard ratio, 1.07; 95% CI, 0.84 to 1.37; P=0.56); or myocardial infarction (13.2% vs. 12.3%; hazard ratio, 1.13; 95% CI, 0.89 to 1.43; P=0.33).

Conclusions.—As an initial management strategy in patients with stable coronary artery disease, PCI did not reduce the risk of death, myocardial infarction, or other major cardiovascular events when added to optimal medical therapy. (ClinicalTrials.gov number, NCT00007657.)

▶ PCI added as an additional strategy to optimal medical management does not reduce risk of death, myocardial infarction, or other major cardiovascular events when compared to optimal medical therapy alone. About one third of patients in the medical therapy–only group will eventually require revascularization for symptoms or for development of an acute coronary syndrome. However, it appears that PCI can be safely deferred until symptoms increase or there is development of acute coronary syndrome. This study has huge implications for cardiology practice in the United States, as approximately 85% of PCIs are performed electively in patients with stable coronary disease.[1]

G. L. Moneta, MD

Reference

1. Feldman DN, Gade CL, Slotwiner AJ; New York State Angioplasty Registry. Comparisons of outcomes of percutaneous coronary interventions in patients of three age groups(<60, 60 to 80, and >80 years) (from the New York State Angioplasty Registry). *Am J Cardiol.* 2006;98:1334-1339.

Enoxaparin versus Unfractionated Heparin in Elective Percutaneous Coronary Intervention

Montalescot G, for the STEEPLE Investigators (Universitaire Pitié-Salpêtrière, Paris; et al)
N Engl J Med 355:1006-1017, 2006

Background.—Despite its limitations, unfractionated heparin has been the standard anticoagulant used during percutaneous coronary intervention (PCI). Several small studies have suggested that intravenous enoxaparin may be a safe and effective alternative. Our primary aim was to assess the safety of enoxaparin as compared with that of unfractionated heparin in elective PCI.

Methods.—In this prospective, open-label, multicenter, randomized trial, we randomly assigned 3528 patients with PCI to receive enoxaparin (0.5 or 0.75 mg per kilogram of body weight) or unfractionated heparin adjusted for activated clotting time, stratified according to the use or nonuse of glycoprotein IIb/IIIa inhibitors. The primary end point was the incidence of major or minor bleeding that was not related to coronary-artery bypass grafting. The main secondary end point was the percentage of patients in whom the target anticoagulation levels were reached.

Results.—Enoxaparin at a dose of 0.5 mg per kilogram was associated with a significant reduction in the rate of non–CABG-related bleeding in the first 48 hours, as compared with unfractionated heparin (5.9% vs. 8.5%; absolute difference, –2.6; 95% confidence interval [CI], –4.7 to –0.6; P=0.01), but the higher enoxaparin dose was not (6.5% vs. 8.5%; absolute difference, –2.0; 95% CI, –4.0 to 0.0; P=0.051). The incidence of major bleeding was significantly reduced in both enoxaparin groups, as compared with the unfractionated heparin group. Target anticoagulation levels were reached in significantly more patients who received enoxaparin (0.5-mg-per-kilogram dose, 79%; 0.75-mg-per-kilogram dose, 92%) than who received unfractionated heparin (20%, P<0.001).

Conclusions.—In elective PCI, a single intravenous bolus of 0.5 mg of enoxaparin per kilogram is associated with reduced rates of bleeding, and a dose of 0.75 mg per kilogram yields rates similar to those for unfractionated heparin, with more predictable anticoagulation levels. The trial was not large enough to provide a definitive comparison of efficacy in the prevention of ischemic events. (ClinicalTrials.gov number, NCT00077844.)

▶ Low–molecular weight heparins provide more reliable anticoagulation and lower bleeding rates than unfractionated heparin in many settings, now apparently also including percutaneous coronary intervention. Despite the fact that PCI in patients with stable coronary disease does not appear to prolong life,[1] I suspect PCI will continue to be performed at a high rate in patients with stable coronary artery disease, given the number of cardiologists out there and patient dissatisfaction with anginal symptoms. Although a single intravenous dose of 0.5 mg/kg of enoxaparin in this study was associated with reduced rates of bleeding, there was a slightly increased death rate in the patients treated with 0.5 mg/kg of enoxaparin. This resulted in early termination of enrollment in that group. The complications in the 0.5 mg/kg enoxaparin group that were considered by the investigators to be possibly related to treatment included rupture of a coronary artery with pericardial tamponade, a cardiac arrest several days after successful PCI, an episode of intracranial hemorrhage, and a periprocedural coronary occlusion after rotoblade dissection. Even though in the final analysis there were no statistical differences between treatment groups, a larger trial is needed to provide more definitive results.

G. L. Moneta, MD

Reference

1. Liakishev AA. Optimal Medical Therapy with or without PCI for Stable Coronary Disease. Results of COURAGE trial. *Kardiologiia.* 2007;47:91.

Correlates and Long-Term Outcomes of Angiographically Proven Stent Thrombosis With Sirolimus- and Paclitaxel-Eluting Stents
Kuchulakanti PK, Chu WW, Torguson R, et al (Washington Hosp Ctr, Washington, DC)
Circulation 113:1108-1113, 2006

Background.—Stent thrombosis (ST) is a serious complication of drug-eluting stent (DES) implantation regardless of the timing (acute, subacute, or late). The correlates of ST with DES are not yet completely elucidated.

Method and Results.—From a total cohort of 2974 consecutive patients treated with DES since April 2003, we identified 38 patients who presented with angiographic evidence of ST (1.27%). The ST occurred acutely in 5 patients, subacutely (≤30 days) in 25 patients, and late (>30 days) in 8 patients. The clinical, angiographic, and procedural variables of these patients were compared with the remaining 2936 consecutive patients who underwent DES implantation and did not experience ST during a follow-up of 12 months. Logistic regression analysis was conducted to determine the correlates of ST. Compared with patients without ST, patients with ST had a higher frequency of diabetes, acute postprocedural renal failure, and chronic renal failure. There were more bifurcation lesions, type C lesions, and a trend for smaller-diameter stents. Discontinuation of clopidogrel was higher in these patients (36.8% versus 10.7%; $P<0.0001$). The mean duration to ST from the stent implantation was 8.9 ± 8.5 days in subacute and 152.7 ± 100.4 days in late thrombosis cases. Mortality was significantly higher in patients with ST compared with those without ST at 6 months (31% versus 3%; $P<0.001$). Multivariate analysis detected cessation of clopidogrel therapy, renal failure, bifurcation lesions, and in-stent restenosis as significant correlates of ST ($P<0.05$).

Conclusions.—ST continues to be a serious complication of contemporary DES use. Careful management is warranted in patients with renal failure and in those undergoing treatment for in-stent restenosis and bifurcations. Special focus on clopidogrel compliance may minimize the incidence of ST after DES implantation.

▶ All procedures have potential complications. All risks for complications vary in how and whether they can be reduced. Animal models suggest that drug-eluting stents decrease rates of re-endothelialization, making the site of a stent a site of potential thrombosis by creating a local "hypercoagulable area." The only factor identified in this study that can be influenced by patients is cessation of Clopidogrel therapy, and the risk of stent thrombosis, while higher initially, never seems to go away. Patients with drug-eluting stents must be educated to the importance of compliance with their medications. It may be that at some point cessation of clopidogrel will no longer affect the tendency for a stent to thrombose. But until we know whether and when that is the case, lifelong clopidogrel therapy seems prudent in patients with drug-eluting stents.

G. L. Moneta, MD

Elevated Placental Growth Factor Levels Are Associated With Adverse Outcomes at Four-Year Follow-Up in Patients With Acute Coronary Syndromes

Lenderink T, for the CAPTURE Investigators (Atrium Med Centre, Heerlen, the Netherlands; et al)
J Am Coll Cardiol 47:307-311, 2006

Objectives.—This study sought to evaluate the predictive value of baseline placental growth factor (PlGF) for long-term cardiovascular events in acute coronary syndromes (ACS).

Background.—A biomarker of vascular inflammation, PlGF is identified as a powerful predictor for short-term outcome in patients with ACS.

Methods.—In 544 patients who were enrolled in the placebo arm of the c7E3 Fab Anti Platelet Therapy in Unstable REfractory angina (CAPTURE)

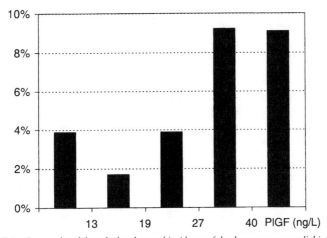

FIGURE 1.—Bar graphs of the calculated annual incidence of death or non-myocardial infarction according to placental growth factor (PlGF) status grouped in quintiles. (Courtesy of Lenderink T, for the CAPTURE Investigators. Elevated placental growth factor levels are associated with adverse outcomes at four-year follow-up in patients with acute coronary syndromes. *J Am Coll Cardiol.* 2006;47:307-311. Copyright 2006 by Elsevier.

trial, PlGF levels were determined as well as markers of myocardial necrosis (troponin T [TnT]), general inflammation (high-sensitivity C-reactive protein [hsCRP]), and platelet activation (soluble CD40 ligand [sCD40L]). Cox proportional hazard regression analyses were applied to evaluate the relationship between biomarkers and the occurrence of all-cause death or nonfatal myocardial infarction during a median follow-up period of four years.

Results.—Patients with PlGF levels in the fourth and fifth quintile (>27 ng/l) had higher mortality than those with lower levels (10.8% vs. 3.2%; hazard ratio [HR], 3.3; 95% confidence interval [CI], 1.6 to 7.1), as well as a higher incidence of the composite end point of death or myocardial infarction (27.6% vs. 11.3% events; HR, 2.6; 95% CI, 1.7 to 3.9). The relationship between PlGF and the composite end point remained significant after adjustment for TnT, sCD40L, and hsCRP (adjusted HR, 3.3; 95% CI, 2.0 to 5.4).

Conclusions.—In patients with ACS, elevated plasma levels of PlGF are associated with adverse cardiac outcomes during long-term follow-up. These data suggest that PlGF as a more specific marker of vascular inflammation should be considered for risk stratification of patients with ACS rather than general markers of inflammation (Fig 1).

▶ Accumulating data suggest that C - reactive protein may not be all that specific in predicting future cardiovascular events in individual patients. Perhaps placental growth factor will serve as a more-specific marker of vascular inflammation and a more-powerful predictor of vascular events. There will undoubtedly be additional studies evaluating the role of placental growth factor versus other markers of inflammation in predicting future cardiovascular events in various subsets of patients with atherosclerosis. The importance of this in the individual patient is unknown. See also this article regarding multiple biomarkers for the prediction of first major cardiovascular events and death.[1]

G. L. Moneta, MD

Reference

1. Lippi G, Salvagno GL, Targher G, Guidi GC. Multiple biomarkers for the prediction of first major cardiovascular events and death. *MedGenMed.* 2007;9:34.

3 Epidemiology

Risk factors for premature peripheral vascular disease: Results for the National Health and Nutritional Survey, 1999-2002
Lane JS, Vittinghoff E, Lane KT, et al (Univ of California, San Francisco)
J Vasc Surg 44:319-325, 2006

Purpose.—Premature peripheral vascular disease (PVD), occurring <60 years of age, is associated with significant cardiovascular morbidity, limb loss, and death. We hypothesized that different risk factors predict the development of PVD in patients <60 years than in patients ≥60 years.

Methods.—To address this question, we conducted a population-based observational study using the National Health and Nutritional Survey (NHANES) data set, which represents the noninstitutionalized civilian population in the United States. From 1999 to 2002, 5083 participants were analyzed as part of the NHANES survey. PVD status was defined by an ankle-brachial index (ABI) of <0.9. Putative risk factors for the development of PVD were collected by physical examination, interview, and laboratory testing. Univariate and multivariate logistic regression analyses were used to evaluate interactions between age strata and the development of PVD.

Results.—Premature PVD was found in 2.1% ± 0.2% of the population <60 years, and PVD was found in 12.0% ± 0.8% of the population ≥60 years. This corresponds to approximately 1.44 million people with premature PVD. Multivariate analysis determined coronary artery disease (odds ratio [OR] 2.90 vs 1.26, $P = .083$) and elevated serum fibrinogen (OR 1.07 vs 1.03, $P = .034$) were stronger predictors of PVD in subjects <60 years than in older subjects. Chronic renal insufficiency (OR 1.02 vs 1.16, $P = .006$) was more highly predictive of PVD in subjects >60 years. Other significant predictors, irrespective of age, in the multivariate model included hypertension (OR 1.99, $P < .001$), smoking (OR 2.22, $P < .001$), and serum homocysteine (OR 1.27, $P = .067$).

Conclusions.—Clinicians should be aware of the high risk of developing premature PVD in patients <60 years with coexisting coronary artery disease or elevated plasma fibrinogen. Routine screening by ABI measurements in high-risk patients would enhance the detection of subclinical premature PVD and allow for secondary intervention.

▶ There is not a lot that is surprising here, although the finding that elevated plasma fibrinogen levels were associated with early detectable PVD would not be at the top of most people's lists. When going to look for PVD, one has to decide who to screen. It doesn't seem practical to send off for homocysteine levels and fibrinogen levels in everyone under 60 years of age because it appears that ABI was only measured once, and therefore, what we really have here is determination of variables that were associated with PVD but not necessarily predictive of future PVD. A primary care physician will likely do more for his or her patients by measuring blood pressure, ankle brachial index, blood glucose levels, and creatinine and asking about smoking than measuring fibrinogen and homocysteine levels in all patients under 60 years of age.

G. L. Moneta, MD

Screening for asymptomatic cardiovascular disease with noninvasive imaging in patients at high-risk and low-risk according to the European Guidelines on Cardiovascular Disease Prevention: The SMART study
Goessens BMB, for the SMART Study Group (Univ Med Ctr, Utrecht, The Netherlands)
J Vasc Surg 43:525-532, 2006

Objective.—To assess the prevalence of atherosclerotic risk factors and to investigate the added value of noninvasive imaging in detecting asymptomatic cardiovascular diseases in patients at low risk and high risk according to the European Guidelines on Cardiovascular Disease Prevention.

Methods.—In the vascular screening program of the University Medical Center Utrecht, patients aged 18 to 79 years who had recently received a diagnosis of manifest vascular disease (coronary heart disease, cerebrovascular disease, abdominal aortic aneurysm, or peripheral arterial disease [PAD]) or had a risk factor (hypertension, hyperlipidemia, or diabetes mellitus) were assessed for atherosclerotic risk factors and (other) arterial diseases by noninvasive means. The European guidelines were applied to quantify the number of high-risk patients.

Results.—Eighty-eight percent of 3950 patients were considered to be at high-risk. More than 80% had hyperlipidemia, approximately 50% had hypertension, 21% had diabetes mellitus, and 31% were current smokers. An asymptomatic reduced ankle-brachial index (≤ 0.90) was most frequently observed in patients with cerebrovascular disease (21%); an asymptomatic abdominal aortic aneurysm (≥ 3.0 cm) in patients with PAD (5%) or cerebrovascular disease (5%); and an asymptomatic carotid stenosis ($\geq 50\%$) in patients with PAD (15%). On the basis of noninvasive measurements, 73 (13%) of 545 patients initially considered as low risk were reclassified as high risk.

Conclusions.—This study confirmed a high prevalence and clustering of modifiable atherosclerotic risk factors in high-risk patients. The yield of noninvasive vascular measurements was relatively low but identified a sizable number of high-risk patients. Standard screening for asymptomatic atherosclerotic disease identified a limited number of vascular abnormalities that necessitated immediate medical attention in patients already identified as high-risk patients.

▶ This is one of the best papers describing the results of screening for cardiovascular disease. Imaging studies, predictably, added little to the evaluation of standard risk factors and very infrequently identified a lesion that required immediate treatment. We used to perform carotid duplex and abdominal aortic aneurysm screening in all patients with peripheral vascular disease, but stopped because the yield seemed too low to justify the effort in an already overburdened vascular laboratory. Blanket screening will remain controversial, as the significance of the yield is truly in the eye of the beholder. However, in the United States, as we all know, imaging studies for screening, with the exception of screening for abdominal aortic aneurysm in selected catagories of patients, are not reimbursed. This fact alone will limit the use of imaging studies for screening. If, however, patients wish to pay for them, I have no objection to screening anyone. People can use their personal funds however they wish.

G. L. Moneta, MD

Physical Activity During Daily Life and Mortality in Patients With Peripheral Arterial Disease
Garg PK, Tian L, Criqui MH, et al (New York Univ; Northwestern Univ, Chicago; Univ of California, San Diego; et al)
Circulation 114:242-248, 2006

Background.—We determined whether patients with lower-extremity peripheral arterial disease (PAD) who are more physically active during daily life have lower mortality rates than PAD patients who are less active.

Method and Results.—Participants were 460 men and women with PAD (mean age 71.9+/-8.4 years) followed up for 57 months (interquartile range 36.6 to 61.9 months). At baseline, participants were interviewed about their physical activity. Vertical accelerometers measured physical activity continuously over 7 days in 225 participants. Analyses were adjusted for age, sex, race, body mass index, hypertension, smoking, comorbidities, total cholesterol, HDL cholesterol, leg symptoms, and ankle-brachial index. At 57-month follow-up, 134 participants (29%) had died, including 75 participants (33%) who wore accelerometers. Higher baseline physical activity levels measured by vertical accelerometer were associated with lower all-cause mortality (P(trend)=0.003). Relative to PAD participants in the highest quartile of accelerometer-measured physical activity, those in the lowest quartile had higher total mortality (hazard ratio 3.48, 95% confidence interval 1.23 to 9.87, P=0.019). Similar results were observed for the combined outcome of cardiovascular events or cardiovascular mortality (P(trend) =0.005). Higher numbers of stair flights climbed during 1 week were associated with lower total mortality (P(trend)=0.035).

Conclusions.—PAD patients with higher physical activity during daily life have reduced mortality and cardiovascular events compared with PAD patients with the lowest physical activity, independent of confounders. Further study is needed to determine whether interventions that increase physical activity during daily life are associated with improved survival in patients with PAD.

▶ It is well known that higher physical activity levels are associated with lower all cause and cardiovascular disease mortality in healthy populations. It appears this is also the case in patients with peripheral arterial disease. Therefore, even if a walking program does not improve patient's claudication distance, it may be patients should be encouraged to increase their physicial activity levels to prolong survival and decrease adverse cardiovascular events.

Gregory L. Moneta, MD

Overweight, Obesity, and Mortality in a Large Prospective Cohort of Persons 50 to 71 Years Old
Adams KF, Schatzkin A, Harris TB, et al (NIH, Bethesda, Md; AARP, Washington, DC)
N Engl J Med 355:763-778, 2006

Background.—Obesity, defined by a body-mass index (BMI) (the weight in kilograms divided by the square of the height in meters) of 30.0 or more, is associated with an increased risk of death, but the relation between overweight (a BMI of 25.0 to 29.9) and the risk of death has been questioned.

Methods.—We prospectively examined BMI in relation to the risk of death from any cause in 527,265 U.S. men and women in the National Institutes of Health–AARP cohort who were 50 to 71 years old at enrollment in 1995–1996. BMI was calculated from self-reported weight and height. Relative risks and 95 percent confidence intervals were adjusted for age, race or ethnic group, level of education, smoking status, physical activity, and alcohol intake. We also conducted alternative analyses to address potential biases related to preexisting chronic disease and smoking status.

Results.—During a maximum follow-up of 10 years through 2005, 61,317 participants (42,173 men and 19,144 women) died. Initial analyses showed an increased risk of death for the highest and lowest categories of BMI among both men and women, in all racial or ethnic groups, and at all ages. When the analysis was restricted to healthy people who had never smoked, the risk of death was associated with both overweight and obesity among men and women. In analyses of BMI during midlife (age of 50 years) among those who had never smoked, the associations became stronger, with the risk of death increasing by 20 to 40 percent among overweight persons and by two to at least three times among obese persons; the risk of death among underweight persons was attenuated.

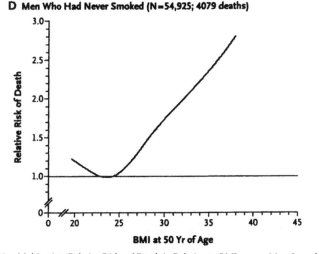

D Men Who Had Never Smoked (N=54,925; 4079 deaths)

BMI at 50 Yr of Age

FIGURE 1.—Multivariate Relative Risks of Death in Relation to BMI among Men. In each panel, the lines are natural cubic splines showing the shape of the dose-response curve for mortality according to BMI on a continuous basis. Relative risks are indicated by solid lines, and 95 percent confidence intervals by dashed lines. Panels A, B, and C (in the original article) are based on current BMI values, whereas Panel D represents BMI at the age of 50 years. The reference point is the midpoint of the reference group (BMI, 23.5 to 24.9) for categorical analyses, with knots placed at the 5th, 25th, 75th, and 95th percentiles of the BMI distribution among all men. The graphic display is truncated at 1 percent and 99 percent of BMI on the basis of the distribution of baseline (current) BMI among all men (Panels A, B, and C [in the original article]) and BMI at the age of 50 years among men who had never smoked (Panel D). All models are adjusted for age, race or ethnic group, level of education, alcohol consumption, and physical activity. The model for all men is adjusted for smoking status and the number of cigarettes smoked per day. The models for men who were former or current smokers are adjusted for the number of cigarettes smoked per day; men for whom information on the number of cigarettes smoked per day was missing were excluded. (Reprinted with permission from Adams KF, Schatzkin A, Harris TB, et al. Overweight, obesity, and mortality in a large prospective cohort of persons 50 to 71 years old. *N Engl J Med.* 2006;355:763-778. Copyright © 2006, Massachusetts Medical Society. All rights reserved.)

Conclusions.—Excess body weight during midlife, including overweight, is associated with an increased risk of death (Figs 1D and 2D).

▶ One of the realities of western civilization is that people tend to gain weight as they age. This article and another article in the *New England Journal of Medicine*[1] suggests that even modest weight gains in middle age are associated with an increased mortality rate. The mechanism for this increased mortality rate in overweight but not obese persons is unknown. It is postulated to be at least partially related to chronic inflammatory states secondary to excess adipose tissue. Whatever the cause, it appears that middle-aged persons will significantly benefit by reversing the tendency for weight gain that accompanies aging. I wonder how long it will be before a warning from the surgeon general is required on all packages of candy bars, potato chips, and other junk foods.

G. L. Moneta, MD

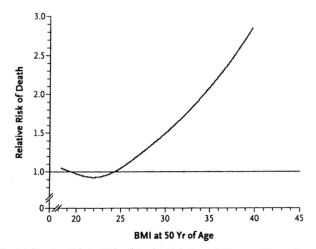

D Women Who Had Never Smoked (N=56,156; 2867 deaths)

BMI at 50 Yr of Age

FIGURE 2.—Multivariate Relative Risks of Death in Relation to BMI among Women. In each panel, the lines are natural cubic splines showing the shape of the dose-response curve for mortality according to BMI on a continuous basis. Relative risks are indicated by solid lines, and 95 percent confidence intervals by dashed lines. Panels A, B, and C (in the original article) are based on current BMI, whereas Panel D represents BMI at the age of 50 years. The reference point is the midpoint of the reference group (BMI, 23.5 to 24.9) for categorical analyses, with knots placed at the 5th, 25th, 75th, and 95th percentiles of the BMI distribution among all women. The graphic display is truncated at 1 percent and 99 percent of BMI on the basis of the distribution of baseline (current) BMI among all women (Panels A, B, and C [in the original article]) and BMI at the age of 50 years among women who had never smoked (Panel D). All models are adjusted for age, race or ethnic group, level of education, alcohol consumption, and physical activity. The model for all women is adjusted for smoking status and the number of cigarettes smoked per day. The models for women who were former or current smokers are adjusted for the number of cigarettes smoked per day; women for whom information on the number of cigarettes smoked per day was missing were excluded. (Courtesy of Adams KF, Schatzkin A, Harris TB, et al. Overweight, obesity, and mortality in a large prospective cohort of persons 50 to 71 years old. *N Engl J Med.* 2006;355:763-778. Copyright © 2006, Massachusetts Medical Society. All rights reserved.)

Reference

1. Jee SH, Sull JW, Park J, et al. Body-mass index and mortality in Korean men and women. *N Engl J Med.* 2006;355:779-787.

Mortality and Cardiac and Vascular Outcomes in Extremely Obese Women

McTigue K, Larson JC, Valoski A, et al (Univ of Pittsburgh, Pa; Fred Hutchinson Cancer Research Ctr, Seattle; Wake Forest Univ, Winston-Salem, NC; et al)
JAMA 296:79-86, 2006

Context.—Obesity, typically measured as body mass index of 30 or higher, has 3 subclasses: obesity 1 (30-34.9); obesity 2 (35-39.9); and extreme obesity (≥40). Extreme obesity is increasing particularly rapidly in the United States, yet its health risks are not well characterized.

Objective.—To determine how cardiovascular and mortality risks differ across clinical weight categories in women, with a focus on extreme obesity.

Design, Setting, and Participants.—We examined incident mortality and cardiovascular outcomes by weight status in 90,185 women recruited from 40 US centers for the Women's Health Initiative Observational Study and followed up for an average of 7.0 years (October 1, 1993 to August 31, 2004).

Main Outcome Measures.—Incidence of mortality, coronary heart disease, diabetes, and hypertension.

Results.—Extreme obesity prevalence differed with race/ethnicity, from 1% among Asian and Pacific Islanders to 10% among black women. All-cause mortality rates per 10,000 person-years were 68.39 (95% confidence interval [CI], 65.26-71.68) for normal body mass index, 71.16 (95% CI, 67.68-74.82) for overweight, 84.47 (95% CI, 78.90-90.42) for obesity 1, 102.85 (95% CI, 92.90-113.86) for obesity 2, and 116.85 (95% CI, 103.36-132.11) for extreme obesity. Analyses adjusted for age, smoking, educational achievement, US region, and physical activity levels showed that weight-related risk for all-cause mortality, coronary heart disease mortality, and coronary heart disease incidence did not differ by race/ethnicity. Adjusted analyses among white and black participants showed positive trends in all-cause mortality and coronary heart disease incidence with increasing weight category. Much of the obesity-related mortality and coronary heart disease risk was mediated by diabetes, hypertension, and hyperlipidemia. In white women, weight-related all-cause mortality risk was modified by age, with obesity conferring less risk among older women.

Conclusions.—Considering obesity as a body mass index of 30 or higher may lead to misinterpretation of individual and population risks. Escalating extreme obesity may exacerbate health effects and costs of the obesity epidemic.

► In my hospital it seems as though there is a 300-lb person in every elevator (but not in the stairwells!). The obesity epidemic is well established. For those of us who take care of patients, it is not surprising that mortality risks can be stratified by level of obesity. Women who are overweight but not obese may be initially comforted by the fact that being overweight was not associated with an increased mortality rate in this study. However, being overweight was associated with an increased incidence of coronary heart disease, and there certainly are considerable morbidity and mortality rates associated with coronary heart disease. It may be that the 7-year period of observation used in this study is insufficient to detect the long-term health effects of just being overweight but not obese.

G. L. Moneta, MD

Multiple Biomarkers for the Prediction of First Major Cardiovascular Events and Death

Wang TJ, Gona P, Larson MG, et al (Framingham Heart Study, Mass; Harvard Med School; Boston Univ; et al)

N Engl J Med 355:2631-2639, 2006

Background.—Few investigations have evaluated the incremental usefulness of multiple biomarkers from distinct biologic pathways for predicting the risk of cardiovascular events.

Methods.—We measured 10 biomarkers in 3209 participants attending a routine examination cycle of the Framingham Heart Study: the levels of C-reactive protein, B-type natriuretic peptide, N-terminal pro–atrial natriuretic peptide, aldosterone, renin, fibrinogen, D-dimer, plasminogen-activator inhibitor type 1, and homocysteine; and the urinary albumin-to-creatinine ratio.

Results.—During follow-up (median, 7.4 years), 207 participants died and 169 had a first major cardiovascular event. In Cox proportional-hazards models adjusting for conventional risk factors, the following biomarkers most strongly predicted the risk of death (each biomarker is followed by the adjusted hazard ratio per 1 SD increment in the log values): B-type natriuretic peptide level (1.40), C-reactive protein level (1.39), the urinary albumin-to-creatinine ratio (1.22), homocysteine level (1.20), and renin level (1.17). The biomarkers that most strongly predicted major cardiovascular events were B-type natriuretic peptide level (adjusted hazard ratio, 1.25 per 1 SD increment in the log values) and the urinary albumin-to-creatinine ratio (1.20). Persons with "multimarker" scores (based on regression coefficients of significant biomarkers) in the highest quintile as compared with those with scores in the lowest two quintiles had elevated risks of death (adjusted hazard ratio, 4.08; P<0.001) and major cardiovascular events (adjusted hazard ratio, 1.84; P=0.02). However, the addition of multimarker scores to conventional risk factors resulted in only small increases in the ability to classify risk, as measured by the C statistic.

Conclusions.—For assessing risk in individual persons, the use of the 10 contemporary biomarkers that we studied adds only moderately to standard risk factors (Fig 1).

▶ There is huge interest in risk stratification of patients for cardiovascular events. This interest has spawned what can be described as a cottage industry of assessment of biomarkers for cardiovascular events. This study confirms that multiple biomarkers are capable of predicting increased cardiovascular risks, but unfortunately they add little to the prediction of risk in individual patients. Routine assessment of biomarkers ofcardiovascular risk does not appear warranted.

G. L. Moneta, MD

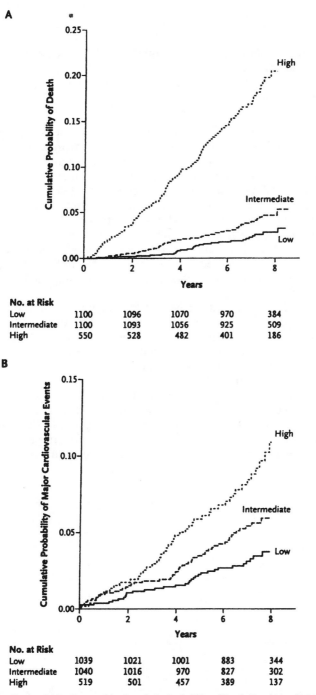

FIGURE 1.—Kaplan–Meier Curves of the Cumulative Probability of Death (Panel A) and Major Cardio-vascular Events (Panel B), According to Category of Multimarker Score. Multimarker scores were classified as low, intermediate, or high, as described in Table 2. (Reprinted by permission of Wang TJ, Gona P, Larson MG, et al. Multiple biomarkers for the prediction of first major cardiovascular events and death. *N Engl J Med.* 2006;355:2631-2639. Copyright © 2006, Massachusetts Medical Society. All rights reserved.)

Anti-Cardiolipin Antibodies and Overall Survival in a Large Cohort: Preliminary Report

Endler G, Marsik C, Jilma B, et al (Med Univ of Vienna)
Clin Chem 52:1040-1044, 2006

Background.—Anti-cardiolipin antibodies have been associated with both arterial and venous thrombosis, but their overall impact on all-cause or vascular mortality is unknown. In this study, we evaluated the influence of anti-cardiolipin antibodies on all-cause and vascular mortality.

Methods.—All individuals who fulfilled the inclusion criteria (completeness of data, no admission from an intensive care unit, unique identification with name and date of birth) and whose anti-cardiolipin antibodies were measured between October 2002 and February 2004 were included in this study (n = 4756; 64% female; median age, 46 years). Death/survival and cause of death were obtained from the Austrian Death Registry. The median observation period was 1.5 years, and the study comprised 7189 person-years.

Results.—During the study period, 184 patients (3.9%) died. There were no associations between either anti-cardiolipin IgM or IgG antibodies and both vascular death and noncancer mortality as outcome variables in a Cox regression analysis adjusted for age and sex. In contrast, the risk of cancer-related mortality was increased 2.6-fold.

Conclusions.—Anti-cardiolipin antibodies are associated with cancer mortality, likely as an epiphenomenon of malignancy, but they are not predictive of vascular mortality or noncancer mortality. Hence, although a clear association between anti-cardiolipin antibodies and (mostly nonfatal) vascular events has been described in the literature, our data indicate that this finding is not necessarily associated with an increase in vascular mortality (Fig 2).

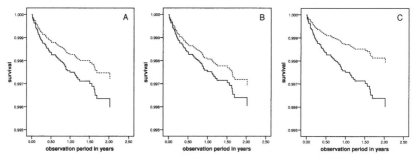

FIGURE 2.—Vascular mortality and anti-cardiolipin antibodies in a Cox regression analysis adjusted for sex and age. Shown are vascular mortality and concentrations of any anti-cardiolipin (either IgG or IgM) antibodies (*A*), IgM anti-cardiolipin antibodies only (*B*); and IgG anti-cardiolipin antibodies only (*C*). In all panels, the *solid line* indicates antibody concentrations at or below the upper reference limit and the *dashed line* indicates antibody concentrations above the upper reference limit. Vascular mortality did not differ significantly in patients with or without increased anti-cardiolipin antibodies. (Courtesy of Endler G, Marsik C, Jilma B, et al. Anti-cardiolipin antibodies and overall survival in a large cohort: preliminary report. *Clin Chem.* 2006;52:1040-1044. Copyright © 2006, The American Association for Clinincal Chemistry.)

▶ The literature describes a clear association between primary nonfatal vascular events and anticardiolipin antibodies. The authors' data indicate that whereas patients with elevated IgM or IgG levels may have an increased incidence of vascular events, it does not appear to affect the vascular-related mortality rate. This study is limited by the fact that anticardiolipin antibody measurements can be affected by interactions with plasma lipids, and lipids were not measured in this study. In addition, a period of observation of a median of 1.5 years per patient is relatively short for mortality observations.

G. L. Moneta, MD

Clopidogrel and Aspirin Versus Aspirin Alone for the Prevention of Atherothrombotic Events
Bhatt DL, for the CHARISMA Investigators (Cleveland Clinic, Ohio; et al)
N Engl J Med 354:1-12, 2006

Background.—Dual antiplatelet therapy with clopidogrel plus low-dose aspirin has not been studied in a broad population of patients at high risk for atherothrombotic events.

Methods.—We randomly assigned 15,603 patients with either clinically evident cardiovascular disease or multiple risk factors to receive clopidogrel (75 mg per day) plus low-dose aspirin (75 to 162 mg per day) or placebo plus low-dose aspirin and followed them for a median of 28 months. The primary efficacy end point was a composite of myocardial infarction, stroke, or death from cardiovascular causes.

Results.—The rate of the primary efficacy end point was 6.8 percent with clopidogrel plus aspirin and 7.3 percent with placebo plus aspirin (relative risk, 0.93; 95 percent confidence interval, 0.83 to 1.05; P=0.22). The respective rate of the principal secondary efficacy end point, which included hospitalizations for ischemic events, was 16.7 percent and 17.9 percent (relative risk, 0.92; 95 percent confidence interval, 0.86 to 0.995; P=0.04), and the rate of severe bleeding was 1.7 percent and 1.3 percent (relative risk, 1.25; 95 percent confidence interval, 0.97 to 1.61 percent; P=0.09). The rate of the primary end point among patients with multiple risk factors was 6.6 percent with clopidogrel and 5.5 percent with placebo (relative risk, 1.2; 95 percent confidence interval, 0.91 to 1.59; P=0.20) and the rate of death from cardiovascular causes also was higher with clopidogrel (3.9 percent vs. 2.2 percent, P=0.01). In the subgroup with clinically evident atherothrombosis, the rate was 6.9 percent with clopidogrel and 7.9 percent with placebo (relative risk, 0.88; 95 percent confidence interval, 0.77 to 0.998; P=0.046).

Conclusions.—In this trial, there was a suggestion of benefit with clopidogrel treatment in patients with symptomatic atherothrombosis and a suggestion of harm in patients with multiple risk factors. Overall, clopidogrel plus aspirin was not significantly more effective than aspirin alone in reduc-

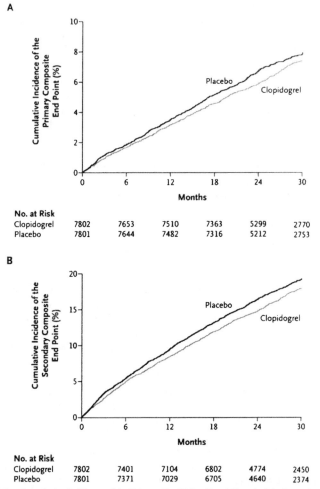

FIGURE 1.—Cumulative Incidence of the Primary End Point (Panel A) and of the Secondary End Point (Panel B). Panel A shows cumulative incidence curves for the primary end point of myocardial infarction, stroke, or death from cardiovascular causes. Cumulative incidence curves are displayed only up to 30 months because the uncertainty of the estimates beyond this point becomes quite large. The number of patients followed after 30 months decreases rapidly to zero, and only 21 primary efficacy events occurred after this time (13 in the clopidogrel group and 8 in the placebo group). Panel B shows cumulative incidence curves for the secondary end point, which included hospitalizations. (Reprinted by permission of Bhatt DL, for the CHARISMA Investigators. Clopidogrel and aspirin versus aspirin alone for the prevention of atherothrombotic events. *N Engl J Med.* 2006;354:1-12. Copyright © 2006, Massachusetts Medical Society. All rights reserved.)

ing the rate of myocardial infarction, stroke, or death from cardiovascular causes. (ClinicalTrials.gov number, NCT00050817.) (Fig 1).

▶ This long-awaited, important trial indicates that dual antiplatelet therapy is no more effective than aspirin alone in reducing rates of cardiovascular death, stroke, and myocardial infarction in patients with stable cardiovascular disease or multiple risk factors. The data suggest potential benefit in symptomatic patients with established vascular disease, but with an increased rate of bleeding. At this point, we can say that dual antiplatelet therapy is not indicated in patients without established vascular disease and that patients with symptomatic vascular disease may have slight benefit, but at an increased risk of bleeding.

G. L. Moneta, MD

Homocysteine Lowering with Folic Acid and B Vitamins in Vascular Disease
Lonn E, for The Heart Outcomes Prevention Evaluation (HOPE) 2 Investigators (McMaster Univ, Hamilton, Ont, Canada; et al)
N Engl J Med 354:1567-1577, 2006

Background.—In observational studies, lower homocysteine levels are associated with lower rates of coronary heart disease and stroke. Folic acid and vitamins B_6 and B_{12} lower homocysteine levels. We assessed whether supplementation reduced the risk of major cardiovascular events in patients with vascular disease.

Methods.—We randomly assigned 5522 patients 55 years of age or older who had vascular disease or diabetes to daily treatment either with the combination of 2.5 mg of folic acid, 50 mg of vitamin B_6, and 1 mg of vitamin B_{12} or with placebo for an average of five years. The primary outcome was a composite of death from cardiovascular causes, myocardial infarction, and stroke.

Results.—Mean plasma homocysteine levels decreased by 2.4 µmol per liter (0.3 mg per liter) in the active-treatment group and increased by 0.8 µmol per liter (0.1 mg per liter) in the placebo group. Primary outcome events occurred in 519 patients (18.8 percent) assigned to active therapy and 547 (19.8 percent) assigned to placebo (relative risk, 0.95; 95 percent confidence interval, 0.84 to 1.07; P=0.41). As compared with placebo, active treatment did not significantly decrease the risk of death from cardiovascular causes (relative risk, 0.96; 95 percent confidence interval, 0.81 to 1.13), myocardial infarction (relative risk, 0.98; 95 percent confidence interval, 0.85 to 1.14), or any of the secondary outcomes. Fewer patients assigned to active treatment than to placebo had a stroke (relative risk, 0.75; 95 percent confidence interval, 0.59 to 0.97). More patients in the active-treatment group were hospitalized for unstable angina (relative risk, 1.24; 95 percent confidence interval, 1.04 to 1.49).

Conclusions.—Supplements combining folic acid and vitamins B_6 and B_{12} did not reduce the risk of major cardiovascular events in patients with vascular disease. (ClinicalTrials.gov number, NCT00106886; Current Controlled Trials number, ISRCTN14017017.)

▶ Multiple trials have now demonstrated a lack of efficacy of supplemental vitamin therapy to decrease cardiovascular events. This is despite documented lowering of homocysteine levels by the vitamin therapy. This discordance between epidemiology and results of clinical trials is similar to that noted for estrogen and antioxidant vitamins. It may be that the epidemiologic data of homocysteine are confused by confounding variables that cannot be completely adjusted for in multivariable analysis. It may, however, simply be that homocysteine is a marker for, but not a cause of, vascular disease.

G. L. Moneta, MD

A Controlled Trial of Homocysteine Lowering and Cognitive Performance
McMahon JA, Green TJ, Skeaff CM, et al (Univ of Otago, Dunedin, New Zealand)
N Engl J Med 354:2764-2772, 2006

Background.—The results of observational studies suggest that plasma homocysteine concentrations are inversely related to cognitive function in older people. Our objective was to test the hypothesis that lowering the plasma homocysteine concentration improves cognitive function in healthy older people.

Methods.—We conducted a two-year, double-blind, placebo-controlled, randomized clinical trial involving 276 healthy participants, 65 years of age or older, with plasma homocysteine concentrations of at least 13 µmol per liter. Homocysteine-lowering treatment was a daily supplement containing folate (1000 µg) and vitamins B_{12} (500 µg) and B_6 (10 mg). Tests of cognition were conducted at baseline and after one and two years of treatment. Treatment effects were adjusted for baseline values, sex, and education.

Results.—On average, during the course of the study, the plasma homocysteine concentration was 4.36 µmol per liter (95 percent confidence interval, 3.81 to 4.91 µmol per liter) lower in the vitamin group than in the placebo group ($P<0.001$). Overall, there were no significant differences between the vitamin and placebo groups in the scores on tests of cognition.

Conclusions.—The results of this trial do not support the hypothesis that homocysteine lowering with B vitamins improves cognitive performance. (Australian Clinical Trials registry number, ACTR NO 12605000030673.)

▶ This study was stimulated by an aging population, and cognitive decline in the elderly is a major public health concern. Elevated homocysteine levels have also been associated with Alzheimer's disease and cognitive decline.[1,2] However, like studies relating homocysteine to vascular disease, treatment of homocysteine levels does not influence the condition with which it is associated. In this study, the follow-up was 2 years. This is a relatively short period, and perhaps long-term effects on cognition of lowering homocysteine levels may have been missed. In addition, this was a healthy population, and slowing of decline in cognitively impaired patients by lowering homocysteine levels has not been ruled out by this study.

G. L. Moneta, MD

References

1. Seshadri S, Beiser A, Selhub J, et al. Plasma homocysteine as a risk factor for dementia and Alzheimer's disease. *N Engl J Med.* 2002;346:476-483.
2. Selhub J, Bagley LC, Miller J, Rosenberg IH. B vitamins, homocysteine, and neurocognitive function in the elderly. *Am J Clin Nutr.* 2000;71:614s-620s.

Risk Factors for Progression of Peripheral Arterial Disease in Large and Small Vessels
Aboyans V, Criqui MH, Denenberg JO, et al (Univ of California, San Diego; Dupuytren Univ, Limoges, France: Harvard Med School; et al)
Circulation 113:2623-2629, 2006

Background.—Data on the natural history of peripheral arterial disease (PAD) are scarce and are focused primarily on clinical symptoms. Using noninvasive tests, we assessed the role of traditional and novel risk factors on PAD progression. We hypothesized that the risk factors for large-vessel PAD (LV-PAD) progression might differ from small-vessel PAD (SV-PAD).

Method and Results.—Between 1990 and 1994, patients seen during the prior 10 years in our vascular laboratories were invited for a new vascular examination. The first assessment provided baseline data, with follow-up data obtained at this study. The highest decile of decline was considered major progression, which was a −0.30 ankle brachial index decrease for LV-PAD and a −0.27 toe brachial index decrease for SV-PAD progression. In addition to traditional risk factors, the roles of high-sensitivity C-reactive protein, serum amyloid-A, lipoprotein(a), and homocysteine were assessed. Over the average follow-up interval of 4.6±2.5 years, the 403 patients showed a significant ankle brachial index and toe brachial index deterioration. In multivariable analysis, current smoking, ratio of total to HDL cholesterol, lipoprotein(a), and high-sensitivity C-reactive protein were related to LV-PAD progression, whereas only diabetes was associated with SV-PAD progression.

Conclusions.—Risk factors contribute differentially to the progression of LV-PAD and SV-PAD. Cigarette smoking, lipids, and inflammation contribute to LV-PAD progression, whereas diabetes was the only significant predictor of SV-PAD progression.

▶ The common observation that diabetic vascular disease is typically more distal than proximal is confirmed in this longitudinal study. Diabetes is a different risk factor from large-vessel risk factors such as smoking and hyperlipidemia. However, control of small-vessel disease or other diabetic complications does not appear related to control of hyperglycemia.

G. L. Moneta, MD

Relation of Inflammation to Peripheral Arterial Disease in the National Health and Nutrition Examination Survey, 1999–2002

Wildman RP, Muntner P, Chen J, et al (Tulane Univ, New Orleans, La; Univ of Pittsburgh, Pa)
Am J Cardiol 96:1579-1583, 2005

The relation between inflammation and peripheral arterial disease (PAD) is not well characterized. This study examined this relation and its consistency across important subgroups in a cross-sectional, nationally representative sample of the adult United States population. C-reactive protein (CRP), fibrinogen, leukocyte count, and PAD were assessed in a sample of 4,787 participants aged ≥40 years in the National Health and Nutrition Examination Survey 1999–2002. PAD was defined as an ankle-brachial blood pressure index <0.9. Graded relations were present between inflammatory markers and PAD. The multivariate adjusted odds ratios of PAD associated with the highest versus the lowest quartile of CRP, fibrinogen, and leukocyte count were 2.14 (95% confidence interval [CI] 1.41 to 3.25), 2.49 (95% CI 1.27 to 4.85), and 1.67 (95% CI 0.84 to 3.31), respectively (each p trend <0.05 across quartiles). Associations between inflammation and PAD were similar across gender, obesity, and diabetic subgroups. However, the odds ratios of PAD for the highest CRP quartile versus the 3 lowest quartiles were 3.10 (95% CI 1.76 to 5.45) for non-Hispanic blacks versus 1.50 (95% CI 0.98 to 2.28) for non-Hispanic whites and 1.11 (95% CI 0.57 to 2.17) for Mexican Americans (p interaction = 0.049) and 5.59 (95% CI 1.82 to 17.17) for patients aged 40 to 54 years versus 2.01 (95% CI 1.13 to 3.58) for patients aged 55 to 69 years and 0.98 (95% CI 0.65 to 1.48) for patients aged ≥70 years (p interaction = 0.018). Odds ratios of PAD for the highest fibrinogen quartile versus the lowest 3 quartiles were 3.26 (95% CI 1.69 to 6.28) for current smokers versus 0.83 (95% CI 0.51 to 1.35) for never smokers (p interaction = 0.006). In conclusion, in the general United States adult population, inflammation is independently associated with PAD.

▶ This article uses several markers of inflammation—CRP, fibrinogen, and leukocyte count—to support the epidemiological association between inflammation and PAD. Although the association is confirmed, it remains to be seen whether inhibiting inflammation will alter the natural history and biology of PAD.

G. L. Moneta, MD

Relationship Between C-Reactive Protein and Subclinical Atherosclerosis: The Dallas Heart Study
Khera A, de Lemos JA, Peshock RM, et al (Univ of Texas, Dallas; Brigham and Women's Hosp, Boston)
Circulation 113:38-43, 2006

Background.—Elevated levels of C-reactive protein (CRP) are associated with increased risk for incident cardiovascular events on the basis of observations from several prospective epidemiological studies. However, less is known regarding the relationship between CRP levels and atherosclerotic burden.

Method and Results.—We measured CRP in 3373 subjects 30 to 65 years of age who were participating in the Dallas Heart Study, a multiethnic, population-based, probability sample. Electron-beam CT scans were used to measure coronary artery calcification (CAC) in 2726 of these subjects, and MRI was used to measure aortic plaque in 2393. CRP levels were associated with most traditional cardiovascular risk factors. Subjects with CAC had higher median CRP levels than those without CAC (men: median, 2.4 versus 1.8 mg/L, $P<0.001$; women: median, 5.2 versus 3.6 mg/L, $P<0.001$), and there was a modest trend toward increasing CRP levels with increased CAC levels in men (P for trend$=0.003$) but not in women (P for trend$=0.08$). Male subjects with aortic plaque also had higher CRP levels than those without (median, 2.3 versus 1.8; $P<0.001$). In multivariate analysis adjusted for traditional cardiovascular risk factors, body mass index, and estrogen and statin medication use, the associations between CRP levels and CAC and CRP levels and aortic plaque were no longer statistically significant.

Conclusions.—In a large, population-based sample, subjects with higher CRP levels had a modest increase in the prevalence of subclinical atherosclerosis, but this association was not independent of traditional cardiovascular risk factors. CRP is a poor predictor of atherosclerotic burden.

▶ Despite several studies reporting the association between CRP and atherosclerosis, this large and robust study fails to show independent association of CRP with atherosclerotic burden. CRP may be related to plaque stability, but the strength of this association—and whether it is mechanistic to cardiovascular events—remains to be seen.

G. L. Moneta, MD

Oxidized Phospholipids Predict the Presence and Progression of Carotid and Femoral Atherosclerosis and Symptomatic Cardiovascular Disease: Five-Year Prospective Results From the Bruneck Study

Tsimikas S, Kiechl S, Willeit J, et al (Univ of California San Diego, La Jolla; St George's Hosp Med School, London; Austrian Academy of Sciences, Innsbruck, Austria; et al)
J Am Coll Cardiol 47:2219-2228, 2006

Objectives.—The purpose of this work was to determine the predictive value of oxidized phospholipids (OxPLs) present on apolipoprotein B-100 particles (apoB) in carotid and femoral atherosclerosis.

Background.—The OxPLs are pro-inflammatory and pro-atherogenic and may be detected using the antibody E06 (OxPL/apoB).

Methods.—The Bruneck study is a prospective population-based survey of 40- to 79-year-old men and women initiated in 1990. Plasma levels of OxPL/apoB and lipoprotein (a) [Lp(a)] were measured in 765 of 826 (92.6%) and 671 of 684 (98.1%) subjects alive in 1995 and 2000, respectively, and correlated with ultrasound measures of carotid and femoral atherosclerosis.

Results.—The distribution of the OxPL/apoB levels was skewed to lower levels and nearly identical to Lp(a) levels. The OxPL/apoB and Lp(a) levels were highly correlated (r = 0.87, p < 0.001), and displayed long-term stability and lacked correlations with most cardiovascular risk factors and lifestyle variables. The number of apolipoprotein (a) kringle IV-2 repeats was inversely related to Lp(a) mass (r = −0.48, p < 0.001) and OxPL/apoB levels (r = −0.46, p < 0.001). In multivariable analysis, OxPL/apoB levels were strongly and significantly associated with the presence, extent, and development (1995 to 2000) of carotid and femoral atherosclerosis and predicted the presence of symptomatic cardiovascular disease. Both OxPL/apoB and Lp(a) levels showed similar associations with atherosclerosis severity and progression, suggesting a common biological influence on atherogenesis.

Conclusions.—This study suggests that pro-inflammatory oxidized phospholipids, present primarily on Lp(a), are significant predictors of the presence and extent of carotid and femoral atherosclerosis, development of new lesions, and increased risk of cardiovascular events. The OxPL biomarkers may provide valuable insights into diagnosing and monitoring cardiovascular disease.

▶ The authors report that oxidized phospholipids on apoB particles predict development of atherosclerotic lesions and cardiovascular events, serving as a new biomarker for atherosclerotic disease. These inflammatory lipids will be important if they are found to be part of the mechanism of the disease or if they can serve as a point of control for medical therapy. Otherwise they may be yet another biomarker with no real practical value. I also suggest this very important article by Wang et al.[1]

G. L. Moneta, MD

Reference

1. Wang TJ, Gona P, Larson MG, et al. Multiple biomarkers for the prediction of first major cardiovascular events and death. *N Engl J Med.* 2006;355:2631-2639.

Hemostatic Factors, Inflammatory Markers, and Progressive Peripheral Atherosclerosis: The Edinburgh Artery Study
Tzoulaki I, Murray GD, Price JF, et al (Univ of Edinburgh, United Kingdom; Univ of Aberdeen, United Kingdom; Univ of Glasgow and Royal Infirmary, United Kingdom)
Am J Epidemiol 163:334-341, 2006

The interplay between inflammatory and hemostatic mechanisms may play a crucial role in the development and progression of atherosclerosis. The authors evaluated the separate and joint associations of hemostatic and inflammatory variables on peripheral atherosclerotic progression in the Edinburgh Artery Study, a population cohort study of 1,592 men and women aged 55–74 years that started in 1987. Levels of fibrinogen, fibrin D-dimer, von Willebrand factor, tissue plasminogen activator antigen, factor VII, prothrombin fragment 1 + 2, urinary fibrinopeptide A, C-reactive protein, and interleukin-6 were measured at baseline. Arm and ankle blood pressures were measured, and atherosclerotic progression was assessed by computing ankle brachial index (ABI) at baseline (1,582 participants) and after 12 years of follow-up (813 participants). Fibrinogen ($p=0.05$) and D-dimer ($p\leq0.05$) were significantly associated with ABI change independently of baseline ABI and cardiovascular disease risk factors. However, these associations were no longer significant when analyses were adjusted for either C-reactive protein or interleukin-6. Moreover, subjects with higher levels of both D-dimer and interleukin-6 at baseline had the greatest ABI decline. In conclusion, fibrinogen and D-dimer, but not other hemostatic factors, were associated with progressive peripheral atherosclerosis. Since D-dimer and fibrinogen are acute phase reactants, these data support the hypothesis that inflammation is more related to atherosclerosis than is hypercoagulation.

▶ In this ambitious study of more than 1,500 men and women serum biomarkers were compared with the ABI at baseline and after 12 years. Increases in fibrinogen, D-dimer, and interleukin-6 were associated with decreases in the ABI. This study uses highly accurate biomarkers, on the one hand, and a crude surrogate for atherosclerosis (ABI) on the other. Of note, mean ABI for all participants went from 1.03 to 1.0 over 12 years. Still, this article supports the hypothesis that inflammation, and also perhaps hypercoagulation, are related to atherogenesis.

G. L. Moneta, MD

Prospective evaluation of the relationship between C-reactive protein, D-dimer and progression of peripheral arterial disease

Musicant SE, Taylor LM Jr, Peters D, et al (Oregon Health & Science Univ, Portland)

J Vasc Surg 43:772-780, 2006

Objective.—Elevated levels of C-reactive protein (CRP) and D-dimer (DD) have been associated with the presence and progression of various forms of atherosclerotic disease, particularly coronary heart disease. We hypothesize that there is a relationship between elevated levels of baseline CRP and DD and progression of peripheral arterial disease (PAD) in patients with symptomatic PAD. The current study is a prospective evaluation of this hypothesis.

Methods.—Between 1996 and 2003, 384 subjects were enrolled in a National Institutes of Health-sponsored blinded, prospective trial evaluating the effects of multiple atherosclerotic risk factors on progression of symptomatic PAD. Baseline levels of CRP and D-dimer were obtained in 332 subjects. Subjects were followed every 6 months with clinical history and exam, ankle-brachial pressure index (ABI), and carotid artery duplex scanning (CDS). The primary study end point was a composite of ABI progression, CDS progression, stroke, myocardial infarction, amputation, and death from cardiovascular disease. Secondary end points included each of the components of the primary end point. The relationship between time to the various endpoints and baseline CRP and DD levels was examined by life-table analysis and Cox proportional hazards analysis.

Results.—Adequate baseline samples for CRP and DD were available in 332 subjects (mean age, 67 years; 57.8% men) with mean follow-up of 38.4 months (range, 1 to 99 months). Mean baseline levels (± SD) for CRP were 0.8 ± 1.14 (range, 0.03 to 13.0), and mean DD levels were 227.4 ± 303.3 (range, 1.9 to 2744.8). Progression, as defined by the primary end point, occurred in 48.5% of subjects. Subjects with elevated CRP (highest tertile) were no more likely to have any of the progression end points than those with the lowest values (lowest tertile) (P = NS, log-rank test, for all comparisons). By univariate analysis, subjects with elevated DD (highest tertile) were significantly more likely to die from any cause compared with subjects with the lowest DD values (lowest tertile) (P = .03, log-rank test). They were, however, no more likely to reach any of the other progression end points, including the primary end point (P = NS, log-rank test for all other comparisons). Multivariate analysis showed that DD level was a significant independent variable associated with occurrence of myocardial infarction (hazard ratio, 2.3; P = .02).

Conclusions.—In subjects with symptomatic PAD, elevated baseline DD, a marker of thrombotic activity, was significantly associated with the occurrence of myocardial infarction. This study did not confirm a relationship between progression of PAD and baseline DD or CRP during the first 3 years. Baseline DD and CRP do not provide useful risk stratification in patients at high risk for progression of symptomatic PAD. Future studies should evaluate serial levels of these markers to assess their utility in predicting progression of symptomatic PAD.

▶ In contradistinction to studies purporting the importance of CRP, often by investigators with a vested interest in a particular assay, these authors failed to find any association between elevated CRP and PAD progression. Elevated D-dimer levels were associated with myocardial infarction, suggesting that this marker of fibrinolysis may be of use in the management of coronary disease but not so useful for PAD management. Larger studies with longer follow-up on PAD progression are required before we completely discard these serum markers.

G. L. Moneta, MD

4 Vascular Lab and Imaging

Optimal Peak Systolic Velocity Threshold at Duplex US for Determining the Need for Carotid Endarterectomy: A Decision Analytic Approach
Heijenbrok-Kal MH, Buskens E, Nederkoorn PJ, et al (Erasmus MC-Univ Med Ctr Rotterdam, the Netherlands; Academic Med Ctr, Amsterdam; Univ Med Ctr Utrecht, the Netherlands; et al)
Radiology 238:480-488, 2006

Purpose.—To determine the optimal peak systolic velocity (PSV) threshold at duplex ultrasonography (US) required to establish the need for carotid endarterectomy in symptomatic patients on the basis of the long-term cost-effectiveness outcomes of diagnostic testing and subsequent treatment.

Materials and Methods.—From January 1997 through January 2000, a prospective medical ethics committee–approved multicenter study was conducted. After giving informed consent, patients with amaurosis fugax, transient ischemic attack, or minor stroke who underwent duplex US and digital subtraction angiography were included in the study. Selective ipsilateral carotid angiograms were obtained in at least three planes. Arteries that were nearly or totally occluded at duplex US were excluded because the PSV cannot be reliably measured in these vessels. Receiver operating characteristic (ROC) curves were constructed for the diagnoses of 70%–99% and 50%–99% stenoses. Optimal likelihood ratios were calculated on the basis of lifetime costs and quality-adjusted life-years derived at cost-effectiveness analysis and the prevalence of disease. The associated optimal sensitivities, specificities, and PSV thresholds were derived from the ROC curves.

Results.—In this clinical study, 350 patients were included. The nonoccluded arteries in a total of 236 patients were assessable for ROC analysis. For the diagnosis of 70%–99% stenosis, the optimal likelihood ratio was 0.21, which was associated with a PSV threshold of 220 cm/sec, a sensitivity of 97% (127 of 131 patients; 95% confidence interval [CI]: 94%, 100%), and a specificity of 48% (50 of 105 patients; 95% CI: 38%, 57%). For the diagnosis of 50%–99% stenosis, the optimal likelihood ratio was 0.38, which was associated with a PSV threshold of 180 cm/sec, a sensitivity of 95% (182 of 191 patients; 95% CI: 92%, 98%), and a specificity of 69% (31 of 45 patients; 95% CI: 55%, 82%).

Conclusion.—On the basis of the lifetime outcomes of diagnostic testing and subsequent treatment, the optimal PSV thresholds for the diagnosis of 70%–99% and 50%–99% carotid artery stenoses in patients with amaurosis fugax, transient ischemic attack, or minor stroke were 220 cm/sec and 180 cm/sec, respectively.

▶ This is the type of analysis needed for the modern practice of carotid interventions. The consequences of detecting a carotid stenosis above a specific threshold level must be considered and interpreted with respect as to whether the patient does or does not have associated symptoms. Peak systolic velocity values suggested here of 220 cm/s for ≤70% stenosis is acceptable for a symptomatic but not an asymptomatic patient. The specificity and positive predictive value is too low for an asymptomatic patient where the therapeutic index for carotid intervention is narrow. I also think that 180 cm/s for 50% stenosis is a bit low even for symptomatic patients because the therapeutic index for carotid endarterectomy for symptomatic patients with 50% to 69% stenosis is not much different than that for patients with high-grade asymptomatic stenosis.

G. L. Moneta, MD

Non-invasive imaging compared with intra-arterial angiography in the diagnosis of symptomatic carotid stenosis: a meta-analysis
Wardlaw JM, for the NHS Research and Development Health Technology Assessment Carotid Stenosis Imaging Group (Univ of Edinburgh, England; et al)
Lancet 367:1503-1512, 2006

Background.—Accurate carotid imaging is important for effective secondary stroke prevention. Non-invasive imaging, now widely available, is replacing intra-arterial angiography for carotid stenosis, but the accuracy remains uncertain despite an extensive literature. We systematically reviewed the accuracy of non-invasive imaging compared with intra-arterial angiography for diagnosing carotid stenosis in patients with carotid territory ischaemic symptoms.

Methods.—We searched for articles published between 1980 and April 2004; included studies comparing non-invasive imaging with intra-arterial angiography that met Standards for Reporting of Diagnostic Accuracy (STARD) criteria; extracted data to calculate sensitivity and specificity of non-invasive imaging, to test for heterogeneity and to perform sensitivity analyses; and categorised percent stenosis by the North American Symptomatic Carotid Endarterectomy Trial (NASCET) method.

Results.—In 41 included studies (2541 patients, 4876 arteries), contrast-enhanced MR angiography was more sensitive (0·94, 95% CI 0·88–0·97) and specific (0·93, 95% CI 0·89–0·96) for 70-99% stenosis than Doppler ultrasound, MR angiography, and CT angiography (sensitivities 0·89, 0·88, 0·76; specificities 0·84, 0·84, 0·94, respectively). Data for 50–69% stenoses and combinations of non-invasive tests were sparse and unreliable. There was heterogeneity between studies and evidence of publication bias.

Interpretation.—Non-invasive tests, used cautiously, could replace intra-arterial carotid angiography for 70–99% stenosis. However, more data are required to determine their accuracy, especially at 50–69% stenoses where the balance of risk and benefit for carotid endarterectomy is particularly narrow, and to explore and overcome heterogeneity. Methodology for evaluating imaging tests should be improved; blinded, prospective studies in clinically relevant patients are essential basic characteristics.

▶ This is an older form of analysis where the authors focus only on the mathematics of generating relative sensitivities and specificities for threshold levels of internal carotid artery stenosis. They do not consider the clinical implications of their conclusions with respect to an individual patient.[1] I agree that duplex is less likely to be accurate to determine a 50% to 60% ICA stenosis than a greater than 70% stenosis. With maximum and minimal velocity, criteria will always be less accurate than criteria that merely determines whether a certain level of stenosis is present.

G. L. Moneta, MD

Reference

1. Heijenbrok-Kal MH, Buskens E, Nederkoorn PJ, van der Graaf Y, Hunink MG. Optimal peak systolic velocity threshold at duplex us for determining the need for carotid endarterectomy: a decision analytic approach. *Radiology.* 2006;238: 480-488.

Safety of Arch Aortography for Assessment of Carotid Arteries

Berczi V, Randall M, Balamurugan R, et al (Northern Gen Hosp, Sheffield, England; Royal Hallamshire Hosp, Sheffield, England)
Eur J Vasc Endovasc Surg 31:3-7, 2006

Purpose.—To retrospectively review the safety of arch aortography and compare complication rates with published figures for selective catheter angiography.

Methods.—The medical records of patients undergoing arch aortography over the last 3 years ($n=311$; 180 male, 131 female; mean±SD age 71.0±9.2 years, range 42–90 years) were retrospectively reviewed. Any periprocedural (0–48 h) complications were recorded. A certified neurologist (MSR/GSV) classified all questionable neurological events.

Results.—There were no focal neurological events or deaths ($n=0$; 0%; CI: 0–0.96%). Non-focal neurological events included mild disorientation ($n=2$; 0.6%; CI: 0.176–2.31) and unequal pupils ($n=1$; 0.3%; CI: 0.056–1.79%). Cardiovascular events included symptomatic hypotension ($n=4$; 1.3%; CI: 0.50–3.25%), angina ($n=1$; 0.3%; CI: 0.056–1.79%) and arrhythmia ($n=4$; 1.3%; CI: 0.50–3.25). There were 27 minor access site complications (8.7%; CI: 6.0–12.3). None of these complications extended hospital stay. None of the arch angiograms had to be followed by selective carotid angiography.

Conclusion.—Arch aortography appears to have a lower neurological complication rate than selective carotid angiography.

▶ I am not sure there is a great need for isolated cathether-based studies intended only to visualize the aortic arch. The status of the internal carotid artery can almost always be assessed noninvasively, as can the aortic arch. I see no advantage of performing an arch aortogram one day to assess the arch for potential carotid stenting and then performing the stent as an entirely separate procedure. That seems to be a procedure designed to favor the surgeon and not the patient. The principal indication for isolated arch aortograms in the modern world is to assess the origins of the great vessels when the combination of physical examination and noninvasive testing had not provided definitive information.

G. L. Moneta, MD

Inflammation in Carotid Atherosclerotic Plaque: A Dynamic Contrast-enhanced MR Imaging Study

Kerwin WS, O'Brien KD, Ferguson MS, et al (Univ of Washington, Seattle; Mountain-Whisper-Light Statistical Consulting, Seattle; VA Puget Sound Health Care System, Seattle)
Radiology 241:459-468, 2006

Purpose.—To prospectively evaluate if there is an association between plaque enhancement at magnetic resonance (MR) imaging and proinflammatory cardiovascular risk factors and plaque content.

Materials and Methods.—This study was performed with informed consent, HIPAA compliance, and institutional review board approval. Contrast agent dynamics within carotid plaques were measured in 30 patients (29 men, one woman; mean age, 67.7 years ± 10.7 [standard deviation]) who were scheduled to undergo carotid endarterectomy. Measurements were based on kinetic modeling of images obtained at 15-second intervals during which a gadolinium-based contrast agent was injected. The time-varying signal intensities within the plaques were used to estimate the fractional plasma volume (v_p) and transfer constant (K^{trans}) of contrast material into the extracellular space. Pearson correlation coefficients were computed between blinded MR measurements and histologic measurements of plaque composition, including macrophages, neovasculature, necrotic core, calcification, loose matrix, and dense fibrous tissue. Correlation coefficients or mean differences were computed regarding clinical markers of cardiovascular risk.

Results.—Analyzable MR images and histologic results were obtained in 27 patients. Measurements of K^{trans} correlated with macrophage ($r = 0.75$, $P < .001$), neovasculature ($r = 0.71$, $P < .001$), and loose matrix ($r = 0.50$, $P = .01$) content. Measurements of v_p correlated with macrophage ($r = 0.54$,

$P = .004$), neovasculature ($r = 0.68$, $P < .001$), and loose matrix ($r = 0.42$, $P = .03$) content. For clinical parameters, significant associations were correlated with K^{trans} only, with decreased high-density lipoprotein levels ($r = -0.66$, $P < .001$) and elevated K^{trans} measurements in smokers compared with nonsmokers (mean, 0.134 min^{-1} vs 0.074 min^{-1}, respectively; $P = .01$).

Conclusion.—The correlations between K^{trans} and histologic markers of inflammation suggest that K^{trans} is a quantitative and noninvasive marker of plaque inflammation, which is further supported by the correlation of K^{trans} with proinflammatory cardiovascular risk factors, decreased high-density lipoprotein levels, and smoking.

▶ The study suggests that K^{trans} may serve as a noninvasive quantitative marker of plaque information. Eventually, MR imaging in quantification of plaque information may allow for serial noninvasive imaging of plaques and evaluation of therapies intended to reduce plaque inflammation.

G. L. Moneta, MD

Comparison of Symptomatic and Asymptomatic Atherosclerotic Carotid Plaque Features with in Vivo MR Imaging
Saam T, Cai J, Ma L, et al (Univ of Washington, Seattle; People's Liberation Army Gen Hosp, Beijing, China; Mountain-Whisper-Light Statistical Consulting, Seattle; et al)
Radiology 240:464-472, 2006

Purpose.—To retrospectively determine if in vivo magnetic resonance (MR) imaging can simultaneously depict differences between symptomatic and asymptomatic carotid atherosclerotic plaque.

Materials and Methods.—Institutional review board approval and informed consent were obtained for this HIPAA-compliant study. Twenty-three patients (21 men, two women; mean age, 66.1 years ± 11.0 [standard deviation]) with unilateral symptomatic carotid disease underwent 1.5-T time-of-flight MR angiography and 1.5-T T1-, intermediate-, and T2-weighted MR imaging. Both carotid arteries were reviewed. One observer recorded quantitative and morphologic information, which included measurement of the area of the lumen, artery wall, and main plaque components; fibrous cap status (thick, thin, or ruptured); American Heart Association (AHA) lesion type (types I–VIII); and location (juxtaluminal vs intraplaque) and type of hemorrhage. Plaques associated with neurologic symptoms and asymptomatic plaques were compared with Wilcoxon signed rank and McNemar tests.

Results.—Compared with asymptomatic plaques, symptomatic plaques had a higher incidence of fibrous cap rupture ($P = .007$), juxtaluminal hemorrhage or thrombus ($P = .039$), type I hemorrhage ($P = .021$), and complicated AHA type VI lesions ($P = .004$) and a lower incidence of uncomplicated AHA type IV and V lesions ($P = .005$). Symptomatic plaques also had larger hemorrhage ($P = .003$) and loose matrix ($P = .014$) areas and a smaller lumen area ($P = .008$). No significant differences between symptomatic and asymptomatic plaques were found for quantitative measurements of the lipid-rich necrotic core, calcification, and the vessel wall or for the occurrence of intraplaque hemorrhage or type II hemorrhage.

Conclusion.—This study revealed significant differences between symptomatic and asymptomatic plaques in the same patient.

▶ We sort of already knew most of this. Mutiple studies, using various techniques, have documented differences between symptomatic and asymptomatic carotid plaques. Not mentioned in the abstract is that the arteries with symptomatic plaques in this study were more narrow, with decreased lumen area ($P = .008$), than arteries with asymtomatic plaques. More patients in longitudinal observations are required to control for stenosis and determine the predictive value of the MR findings associated with plaques that were symptomatic. The big questions are what changes are present before symptoms develop and what changes predict symptoms. This would allow for better selection of patients for prophylactic carotid interventions.

G. L. Moneta, MD

A modified calculation of ankle-brachial pressure index is far more sensitive in the detection of peripheral arterial disease
Schröder F, Diehm N, Kareem S, et al (Klinikum Karlsbad-Langensteinbach, Germany; Ruprecht-Karls Univ of Heidelberg, Germany; Univ of Bern, Switzerland)
J Vasc Surg 44:531-536, 2006

Background.—Ankle-brachial pressure index (ABI) is a simple, inexpensive, and useful tool in the detection of peripheral arterial occlusive disease (PAD). The current guidelines published by the American Heart Association define ABI as the quotient of the higher of the systolic blood pressures (SBPs) of the two ankle arteries of that limb (either the anterior tibial artery or the posterior tibial artery) and the higher of the two brachial SBPs of the upper limbs. We hypothesized that considering the lower of the two ankle arterial SBPs of a side as the numerator and the higher of the brachial SBPs as the denominator would increase its diagnostic yield.

Methods.—The former method of eliciting ABI was termed as high ankle pressure (HAP) and the latter low ankle pressure (LAP). ABI was assessed in 216 subjects and calculated according to the HAP and the LAP method. ABI findings were confirmed by arterial duplex ultrasonography. A significant arterial stenosis was assumed if ABI was <0.9.

Results.—LAP had a sensitivity of 0.89 and a specificity of 0.93. The HAP method had a sensitivity of 0.68 and a specificity of 0.99. McNemar's test to compare the results of both methods demonstrated a two-tailed $P < .0001$, indicating a highly significant difference between both measurement methods.

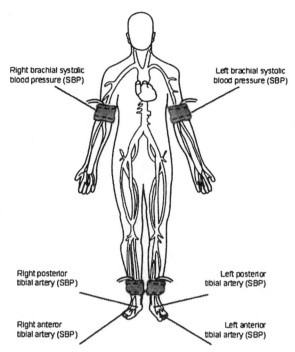

Right brachial systolic blood pressure (SBP)

Left brachial systolic blood pressure (SBP)

Right posterior tibial artery (SBP)

Left posterior tibial artery (SBP)

Right anteror tibial artery (SBP)

Left anterior tibial artery (SBP)

FIGURE 1.—Measurement of ABI as per the current protocol, the HAP method: ABI of right side = higher of the right ankle arterial SBP (mm Hg)/higher of the two brachial SBP (mm Hg). ABI of left side = higher of the left ankle arterial SBP (mm Hg)/higher of the two brachial SBP (mm Hg). Measurement of the ABI by the LAP method: ABI of right side = lower of the two right ankle SBP (mm Hg)/higher of the two brachial SBP (mm Hg). ABI of left side = lower of the two left ankle SBP (mm Hg)/higher of the two brachial SBP (mm Hg). (Reprinted by permission of the publisher from Schröder F, Diehm N, Kareem S, et al. A modified calculation of ankle-brachial pressure index is far more sensitive in the detection of peripheral arterial disease. *J Vasc Surg.* 2006;44:531-536. Copyright 2006 by Elsevier.)

Conclusions.—LAP is the superior method of calculating ABI to identify PAD. This result is of great interest for epidemiologic studies applying ABI measurements to detect PAD and assessing patients' cardiovascular risk (Fig 1).

▶ This method of calculating ankle brachial index (ABI) (ie, using the lowest ankle pressure) is probably more accurate for patients with diabetes with a greater prevalence of infrageniculate arterial disease. In this study there were 23 patients who had peripheral arterial disease detected by using the lowest ankle pressure but who also had normal ankle brachial indices using the highest ankle brachial pressure. Twenty-two of the 23 had duplex-determined infrageniculate occlusive disease.

G. L. Moneta, MD

Heritability of the Ankle-Brachial Index: The Framingham Offspring Study

Murabito JM, Guo C-Y, Fox CS, et al (Natl Heart, Lung, and Blood Inst, Framingham, Mass; Boston Univ; Harvard Med School)
Am J Epidemiol 164:963-968, 2006

The ankle-brachial blood pressure index (ABI) is a widely utilized measure for detecting peripheral arterial disease. Genetic contributions to variation in ABI are largely unknown. The authors sought to estimate ABI heritability in a community-based sample. From 1995 to 1998, ABI was measured in 1,097 men and 1,189 women (mean age = 57 years; range, 29–85 years) from 999 families in the Framingham Offspring cohort. Correlation coefficients for sibling pairs were calculated using the family correlations (FCOR) procedure in S.A.G.E. (Case Western Reserve University, Cleveland, Ohio). The heritability of ABI was estimated using variance-components methods in SOLAR (Southwest Foundation for Biomedical Research, San Antonio, Texas). Analyses were performed on normalized crude ABI and on normalized residuals from multiple linear regression analyses in SAS (SAS Institute, Inc., Cary, North Carolina) that adjusted for age, sex, smoking, diabetes, hypertension, ratio of total cholesterol to high density lipoprotein cholesterol, log triglyceride level, and body mass index. The mean ABI was 1.1 (range, 0.4–1.4). The age- and sex-adjusted and multivariable-adjusted sibling-pair correlation coefficients for normalized ABI were 0.15 and 0.11, respectively, resulting in heritability estimates of 0.30 and 0.22. Crude, age- and sex-adjusted, and multivariable-adjusted heritabilities for normalized ABI estimated using variance-components analysis were 0.27 (standard error, 0.06), 0.30 (standard error, 0.06), and 0.21 (standard error, 0.06), respectively (all p values < 0.0001). A modest proportion of the variability in ABI is explained by genetic factors.

▶ This is complicated math in an indirect way of saying there may be inherited components to atherosclerosis, not very surprising to those of us who take care of patients. I guess if you have a bad family history of atherosclerosis, you can be comforted a bit by this article. It suggests, to my reading, that a person's genetic makeup contributes modestly to the ultimate severity of atherosclerosis later in life. Therefore, even if you have a bad family history you may still do well with appropriate risk factor modification. History is not necessarily going to repeat itself.

G. L. Moneta, MD

Duplex ultrasound criteria for femorofemoral bypass revision

Stone PA, Armstrong PA, Bandyk DF, et al (Univ of South Florida, Tampa)

J Vasc Surg 44:496-502, 2006

Purpose.—This study was conducted to evaluate the impact of duplex ultrasound surveillance on the patency of femorofemoral bypasses performed for symptomatic peripheral arterial occlusive disease (PAOD).

Methods.—A retrospective review was conducted of 108 patients (78 men, 30 women) with a mean age of 62 ± 10 years who underwent femorofemoral prosthetic (n = 100) or vein (n = 8) bypass grafting for symptomatic PAOD (claudication, 38%; rest pain, 41%; tissue loss, 11%; infection, 10%) during a 10-year period. Prior or concomitant inflow iliac artery stenting was performed in 26 patients (24%), and a redo femorofemoral bypass was performed in 19 patients (18%). Duplex ultrasound surveillance of the reconstruction was performed at 6-month intervals to assess patency, graft (midgraft peak systolic flow velocity) hemodynamics, and identify inflow or outflow stenotic lesions. Repair was recommended for a stenosis with a peak systolic velocity (PSV) >300 cm/s and a PSV ratio >3.5. Life-table analysis was used to estimate primary, assisted-primary, and secondary graft patency.

Results.—During a mean 40-month follow-up (range, 2 to 120 months), 31 bypasses (29%) were revised: 19 duplex-detected stenosis involving the inflow iliac artery (n = 15) or anastomotic stenosis (n = 4), or both, 11 for graft thrombosis, and 1 for graft infection. Abnormal inflow iliac (PSV >300

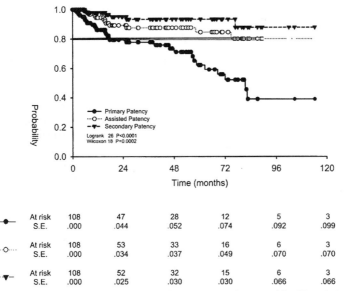

FIGURE 2.—Primary, assisted-primary, and secondary patency (Kaplan-Meier life-table analysis) of 108 femorofemoral bypass grafts, followed by duplex ultrasound surveillance. (Reprinted by permission of the publisher from Stone PA, Armstrong PA, Bandyk DF, et al. Duplex ultrasound criteria for femorofemoral bypass revision. *J Vasc Surg*. 2006;44:496-502. Copyright 2006 by Elsevier.)

cm/s) hemodynamics or a mid-graft PSV <60 cm/s was measured in eight of 11 grafts before thrombosis. Mean time to revision was 30 ± 17 months. The primary graft patency at 1, 3, and 5 years was 86%, 78%, and 62%, respectively. Correction of duplex-detected stenosis resulted in assisted-primary patency of 95% at 1 year and 88% at 3 and 5 years ($P < .0001$, log-rank). Secondary graft patency was 98% at 1 year and 93% at 3 and 5 years.

Conclusions.—Vascular laboratory surveillance after femorofemoral bypass that included duplex ultrasound imaging of the inflow iliac artery and graft accurately identified failing grafts. A duplex-detected identified stenosis with a PSV >300 cm/s correlated with failure, and repair of identified lesions was associated with excellent 5-year patency (Fig 2).

▶ An assisted primary patency rate of 88% at 5 years for femorofemoral grafts performed primarily for occlusive disease is amazing. Note that no graft failed when the mid graft peak systolic velocity was greater than 60 cm/s and no stenoses were identifed under those circumstances. I doubt there are all that many femorofemoral grafts performed for occlusive disease anymore. However, the data here seem sufficiently strong to recommend repair when anastomotic or inflow stenosis is associated with a peak systolic velocity >300 cm/s.

G. L. Moneta, MD

Duplex Guided Balloon Angioplasty of Failing Infrainguinal Bypass Grafts
Marks NA, Hingorani AP, Ascher E (Maimonides Med Ctr, Brooklyn, NY)
Eur J Vasc Endovasc Surg 32:176-181, 2006

Objective.—To assess the results of angioplasty and stent placement under duplex guidance for failing grafts.

Methods.—Over 22 months, 25 patients (72% males) with a mean age of 74±10 years presented to our institution with a failing infrainguinal bypass. The site of the most significant stenotic lesion was in the inflow in four cases, conduit in 18 cases and at the outflow in 11 cases. All arterial (20) or graft (13) entry sites cannulations were performed under direct duplex visualization. Duplex scanning was the sole imaging modality used to manipulate the guide wire and directional catheters from the ipsilateral CFA to a site beyond the most distal stenotic lesion. Selection and placement of balloons and stents were also guided by duplex. In 11 cases (33%), the contralateral CFA was used as the entry site and a standard approach (fluoroscopy and contrast material) was employed. Completion duplex exams were obtained in all cases.

Results.—The overall technical success was 97% (32/33 cases). In only one case, the outflow stenotic lesion in the plantar artery could not be traversed with the guidewire due to extreme tortuosity. Overall local complications rate was 6% (two cases). One vein bypass pseudoaneurysm caused by rupture with a cutting balloon was repaired by patch angioplasty and one SFA pseudoaneurysm at the puncture site required open repair. Overall 30-day survival rate was 100%. Overall 6-month limb salvage and primary patency rates were 100 and 69%, respectively.

Conclusions.—Duplex guided endovascular therapy is an effective modality for the treatment of failing infrainguinal arterial bypasses.

▶ I suspect at least part of the reason this sort of thing is not performed more often is because most of us do not have the technical support that Marks and her colleagues provide the vascular surgeons at Maimonides. A 6-month primary patency rate of 69% seems somewhat low compared with what would be expected with a surgical reconstruction. But the numbers are too small to know whether that reflects a problem with US guidance, a problem with technique (3 patients had stenoses at puncture sites in the vein graft, a technique not generally recommended), or a problem with suboptimal vein grafts to work with, or the fact that angioplasty just doesn't work as well as surgical revisions in the long run.

G. L. Moneta, MD

Vessel Wall Calcifications at Multi–Detector Row CT Angiography in Patients with Peripheral Arterial Disease: Effect on Clinical Utility and Clinical Predictors

Ouwendijk R, Kock MCJM, van Dijk LC, et al (Erasmus MC Rotterdam, the Netherlands; Harvard School of Public Health, Boston)
Radiology 241:603-608, 2006

Purpose.—To evaluate retrospectively the effect of vessel wall calcifications on the clinical utility of multi-detector row computed tomographic (CT) angiography performed in patients with peripheral arterial disease and to identify clinical predictors for the presence of vessel wall calcifications.

Materials and Methods.—The study was approved by the hospital institutional review board, and informed consent was obtained from all patients. For this study the authors included patients from two randomized controlled trials that measured the costs and effects of diagnostic imaging in patients with peripheral arterial disease. All patients underwent CT angiography and were followed up for 6 months. Clinical utility was measured on the basis of therapeutic confidence (rated on a 10-point scale) in the results of initial CT angiography and the need for additional vascular imaging. Univariable and multivariable logistic and linear regression analysis and the area under the receiver operating characteristic curve were used to evaluate the effect of vessel wall calcifications on the clinical utility of CT angiography and the use of patient characteristics to predict the number of calcified segments at CT angiography.

Results.—A total of 145 patients were included (mean age, 64 years; 70% men). The authors found that the number of calcified segments was a significant predictor of the need for additional imaging ($P = .001$) and of the confidence scores ($P < .001$). The number of calcified segments discriminated between patients who required additional imaging after CT angiography and those who did not (area under the receiver operating characteristic curve, 0.66; 95% confidence interval: 0.54, 0.77). Age, diabetes mellitus, and cardiac disease were significant predictors of the number of calcified segments in both the univariable and multivariable analyses ($P < .05$).

Conclusion.—Vessel wall calcifications decrease the clinical utility of CT angiography in patients with peripheral arterial disease. Diabetes mellitus, cardiac disease, and elderly age (older than 84 years) are independently predictive for the presence of vessel wall calcifications.

▶ All imaging techniques have advantages and disadvantages. A clear disadvantage of CTA is evaluation of small, heavily calcified arteries. The study suggests that, despite its lower cost and noninvasive nature, other forms of arterial imaging such as MRA or contrasted angiography should be considered in patients with diabetes, heart disease, and advanced age who require operative intervention of smaller arteries.

G. L. Moneta, MD

Preoperative Multidetector Computed Tomography Evaluation of the Artery of Adamkiewicz and its Origin
Takase K, Akasaka J, Sawamura Y, et al (Tohoku Univ, Japan; Yamagata Univ, Japan; Ishinomaki Red Cross Hosp, Japan)
J Comput Assist Tomogr 30:716-722, 2006

Objective.—To assess the usefulness of MDCT in the preoperative evaluation of the artery of Adamkiewicz (ARM) and its parent artery.

Methods.—Ten patients with thoracoabdominal vascular diseases underwent MDCT of the entire aorta and iliac arteries. The visualization of the ARM, and its branching level and site of origin, and the continuity of the intercostal/lumbar arteries with the ARM were investigated.

Results.—In 9 of the 10 patients, the ARM was clearly visualized. The entire length from the intercostal/lumbar arteries to the ARM could be traced in 8 of the 10 patients. Surgical treatment or stentgraft insertion was based on a consideration of the vascular supply to the ARM. No postoperative ischemic spinal complications occurred.

Conclusions.—MDCT permits the evaluation of the ARM for its entire length and provides information on the intercostal and lumbar arteries and entire aorta (Fig 2C).

▶ It makes sense that identification of a patent artery of Adamkiewicz, and its parent vessel, may be important in planning thoracoabdominal aneurysm repair. This may allow targeted preservation or reattachment of specific intercostal or lumbar vessels. It may also be equally important to know which pa-

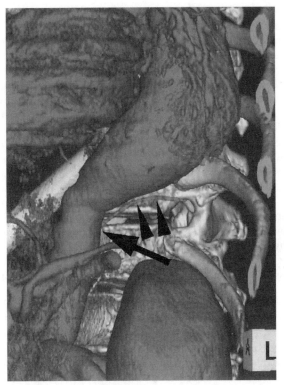

FIGURE 2.—C, Magnified VR image of the lower part of the thoracic aortic aneurysm (80 degrees of left anterior lateral oblique position). (Courtesy of Takase K, Akasaka J, Sawamura Y, et al. Preoperative multidetector computed tomography evaluation of the artery of Adamkiewicz and its origin. *J Comput Assist Tomogr.* 2006;30:716-722.)

tients have occluded parent vessels to the artery of Adamkiewicz. Perhaps in such cases reattachment or preservation or intercostal lumbar vessels is not necessary in thoracoabdominal aneurysm repair. Equally possible, however, is that reattachment of additional vessels to preserve collateral flow would be required.

G. L. Moneta, MD

Magnetic resonance angiography and neuromonitoring to assess spinal cord blood supply in thoracic and thoracoabdominal aortic aneurysm surgery

Nijenhuis RJ, Jacobs MJ, Schurink GW, et al (Maastricht Univ, The Netherlands; Aachen Univ, The Netherlands)
J Vasc Surg 45:71-78, 2007

Objective.—Preoperative knowledge of the blood-supplying trajectory to the spinal cord is of interest, because spinal cord ischemia may occur during thoracic aortic aneurysm (TAA) and thoracoabdominal aortic aneurysm (TAAA) repair and possibly leads to paraplegia. The Adamkiewicz artery (AKA) is considered to be the most important blood supplier of the thoracolumbar spinal cord and has therefore been the focus in preoperative diagnostic imaging. However, in TAA(A) patients, the blood supply to the spinal cord may strongly depend on (intersegmental) collateral circulation, because many segmental arteries are occluded as a result of atherosclerosis. Therefore, the importance of preserving the segmental artery supplying the AKA (SA-AKA) is debated. Here it was investigated whether (1) the AKA and its segmental supplier can be imaged by using magnetic resonance (MR) angiography and (2) aortic cross-clamping of the SA-AKA influences intraoperative spinal cord function, monitored by motor evoked potentials (MEPs).

Methods.—Preoperative MR angiography was performed to localize the SA-AKA and the AKA in 60 patients (19 TAA, 7 TAAA I, 18 TAAA II, 9 TAAA III, and 7 TAAA IV). Spinal cord function was monitored during surgery by using MEPs. When MEPs indicated critical ischemia, the SA-AKA was selectively reattached. To test whether aortic cross-clamping of the SA-AKA was associated with MEP decline, the Fisher statistical exactness test was applied.

Results.—The AKA and SA-AKA could be localized in all 60 (100%) patients between vertebral levels T8 and L2 (72% left sided). In 44 (73%) patients, the SA-AKA was cross-clamped, which led in 32% (14/44) of cases to MEP decline. Reattachment of the preoperatively localized SA-AKA reestablished MEPs and, thus, spinal cord function in 12 of 14 cases. When the SA-AKA was outside the area cross-clamped, the MEPs always remained stable. A significant association ($P < .01$) was found between the location of the SA-AKA relative to the aortic cross-clamps and the MEPs.

Conclusions.—The AKA can be localized before surgery in 100% of TAA (A) patients by using MR angiography. Location of the SA-AKA outside the cross-clamped aortic area is attended with stable MEPs. Interestingly, it was found that in most patients in whom the SA-AKA was cross-clamped, MEPs were not affected, thus indicating sufficient collateral blood supply to maintain spinal cord integrity. Nevertheless, preoperative knowledge of SA-AKA location is of importance, because in 32% of patients, spinal cord function was dependent on this supplier. Revascularization of the SA-AKA can thereby reverse spinal cord dysfunction.

▶ This article addresses some of the questions posed in another important article.[1] Both CTA and MRA can be used to locate the segmental artery supplying the artery of Adamkiewicz. This article was presented before the Society of Vascular Surgery had comments from the floor by some very experienced thoracoabdominal aneurysm surgeons that are quite insightful. As pointed out by Dr Cambria, one drawback of MR as opposed to CTA is that MR does not allow localization of aortic thrombus. It will be nice to know if the segment of aorta supplying the artery of Adamkiewicz is covered with thrombus. Perhaps that means intercostals from elsewhere need to be reimplanted or special attention be made to preserving hypogastric arteries, as suggested by Professor Sandman.

G. L. Moneta, MD

Reference

1. Nojiri J, Matsumoto K, Kato A, et al. The Adamkiewicz artery: demonstration by intra-arterial computed tomographic angiography. *Eur J Cardiothorac Surg.* 2007;31:249-255.

Abdominal Aortic Aneurysm: Can the Arterial Phase at CT Evaluation after Endovascular Repair Be Eliminated to Reduce Radiation Dose?
Macari M, Chandarana H, Schmidt B, et al (New York Univ; Siemens Med Solutions, Malvern, Pa)
Radiology 241:908-914, 2006

Purpose.—To retrospectively determine if arterial phase computed tomographic (CT) imaging is necessary for follow-up imaging of patients who have undergone endovascular stent-graft therapy for abdominal aortic aneurysm.

Materials and Methods.—This HIPAA-compliant study was exempt from institutional review board approval; informed patient consent was waived. Eighty-five patients (66 men, 19 women; mean age, 66 years; range, 45–81 years) underwent 110 multidetector CT examinations after endovascular repair of abdominal aortic aneurysms. Nonenhanced CT images were obtained. Intravenous contrast material was then injected at 4 mL/sec, and arterial and venous phase (60 seconds) CT images were obtained. The nonenhanced and venous phase images were evaluated to determine if an endoleak was present. Subsequently, arterial phase images were analyzed. The effective dose was calculated. Ninety-five percent confidence intervals as indicators of how often arterial phase imaging would contribute to the diagnosis of endoleak were determined.

Results.—Twenty-eight type II endoleaks were detected by using combined nonenhanced and venous phase acquisitions. Twenty-five of the 28 endoleaks were also visualized during the arterial phase. Three type II endoleaks were seen only during the venous phase. The arterial phase images depicted no additional endoleaks. Seventy-eight CT examinations performed in 67 patients revealed no endoleak during the venous phase. The arterial phase images also depicted no endoleaks at these examinations. Thus, for no more than 3.1% of all examinations, there was 95% confidence that arterial phase imaging would depict an endoleak missed at venous phase imaging. Arterial phase imaging contributed to a mean of 36.5% of the effective dose delivered.

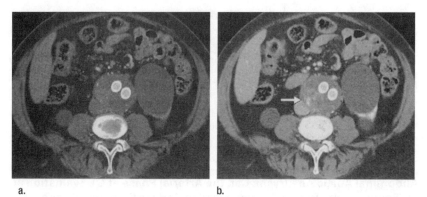

a.   b.

FIGURE 3.—Type II endoleak seen only during venous phase in 72-year-old man. (a) Transverse arterial phase CT image shows no evidence of endoleak. (b) Transverse venous phase CT image shows multiple foci of enhancement (arrow) to the right of the graft. The foci can be traced from a back-bleeding lumbar artery. (Courtesy of Macari M, Chandarana H, Schmidt B. Abdominal aortic aneurysm: can the arterial phase at CT evaluation after endovascular repair be eliminated to reduce radiation dose? *Radiology.* 2006;241:908-914. Radiological Society of North America.)

Conclusion.—Study results indicate that arterial phase imaging may not be necessary for the routine detection of endoleaks. Radiation exposure can be decreased by eliminating this phase (Fig 3).

▶ The radiation administered during a diagnostic CT scan is associated with low, but not zero, health risks. This radiation has been linked to an increase in life-long risk of cancer.[1] Because type 2 endoleaks are relatively benign, the increased radiation dose of arterial-phase acquisitions does not seem warranted. Additional data are required to know whether the arterial-phase acquisitions may, however, remain necessary to detect small type 1 or type 3 endoleaks. Of course, the best way to reduce the radiation associated with a CT scan is to use alternative imaging methods for follow-up of abdominal aortic aneurysm stent grafts.[2-4]

G. L. Moneta, MD

Reference

1. Brenner DJ, Elliston CD. Estimated radiation risks potentially associated with full-body CT screening. *Radiology* 2004;232:736-738.
2. van der Laan MJ, Bartels LW, Viergever MA, Blankensteijn JD. Computed tomography versus magnetic resonance imaging of endoleaks after EVAR. *Eur J Vasc Endovasc Surg.* 2006;32:361-365.
3. Sandford RM, Bown MJ, Fishwick G, et al. Duplex ultrasound scanning is reliable in the detection of endoleak following endovascular aneurysm repair. *Eur J Vasc Endovasc Surg.* 2006;32:537-541.
4. Henao EA, Hodge MD, Felkai DD, et al. Contrast-enhanced duplex surveillance after endovascular abdominal aortic aneurysm repair: improved efficacy using a continuous infusion technique. *J Vasc Surg.* 2006;43:259-264.

Computed Tomography versus Magnetic Resonance Imaging of Endoleaks after EVAR

van der Laan MJ, Bartels LW, Viergever MA, et al (Univ Med Ctr, Utrecht, The Netherlands; St Radboud Univ, Nijmegen, The Netherlands)
Eur J Vasc Endovasc Surg 32:361-365, 2006

Aim.—The aim of study was to compare the sensitivity of MRI and CTA for endoleak detection and classification after EVAR.

Patients and Methods.—Twenty-eight patients, between 2 days and 65 months after EVAR, were evaluated with both CT and MRI. Twenty-five patients had an Ancure graft and the other three had an Excluder. The MRI protocol for endoleak evaluation included: a T1-weighted spin echo, a high-resolution 3D CE-MRA, and a post-contrast T1-weighted spin echo. In total 40 ml Gadolinium was administered. The CT protocol consisted of a blank survey followed by a spiral CT angiography (CTA) using 140 ml of Ultravist. An experienced, blinded observer evaluated all CTs and MRIs.

Results.—Using MRI and MRA techniques significantly more endoleaks (23/35) were detected than with CTA (11/35) ($p=0.01$, Chi-Square). CT could not determine the type of endoleak in 3 of the 11 endoleaks detected and was uncertain in one. MRI was uncertain about the type in 14 of the 23 endoleaks detected. All endoleaks visible on CT were visible by MRI as well.

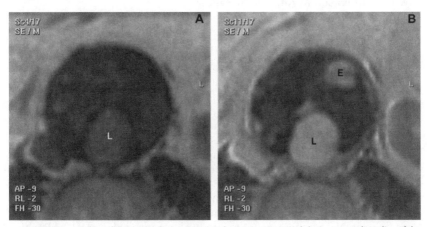

FIGURE 1.—A slice of T_1-weighted pre-contrast enhancement scan and the corresponding slice of the T_1-weighted post-contrast enhancement scan demonstrating an endoleak: L; denotes the graft lumen. E; denotes the endoleak. (Reprinted by permission of the publisher from van der Laan MJ, Bartels LW, Viergever MA, et al. Computed tomography versus magnetic resonance imaging of endoleaks after EVAR. *Eur J Vasc Endovasc Surg.* 2006;32:361-365.)

Conclusions.—MRI techniques are more sensitive for the detection of endoleak after endovascular AAA repair than CT (Fig 1).

▶ Nitinol-based endografts are MR compatible, but some signal dropout is observed with fully supported endografts. Despite this, MR found more endoleaks than CT, but the additional leaks detected by MR were type 2 leaks or leaks of unknown origin and, therefore, of unknown significance. My guess is that US and perhaps devices to measure intrasac pressure will eventually supplant CT for routine follow-up of abdominal aortic aneurysm endografts. MR will be used selectively but not much.

For further reading on this topic I suggest these articles.[1,2]

G. L. Moneta, MD

References

1. Sandford RM, Bown MJ, Fishwick G, et al. Duplex ultrasound scanning is reliable in the detection of endoleak following endovascular aneurysm repair. *Eur J Vasc Endovas Surg.* 2006;32:537-541.
2. Henao EA, Hodge MD, Felhai DD, et al. Contrast-enhanced duplex surveillance after endovascular abdominal aortic aneurysm repair: improved efficacy using a continuous infusion technique. *J Vasc Surg.* 2006;43:259-264.

Duplex Ultrasound Scanning is Reliable in the Detection of Endoleak Following Endovascular Aneurysm Repair

Sandford RM, Bown MJ, Fishwick G, et al (Univ of Leicester, England)
Eur J Vasc Endovasc Surg 32:537-541, 2006

Objective.—To investigate the value of duplex ultrasound scanning (DUSS) in the routine follow up of patients following EVAR.

Methods.—Imaging was reviewed for 310 consecutive patients undergoing EVAR at a single centre. Concurrent ultrasound and CT scans were defined as having occurred within 6 months of each other. There were 244 paired concurrent DUSS and CT scans which were used for further analysis. These modalities were compared with respect to sensitivity, specificity, positive and negative predictive values and level of agreement (by Kappa statistics) using CT as the 'gold standard'.

Results.—DUSS failed to detect a number of endoleaks which were seen on CT and the sensitivity of this test was therefore poor (67%). However, the specificity of DUSS compared more favourably with a value of 91%. Positive predictive values ranged from 33–100% but negative predictive values were more reliable with values of 91–100% at all time points post operatively. There were no type I leaks, or endoleaks requiring intervention which were missed on DUSS. Overall, there was a 'fair' level of agreement between the two imaging modalities using Kappa statistics.

Conclusion.—Although DUSS is not as sensitive as CT scanning in the detection of endoleak, no leaks requiring intervention were missed on DUSS in this study. DUSS is much cheaper than CT and avoids high doses of radiation. DUSS therefore remains a valuable method of follow up after EVAR and can reduce the need for repeated CT scans.

▶ As we come to worry less and less about type 2 endoleaks and endografts that are implanted in younger patients, duplex is very likely to assume a greater role in follow-up of patients with endografts in their abdominal aorta. Concerns over radiation exposure and expense of multiple CT scans over many years demand a less expensive and less toxic method of follow-up. If the duplex scan of the aortic endograft is of good quality and the abdominal aortic aneurysm is stable or shrinking and a plain film suggests the stent is not migrating, then a CT scan will not likely be considered necessary in the future for follow-up of aortic endografts.

G. L. Moneta, MD

Contrast-enhanced Duplex surveillance after endovascular abdominal aortic aneurysm repair: Improved efficacy using a continuous infusion technique
Henao EA, Hodge MD, Felkai DD, et al (Baylor College of Medicine; Methodist Hosp, Houston; Michael E DeBakey Veterans Affairs Med Ctr, Houston)
J Vasc Surg 43:259-264, 2006

Introduction.—Currently, postoperative endoleak surveillance after endovascular aortic aneurysm repair (EVAR) is primarily done by computed tomography (CT). The purpose of this study was to determine the efficacy of contrast-enhanced ultrasonography scans to detect endoleaks by using a novel infusion method and compare these findings with those of CT angiography (CTA).

Methods.—Twenty male patients (mean age, 70.4 years) underwent surveillance utilizing both CTA and contrast-enhanced color Duplex imaging. One 3-mL vial of Optison (Perfluten Protein A microspheres for injection) and 57 mL normal saline, for a total of 60 mL, were administered to each patient as a continuous infusion at 4 mL/min via a peripheral vein. Each study was optimized with harmonic imaging, and a reduced mechanical index of 0.4 to 0.5, compression of 1 to 3, and a focal zone below the aorta to minimize microsphere rupture. One minute was allowed from the time of infusion to the appearance of contrast in the endograft. Flow was evaluated within the lumen of the graft and its components, as was the presence or absence of endoleaks. Findings were compared with standard color-flow Duplex imaging and CT utilizing CTA reconstruction protocols.

Results.—All patients evaluated had modular endografts implanted for elective aneurysm repair. Contrast-enhanced duplex scans identified nine endoleaks: one type I and eight type II. No additional endoleaks were seen on CTA. However, CTA failed to recognize three type II endoleaks seen by contrast-enhanced ultrasound. The continuous infusion method allowed for longer and more detailed imaging. An average of 46.8 mL of the contrast infusion solution was used per patient.

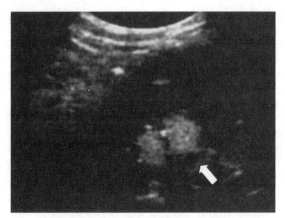

FIGURE 3.—A cross-sectional contrast-enhanced ultrasound image of the iliac limbs of an aortic stent demonstrates a type II endoleak *(arrow)* in the posterior sac. (Reprinted by permission of the publisher from Henao EA, Hodge MD, Felkai DD, et al. Contrast enhanced duplex surveillance after endovascular abdominal aortic aneurysm repair: improved efficacy using a continuous infusion technique. *J Vasc Surg.* 2006;43:259-264. Copyright 2006 by Elsevier.)

Conclusions.—Contrast enhanced Duplex ultrasonography accurately demonstrates endoleaks after EVAR and may be considered as a primary surveillance modality. Continuous infusion permits longer imaging time (Fig 3).

▶ Microspheres to enhance US imaging have been around for a while now but have not really caught on. Despite the fact they are thought to be useful by those who write about them, and this article is no exception, I suspect the problem is logistics. Microspheres turn a noninvasive test into one requiring intravenous infusion and, as far as I know, laboratories are not reimbursed for the cost of the contrast agent or the effort required to administer it. In addition, the microspheres may not add all that much of practical importance.

G. L. Moneta, MD

Multidetector Computed Tomography for Acute Pulmonary Embolism
Stein PD, for the PIOPED II Investigators (St Joseph Mercy Oakland Hosp, Pontiac, Mich; et al)
N Engl J Med 354:2317-2327, 2006

Background.—The accuracy of multidetector computed tomographic angiography (CTA) for the diagnosis of acute pulmonary embolism has not been determined conclusively.

Methods.—The Prospective Investigation of Pulmonary Embolism Diagnosis II trial was a prospective, multicenter investigation of the accuracy of multidetector CTA alone and combined with venous-phase imaging (CTA–CTV) for the diagnosis of acute pulmonary embolism. We used a composite reference test to confirm or rule out the diagnosis of pulmonary embolism.

Results.—Among 824 patients with a reference diagnosis and a completed CT study, CTA was inconclusive in 51 because of poor image quality. Excluding such inconclusive studies, the sensitivity of CTA was 83 percent and the specificity was 96 percent. Positive predictive values were 96 percent with a concordantly high or low probability on clinical assessment, 92 percent with an intermediate probability on clinical assessment, and nondiagnostic if clinical probability was discordant. CTA–CTV was inconclusive in 87 of 824 patients because the image quality of either CTA or CTV was poor. The sensitivity of CTA–CTV for pulmonary embolism was 90 percent, and specificity was 95 percent. CTA–CTV was also nondiagnostic with a discordant clinical probability.

Conclusions.—In patients with suspected pulmonary embolism, multidetector CTA–CTV has a higher diagnostic sensitivity than does CTA alone, with similar specificity. The predictive value of either CTA or CTA–CTV is high with a concordant clinical assessment, but additional testing is necessary when the clinical probability is inconsistent with the imaging results.

▶ It is important to read the "fine print" of this article. My takeaway from this article—CTA-CTV is positive and the clinical probability of pulmonary embolism is high and the patient has a pulmonary embolism with sufficient positive predictive value to go ahead and treat. If the CTA-CTV is negative and clinical probability is low, then the negative predictive value is sufficiently high that it is not necessary to treat for pulmonary embolism. If CTA-CTV is of poor quality or the results of CTA-CTV and clinical probability are discoordinate, then a pulmonary angiogram is still required.

G. L. Moneta, MD

5 Perioperative Considerations

Should Major Vascular Surgery Be Delayed Because of Preoperative Cardiac Testing in Intermediate-Risk Patients Receiving Beta-Blocker Therapy With Tight Heart Rate Control?

Poldermans D, for the Dutch Echocardiographic Cardiac Risk Evaluation Applying Stress Echo Study Group (Erasmus Med Ctr, Rotterdam, the Netherlands; et al)

J Am Coll Cardiol 48:964-969, 2006

Objectives.—The purpose of this study was to assess the value of preoperative cardiac testing in intermediate-risk patients receiving beta-blocker therapy with tight heart rate (HR) control scheduled for major vascular surgery.

Background.—Treatment guidelines of the American College of Cardiology/American Heart Association recommend cardiac testing in these patients to identify subjects at increased risk. This policy delays surgery, even though test results might be redundant and beta-blockers with tight HR control provide sufficient myocardial protection. Furthermore, the benefit of revascularization in high-risk patients is ill-defined.

Methods.—All 1,476 screened patients were stratified into low-risk (0 risk factors), intermediate-risk (1 to 2 risk factors), and high-risk ($\geq$3 risk factors). All patients received beta-blockers. The 770 intermediate-risk patients were randomly assigned to cardiac stress-testing (n = 386) or no testing. Test results influenced management. In patients with ischemia, physicians aimed to control HR below the ischemic threshold. Those with extensive stress-induced ischemia were considered for revascularization. The primary end point was cardiac death or myocardial infarction at 30-days after surgery.

Results.—Testing showed no ischemia in 287 patients (74%); limited ischemia in 65 patients (17%), and extensive ischemia in 34 patients (8.8%). Of 34 patients with extensive ischemia, revascularization before surgery was feasible in 12 patients (35%). Patients assigned to no testing had similar incidence of the primary end point as those assigned to testing (1.8% vs. 2.3%; odds ratio [OR] 0.78; 95% confidence interval [CI] 0.28 to 2.1; p = 0.62). The strategy of no testing brought surgery almost 3 weeks forward. Regardless of allocated strategy, patients with a HR <65 beats/min had lower risk than the remaining patients (1.3% vs. 5.2%; OR 0.24; 95% CI 0.09 to 0.66; p = 0.003).

Conclusions.—Cardiac testing can safely be omitted in intermediate-risk patients, provided that beta-blockers aiming at tight HR control are prescribed.

▶ This article challenges the old paradigm that stable patients with intermediate risk factors for myocardial ischemia should be risk stratified and undergo preoperative testing if they have multiple clinical risk factors. More and more evidence along the lines of this article suggests that routine preoperative noninvasive cardiac testing is not needed for intermediate-risk patients. Perioperative medical therapy is now replacing perioperative myocardial imaging as a more effective method to decrease perioperative cardiac-related morbidity and mortality.

G. L. Moneta, MD

Perioperative myocardial ischemic injury in high-risk vascular surgery patients: Incidence and clinical significance in a prospective clinical trial
Mackey WC, Fleisher LA, Haider S, et al (Tufts-New England Med Ctr, Boston; Univ of Pennsylvania, Philadelphia; Pfizer Inc, New London, Conn; et al)
J Vasc Surg 43:533-538, 2006

Objective.—The purpose of this study was to assess prospectively the incidence, health care resource utilization, and economic burden associated with perioperative myocardial ischemic injury (PMII) in high-risk patients undergoing noncardiac vascular surgery.

Methods.—Two hundred thirty-six patients consented to participate in a pharmacoeconomic substudy as part of a randomized, multicenter clinical trial. Patients were assessed for myocardial ischemic injury by using clinical, biochemical, and electrocardiographic criteria. PMII was defined as fatal or nonfatal myocardial infarction, new or worsened congestive heart failure, or new arrhythmias. Resource utilization parameters were compared for patients with and without PMII. Patients underwent the following index procedures: open abdominal aortic aneurysm repair (n = 44), bypass for aortoiliac disease (n = 29), bypass for femoropopliteal disease (n = 62), bypass for femorotibial disease (n = 71), extra-anatomic bypass (n = 23), and miscellaneous (n = 7). Patients undergoing carotid endarterectomy or only endovascular interventions were excluded. The incremental cost of PMII was estimated by applying the average costs (adjusted to 2004 US dollars) of the hospital ward ($700.00/d) or intensive care unit ($2500.00/d) to the length of stay differences for patients with and without PMII.

Results.—The overall mortality was 3.4% (8/236), and 7 of 8 deaths were related to PMII. PMII occurred in 42 (17.8%) of 236 patients: 22 myocardial infarctions, 11 congestive heart failures, and 12 new arrhythmias (3 patients had 2 PMII events). There was no evidence of differences in the incidence of PMII among the various index procedures. PMII was associated with a dramatic increase in resource utilization. The mean length of stay was 16.8 and 10.0 days for patients with and without PMII, respectively ($P <$ .001). Intensive care unit care was required by 35 (83.3%) of 42 patients with and 121 (62.4%) of 194 patients without PMII ($P < .009$). The mean intensive care unit length of stay was 6.6 and 3.7 days for patients with and without PMII, respectively ($P < .009$). Ten (23.8%) of 42 patients with and 20 (10.3%) of 194 patients without PMII returned to the emergency department for care after discharge ($P < .02$).

Conclusions.—In modern vascular surgery practice, PMII remains common despite the availability of β-blockers and other preventative strategies. PMII is associated with dramatic increases in resource utilization and cost. The increase in resource utilization associated with PMII resulted in an estimated incremental cost per patient of $9980.00. If 250,000 high-risk open vascular operations are performed annually in the United States, the economic burden of PMII in these procedures alone approximates $444 million. Strategies to decrease PMII incidence and severity should be evaluated in large-scale prospective trials.

▶ Myocardial ischemic events happen after vascular surgery. They are, however, not reduced by screening for catheter or open surgical revascularization[1]) but can be decreased by β-blockers[2]. The huge cost of a perioperative myocardial ischemic event documented in this article should catch the attention of hospital administrators everywhere. From a patient care, and a financial perspective, it absolutely makes sense for all hospitals to institute protocols for β-blocker therapy in high- to intermediate-risk surgical patients.

G. L. Moneta, MD

References

1. McFalls EO, Ward HB, Moritz TE, et al. Coronary-artery revascularization before elective major vascular surgery. *N Engl J Med*. 2004;351:2795-2804.
2. Lindenauer PK, Pekow P, Wang K, Mamidi DK, Gutierrez B, Benjamin EM. Perioperative beta-blocker therapy and mortality after major noncardiac surgery. *N Engl J Med*. 2005;353:349-361.

The effects of the type of anesthesia on outcomes of lower extremity infrainguinal bypass
Singh N, Sidawy AN, Dezee K, et al (VA Med Ctr, Washington, DC; Washington Hosp Ctr, Washington, DC; George Washington Univ, Washington, DC)
J Vasc Surg 44:964-970, 2006

Objective.—Three main types of anesthesia are used for infrainguinal bypass: general endotracheal anesthesia (GETA), spinal anesthesia (SA), and epidural anesthesia (EA). We analyzed a large clinical database to determine whether the type of anesthesia had any effect on clinical outcomes in lower extremity bypass.

Methods.—This study is an analysis of a prospectively collected database by the National Surgical Quality Improvement Program (NSQIP) of the Veterans Affairs Medical Centers. All patients from 1995 to 2003 in the NSQIP database who underwent infrainguinal arterial bypass were identified via Current Procedural Terminology codes. The 30-day morbidity and mortality outcomes for various types of anesthesia were compared by using univariate analysis and multivariate logistic regression to control for confounders.

Results.—The NSQIP database identified 14,788 patients (GETA, 9757 patients; SA, 2848 patients; EA, 2183 patients) who underwent a lower extremity infrainguinal arterial bypass during the study period. Almost all patients (99%) were men, and the mean age was 65.8 years. The type of anesthesia significantly affected graft failure at 30 days. Compared with SA, the odds of graft failure were higher for GETA (odds ratio, 1.43; 95% confidence interval [CI], 1.16-1.77; $P = .001$). There was no statistically significant difference in 30-day graft failure between EA and SA. Regarding cardiac events, defined as postoperative myocardial infarction or cardiac arrest, patients with normal functional status (activities of daily living independence) and no history of congestive heart failure or stroke did worse with GETA than with SA (odds ratio, 1.8; 95% CI, 1.32-2.48; $P < .0001$). There was no statistically significant difference between EA and SA in the incidence of cardiac events. GETA, when compared with SA and EA, was associated with more cases of postoperative pneumonia (odds ratio: 2.2 [95% CI, 1.1-4.4; $P = .034$]). There was no significant difference between EA and SA with regard to postoperative pneumonia. Compared with SA, GETA was associated with an increased odds of returning to the operating room (odds ratio, 1.40; 95% CI, 1.20-1.64; $P < .001$), as was EA (odds ratio, 1.17; 95% CI, 1.05-1.31; $P = .005$). GETA was associated with a longer surgical length of stay on univariate analysis, but not after controlling for confounders. There was no significant difference in 30-day mortality among the three groups with univariate or multivariate analyses.

Conclusions.—Although GETA is the most common type of anesthesia used in infrainguinal bypasses, our results suggest that it is not the best strategy, because it is associated with significantly worse morbidity than regional techniques.

▶ This is a controversial area. However, there are enough articles indicating improved outcomes with epidural or spinal anesthesia versus general anesthesia in patients undergoing infrainguinal reconstruction that these regional techniques should be strongly considered in patients undergoing lower extremity revascularization. Although the mortality rate is no different, complications are increased with general anesthesia and complications negatively affect patients and the hospital's bottom line.[1]

G. L. Moneta, MD

Reference

1. Mackey WC, Fleisher LA, Haider S, et al. Perioperative myocardial ischemic injury in high-risk vascular surgery patients: incidence and clinical significance in a prospective clinical trial. J Vasc Surg. 2006;43:533-538.

Influence of perioperative blood glucose levels on outcome after infrainguinal bypass surgery in patients with diabetes

Malmstedt J, Wahlberg E, Jörneskog G, et al (Karolinska Univ, Stockholm; Danderyd Univ, Stockholm)
Br J Surg 93:1360-1367, 2006

Background.—High glucose levels are associated with increased morbidity and mortality after coronary surgery and in intensive care. The influence of perioperative hyperglycaemia on the outcome after infrainguinal bypass surgery among diabetic patients is largely unknown. The aim was to determine whether high perioperative glucose levels were associated with increased morbidity after infrainguinal bypass surgery.

Methods.—Ninety-one consecutive diabetic patients undergoing primary infrainguinal bypass surgery were identified from a prospective vascular registry. Risk factors, indication for surgery, operative details and outcome data were extracted from the medical records. Exposure to perioperative hyperglycaemia was measured using the area under the curve (AUC) method; the AUC was calculated using all blood glucose readings during the first 48 h after surgery.

Results.—Multivariable analysis showed that the AUC for glucose (odds ratio (OR) 13.35, first *versus* fourth quartile), renal insufficiency (OR 4.77)

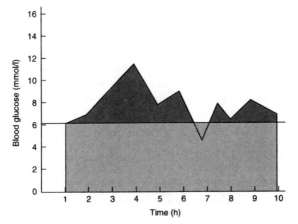

FIGURE 1.—Area under the curve (AUC) method for blood glucose values above 6.1 mmol/l. Exposure to hypoglycaemia is represented by the dark shaded area. The total AUC (dark plus light shaded areas) is used for comparisons between blood glucose levels. (Courtesy of Malmstedt J, Wahlberg E, Jörneskog G. Influence of perioperative blood glucose levels on outcome after infrainguinal bypass surgery in patients with diabetes. *Br J Surg*. 2006;93:1360-1367. Reprinted by permission of Blackwell Publishing.)

and infected foot ulcer (OR 3.38) was significantly associated with poor outcome (death, major amputation or graft occlusion at 90 days). Similarly, the AUC for glucose (OR 14.45, first versus fourth quartile), female sex (OR 3.49) and tissue loss as indication (OR 3.30) was associated with surgical wound complications at 30 days.

Conclusion.—Poor perioperative glycaemic control was associated with an unfavourable outcome after infrainguinal bypass surgery in diabetic patients (Fig 1).

▶ Adverse effects of hypoglycemia in the perioperative period are impaired coagulation, impaired hemoglobin function, and decreased opsonization. Leukocyte function is also impaired, with impaired phagocytosis and chemoattraction to bacteria. There is no agreement on what is an optimal postoperative blood glucose level in a patient with diabetes. However, on the basis of this study and the bulk of the literature, it would seem that keeping blood glucose levels as close to normal as possible in the perioperative period should be the goal.

G. L. Moneta, MD

Plasma N-terminal pro-B-type natriuretic peptide as long-term prognostic marker after major vascular surgery
Feringa HHH, Schouten O, Dunkelgrun M, et al (Erasmus MC, Rotterdam, The Netherlands; Leiden Univ, The Netherlands; Univ of Nebraska, Omaha)
Heart 93:226-231, 2007

Objective.—To assess the long-term prognostic value of plasma N-terminal pro-B-type natriuretic peptide (NT-proBNP) after major vascular surgery.

Design.—A single-centre prospective cohort study.

Patients.—335 patients who underwent abdominal aortic aneurysm repair or lower extremity bypass surgery.

Interventions.—Prior to surgery, baseline NT-proBNP level was measured. Patients were also evaluated for cardiac risk factors according to the Revised Cardiac Risk Index. Dobutamine stress echocardiography (DSE) was performed to detect stress-induced myocardial ischaemia.

Main Outcome Measures.—The prognostic value of NT-proBNP was evaluated for the endpoints all-cause mortality and major adverse cardiac events (MACE) during long-term follow-up.

Results.—In this patient cohort (mean age: 62 years, 76% male), median NT-proBNP level was 186 ng/l (interquartile range: 65–444 ng/l). During a mean follow-up of 14 (SD 6) months, 49 patients (15%) died and 50 (15%) experienced a MACE. Using receiver operating characteristic curve analysis for 6-month mortality and MACE, NT-proBNP had the greatest area under the curve compared with cardiac risk score and DSE. In addition, an NT-proBNP level of 319 ng/l was identified as the optimal cut-off value to predict 6-month mortality and MACE. After adjustment for age, cardiac risk

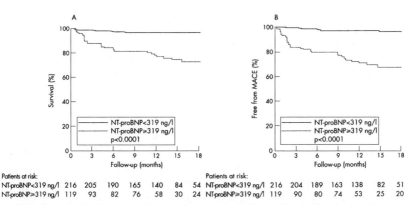

FIGURE 2.—Kaplan-Meier curves showing the cumulative incidence of death (A) and major adverse cardiac events (B) during follow-up, according to N-terminal pro-B-type natriuretic peptide level. MACE, major adverse cardiac events. (Courtesy of Feringa HHH, Schouten O, Dunkelgrun M, et al. Plasma N-terminal pro-B-type natriuretic peptide as long-term prognostic marker after major vascular surgery. *Heart.* 2007;93:226-231. Reprinted with permission from the BMJ Publishing Group.)

score, DSE results and cardioprotective medication, NT-proBNP ≥319 ng/l was associated with a hazard ratio of 4.0 for all-cause mortality (95% CI: 1.8 to 8.9) and with a hazard ratio of 10.9 for MACE (95% CI: 4.1 to 27.9).

Conclusion.—Preoperative NT-proBNP level is a strong predictor of long-term mortality and major adverse cardiac events after major non-cardiac vascular surgery (Fig 2).

▶ Natriuretic peptides are indigenous cardiac hormones. NT-pro-BNP is synthesized in ventricular muscle and released in response to wall stress.[1] Given the relatively poor track record of other markers of cardiac risk in vascular surgical patients, this cardiac hormone deserves additional study both as a predictor of perioperative risk and a predictor of long-term mortality in vascular surgical patients.[2]

G. L. Moneta, MD

Reference

1. Yoshimura M, Yasue H, Okumura K, et al. Different secretion patterns of atrial natriuretic peptide in patients with congestive heart failure. *Circulation* 1993;87: 464-469.
2. Feringa HH, Bax JJ, Elhendy A, et al. Association of plasma N-terminal pro-B-type natriuretic peptide with postoperative cardiac events in patients undergoing surgery for abdominal aortic aneurysm or leg bypass. *Am J Cardiol.* 2006;98:111-115.

Association of Plasma N-Terminal Pro-B-Type Natriuretic Peptide With Postoperative Cardiac Events in Patients Undergoing Surgery for Abdominal Aortic Aneurysm or Leg Bypass

Feringa HHH, Bax JJ, Elhendy A, et al (Erasmus Med College, Rotterdam, The Netherlands; Leiden Univ, The Netherlands; Univ of Nebraska, Omaha)
Am J Cardiol 98:111-115, 2006

Postoperative cardiac events are related to myocardial ischemia and reduced left ventricular function. The utility of N-terminal–pro-B-type natriuretic peptide (NT–pro-BNP) for preoperative cardiac risk evaluation has not been evaluated. The objective of this study was to assess whether plasma NT–pro-BNP predicts postoperative cardiac events in patients who undergo major vascular surgery in addition to clinical and dobutamine stress echocardiographic data. One hundred seventy consecutive patients scheduled for major noncardiac vascular surgery were prospectively evaluated by dobutamine stress echocardiographic and NT–pro-BNP measurements. Multivariable logistic regression analysis was performed to evaluate the predictors of cardiac death and nonfatal myocardial infarction during a follow-up of 30-days. Receiver-operating characteristic analysis was performed to determine the optimal cut-off value of NT–pro-BNP to predict outcome. Patients' mean age was 59 ± 13 years, and 71% were men. The median NT–pro-BNP level was 110 pg/ml (interquartile range 42 to 389). Cardiac events occurred

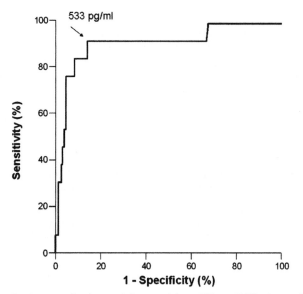

FIGURE 2.—Receiver-operating characteristic curve of plasma NT–pro-BNP levels to predict postoperative cardiac events. Sensitivity and 1 − specificity are plotted for various NT–pro-BNP levels. The ideal cut-off value is indicated by the *arrow*. (Courtesy of Cardiology, Feringa HHH, Bax JJ, Elhendy A, et al. Association of plasma N-terminal pro-B-type natriuretic peptide with postoperative cardiac events in patients undergoing surgery for abdominal aortic aneurysm or leg bypass. *Am J Cardiol.* 2006;98:111-115. Copyright 2006, with permission from Excerpta Medica Inc.)

in 2 of 144 patients (1.4%) with NT–pro-BNP <533 pg/ml (i.e., the optimal cut-off value to predict cardiac events) and in 11 of 26 patients (42%) with NT–pro-BNP ≥533 pg/ml (unadjusted odds ratio 52, 95% confidence interval 11 to 256, p <0.0001). After adjustment for cardiac risk factors and dobutamine stress echocardiographic results, NT–pro-BNP remained significantly associated with cardiac events (adjusted odds ratio 17, 95% confidence interval 3 to 106, p = 0.002). In conclusion, in patients scheduled for major vascular surgery, elevated plasma NT–pro-BNP levels are independently associated with an increased risk for postoperative cardiac events. Further studies in a larger number of patients are required to confirm these findings (Fig 2).

▶ NT-pro-BNP elevations are known to be associated with increased risk of ischemic myocardial events. Therefore, the authors' findings are not all that surprising. The increased use of statins and β-blockers in the greater than 533 μg/mL NT-pro-BNP group adds strength to the authors' conclusions that NT-pro-BNP levels may be a better marker for perioperative cardiac risks than clinical assessment alone.

G. L. Moneta, MD

Elevated C-reactive protein levels are associated with postoperative events in patients undergoing lower extremity vein bypass surgery
Owens CD, Ridker PM, Belkin M, et al (Brigham and Women's Hosp, Boston; Beth Israel Deaconess Med Ctr, Boston)
J Vasc Surg 45:2-9, 2007

Objectives.—Inflammatory markers such as high-sensitivity C-reactive protein (hsCRP) are associated with an increased risk of cardiovascular events and with the severity of peripheral arterial disease. The effects of inflammation on the development of vein graft disease remain speculative. We hypothesized that high levels of inflammatory markers would identify patients at increased risk for adverse events (graft failure, major cardiovascular events) after lower extremity bypass surgery.

Methods.—Patients (n = 91) scheduled to undergo lower extremity bypass using autogenous vein were enrolled into a prospective study at two institutions. Exclusion criteria included the presence of major infection. A baseline plasma sample was obtained on the morning of lower extremity bypass. Biomarkers for inflammation included hsCRP, fibrinogen, and serum amyloid A (SAA). Values between patients with and without critical limb ischemia were compared. Proportions of events among dichotomized populations (upper limit of normal of each laboratory assay) were compared by log-rank test.

Results.—Of the patients undergoing lower extremity bypass, 69% were men, 53% were diabetic, 81% were smokers, and their mean ankle-brachial index was 0.51 ± 0.19. The indication for lower extremity bypass was critical limb ischemia in 55%. There were no perioperative deaths and two early graft occlusions. During a mean follow-up of 342 days (range, 36-694 days) there were four deaths, 27 graft-related events, and 10 other cardiovascular events. No relationships were found between events and demographics, comorbidities, baseline ankle-brachial index, or statin use. High-sensitivity CRP ($P = .005$), fibrinogen ($P < .001$), and SAA ($P = .0001$) levels were associated with critical limb ischemia at presentation. Among patients with an elevated hsCRP (>5 mg/L) immediately before surgery, major postoperative vascular events occurred in 60% (21/35), compared with a 32% (18/56) rate in those with a baseline CRP <5 mg/L ($P = .004$, log-rank test). On multivariable analysis, only elevated hsCRP correlated with adverse graft-related or cardiovascular events ($P = .018$).

Conclusions.—The inflammatory biomarkers of hsCRP, fibrinogen, and SAA correlate with peripheral arterial disease severity at presentation in patients undergoing lower extremity bypass. Patients with elevated hsCRP are at increased risk for postoperative vascular events, most of which are related to the vein graft. These findings suggest a potential relationship between inflammation and outcomes after lower extremity vein bypass surgery.

▶ Despite all the data on C-reactive protein in the cardiology literature over the last 20 years, its clinical impact has been relatively minimal. This study may be an exception in that most of the adverse events predicted by C-reactive protein levels in this study were related to the vein graft itself. Perhaps C-reactive protein levels can help identify which patients with vein grafts placed for critical limb ischemia will be at highest risk for a graft-related event. Perhaps such patients should be more intensely monitored with respect to their grafts postoperatively. However, I don't think,we will see C-reactive protein levels in patients with critical limb ischemia as an exclusion criteria for revascularization.

G. L. Moneta, MD

Effects of Statins on Renal Function After Aortic Cross Clamping During Major Vascular Surgery
Schouten O, Kok NFM, Boersma E, et al (Erasmus Med Ctr, Rotterdam, The Netherlands; Leiden Univ, The Netherlands)
Am J Cardiol 97:1383-1385, 2006

Ischemic reperfusion injury is an important cause of renal dysfunction after major vascular surgery and increases postoperative morbidity and mortality. The aim of the present study was to assess the effect of statins on renal function in patients at high risk for renal dysfunction, that is, those who underwent suprarenal aortic cross clamping-declamping. Seventy-seven patients (28 statin users, 57 men; mean age 69 ± 8 years) with normal preoperative renal function requiring suprarenal aortic cross clamping-declamping during vascular surgery from 1995 to 2005 were studied. Creatinine levels were obtained before surgery and on days 1, 2, 3, 7, and 30 after surgery. An analysis-of-variance model for repeated measurements was applied to compare creatinine levels between statin users and nonusers,

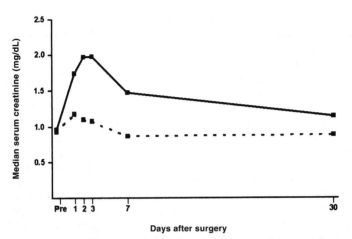

Days after surgery

FIGURE 1.—Median creatinine levels preoperatively and 1, 2, 3, 7, and 30 days after surgery in statin users (*dashed line*) and nonusers (*solid line*), p <0.01 (analysis of variance for repeated measurements). (Courtesy of Schouten O, Kok NFM, Boersma E, et al: Effects of statins on renal function after aortic cross clamping during major vascular surgery. *Am J Cardiol.* 2006;97:1383-1385, with permission from Excerpta Medica Inc.)

with adjustment for clamping time and blood loss. There were no differences in baseline clinical characteristics, preoperative creatinine levels (0.93 vs 0.96 mg/dl, p = 0.59), and glomerular filtration rate (79 vs 73 ml/min, p = 0.1). Postoperative creatinine levels during the 30 days after surgery were significantly lower in statin users than in nonusers (analysis-of-variance p <0.01, 1.17 vs 1.98 mg/dl). Postoperative hemodialysis was required (temporarily) in 7 patients (9.1%), all statin nonusers. These findings suggest an association between statin use and preserved renal function after suprarenal aortic clamping (Fig 1).

▶ Renal protective effects of statins have been demonstrated in animal models and are thought to reflect the moderating influence of statins on endothelial ischemic dysfunction and inflammation. Further work is required to determine when statins must be initiated before aortic clamping and what are optimal doses to minimize ischemia-induced renal dysfunction.

G. L. Moneta, MD

Aggressive Management of Nonocclusive Ischemic Colitis Following Aortic Reconstruction
Menegaux F, Trésallet C, Kieffer E, et al (Université Pierre et Marie Curie (Paris VI))
Arch Surg 141:678-682, 2006

Hypothesis.—Under standard conditions following aortic reconstruction, nonocclusive ischemic colitis (IC) type 1 (mucosal ischemia) and type 2 (mucosal and muscularis ischemia) can be managed nonoperatively, whereas type 3 (transmural ischemia) requires emergency surgery. Our objective was to standardize the surgical approach for IC complicating aortic reconstruction.

Design.—Retrospective cohort study.

Setting.—General surgery, vascular surgery, anesthesiology, and critical care units in a university-affiliated hospital.

Methods.—From January 5, 1997, to December 15, 2003, 49 cases of IC complicating aortic reconstruction were diagnosed (rate, 2.7%). Nonoperative management was used for patients with type 1 or type 2 without multiple organ failure (MOF). All patients with type 3 or with type 2 with MOF underwent urgent resection of the ischemic colon without anastomosis.

Results.—Immediate surgery was performed on 24 patients (49.0%). Nineteen (76.0%) of 25 patients without MOF and with transient endoscopic findings underwent secondary surgery for progression to final IC type 3 (16 patients) or to final IC type 2 with MOF (3 patients). Twenty-three (53.5%) of 43 patients died after colorectal resection (overall mortality, 46.9%). Factors causing significant risk of death were surgery, MOF, final IC type, and amount of perioperative transfusion. The mortality was 57.1% for final IC type 3, 37.5% for final IC type 2 with MOF, and 0% for final IC type 1 or type 2 without MOF.

Conclusions.—Selective management of postoperative IC, based on MOF and the degree of ischemia, is the suggested course of action. For patients with mild ischemia and MOF, an aggressive approach is recommended.

▶ The true incidence of any type of colon ischemia after aortic surgery is likely highly underestimated in this series. However, the idea that is interesting in this article is that the authors advocate colon resection in the presence of multiorgan failure even if there is no transmural colonic necrosis. Focusing on the functional and not just the anatomic consequences of colon ischemia after aortic surgery may improve the outcomes of this highly morbid complication. The down side is that there are not enough patients in this series to tell us what degree of multiorgan failure is enough to merit colon resection in the absence of transmural necrosis.

G. L. Moneta, MD

Plasma D-Lactate as a Potential Early Marker for Colon Ischaemia After Open Aortic Reconstruction

Assadian A, Assadian O. Senekowitsch C, et al (Wilhelminenspital Vienna; Med Univ Vienna; Ludwig Boltzmann Inst for Experimental and Clinical Traumatology and Research Ctr of the Allegemeine Unfallversicherungsanstallt (AUVA), Vienna)
Eur J Vasc Endovasc Surg 31:470-474, 2006

Background and Aim.—The breakdown of mucosal barrier function due to intestinal hypo-perfusion is the earliest dysfunction of ischaemic colitis. Severe colon ischaemia after aortic reconstruction is associated with mortal-

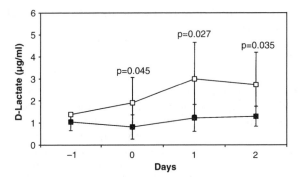

FIGURE 1.—Plasma D-lactate concentrations in patients undergoing aortic surgery. Open squares represent D-lactate concentrations in patients developing histologically proven ischemic colitis; filled squares represent D-lactate concentrations in patients without ischemic colitis. Data are presented as mean±SD. P values represent significance level *versus* corresponding group without ischaemic colitis. (Reprinted by permission of the publisher from Assadian A, Assadian O, Senekowitsch C, et al. Plasma D-lactate as a potential early marker for colon ischaemia after open aortic reconstruction. *Eur J Vasc Endosvasc Surg.* 2006;31:470-474.)

ity rates up to 90%. Therefore, early detection and treatment of patients with extensive ischaemic colitis is of crucial importance. In experimental studies, both D-lactate and bacterial endotoxin have been reported as markers of intestinal mucosal barrier impairment. However, evidence of their value in clinical practice is lacking. The aim of this pilot prospective cohort study was to assess the association between ischaemia of the colon (assessed histologically) and plasma levels of D-lactate and endotoxin in patients undergoing open aortic reconstruction.

Patients and Methods.—Twelve consecutive patients underwent surgery between February and April 2003. Six patients underwent emergency surgery and six patients elective aortic surgery. D-Lactate and endotoxin levels were measured in blood samples collected according to a standardised protocol. For histological examination biopsies were obtained by sigmoidoscopy on days 4–6 after surgery, or earlier if indicated clinically.

Results.—As early as 2 h postoperatively, elevated plasma levels of D-lactate were measured in patients with histologically proven ischaemic colitis. The peak of D-lactate elevation was on postoperative days 1 and 2. Concentration of plasma endotoxin was not significantly different in patients with or without ischaemic colitis.

Conclusion.—Our data suggest that plasma D-lactate levels are a useful marker for early detection of ischaemic colitis secondary to aortic surgery (Fig 1).

▶ Obviously no definitive conclusions can be made from this small pilot study. However, the fact that D-lactate levels were elevated in patients with clinically important colon ischemia before their clinical decline and were not elevated in patients without colonic ischemia suggests a potentially important role for this serum marker in patients who have had aortic reconstruction.

G. L. Moneta, MD

The prevalence of thrombophilia in patients with symptomatic peripheral vascular disease

Vig S, Chitolie A, Bevan D, et al (St George's Hosp, London)

Br J Surg 93:577-581, 2006

Background.—The aim of this prospective study was to establish the prevalence of thrombophilia and hyperhomocysteinaemia using a comprehensive screen in patients with peripheral vascular disease.

Methods.—A total of 150 patients with peripheral vascular disease (with an ankle brachial pressure index of less than 0·8) underwent thrombophilia screening (protein C and protein S, antithrombin, lupus anticoagulant, activated protein C resistance and factor V Leiden and prothrombin mutations). Fasting homocysteine assays were also performed.

Results.—A thrombophilia defect was found in 41 patients (27·3 per cent). The commonest was protein S deficiency, found in 17 patients (11·3 per cent). Others included factor V Leiden mutation, found in 10 (6·7 per cent) and protein C deficiency, found in six (4·0 per cent). Lupus anticoagulant and prothrombin mutation were both found in six (4.0 per cent). One patient had an antithrombin deficiency. Only the presence of critical ischaemia was associated with a positive thrombophilia screen on single variable analysis ($P = 0·03$). Hyperhomocysteinaemia was present in over a third of the study group (37·3 per cent): 45 defined as moderate and 11 as intermediate.

Conclusion.—A quarter of patients with peripheral vascular disease had evidence of thrombophilia, and a third had hyperhomocysteinaemia.

▶ I think we already knew patients with symptomatic vascular disease have an elevated prevalence of a thrombophilia of some sort. I am still not sure what to do with the information. Certainly warfarin therapy has not been conclusively demonstrated to reduce perioperative or long-term graft failure in the patient with thrombophilia.[1]

G. L. Moneta, MD

Reference

1. Lam EY, Taylor LM Jr, Landry GJ, Porter JM, Moneta GL. Relationship between antiphospholipid antibodies and progression of lower extremity arterial occlusive disease after lower extremity bypass operations. *J Vasc Surg.* 2001;33:976-982.

Anaphylactoid reactions to Dextran 40 and 70: Reports to the United States Food and Drug Administration, 1969 to 2004

Zinderman CE, Landow L, Wise RP (Food and Drug Administratration, Bethesda, Md; Office of Blood Research and Review, Bethesda, Md)
J Vasc Surg 43:1004-1009, 2006

Background.—Clinical dextrans, such as Dextran 40 and Dextran 70, are associated with anaphylactoid reactions caused by dextran-reactive immunoglobulin G antibodies. When infused immediately before clinical dextrans, dextran 1 significantly reduces the incidence of severe anaphylactoid reactions. The objective of the study was to describe the frequency and characteristics of reports submitted to the United States Food and Drug Administration (FDA) for anaphylaxis or anaphylactoid events after clinical dextran administration.

Methods.—We searched the FDA's Adverse Event Reporting System for reports associated with a clinical dextran and describing anaphylaxis/anaphylactoid reactions. Our case definition for a probable anaphylaxis/anaphylactoid event required signs or symptoms from at least two body systems, with at least one sign or symptom being hypotension, vasodilation, or respiratory difficulty, and onset within 60 minutes. Other reports were considered possible cases if the reporter specifically described the reaction as anaphylaxis or an anaphylactoid reaction. Premier RxMarket Advisor provided estimates of total US hospitalizations with clinical dextran or dextran 1 administration from 2000 to 2004, based on discharge billing data from a sample of US hospitals. The IMS National Sales Perspective provided estimates of total doses of dextrans sold in the United States from 1999 to 2004, based on volumes of dextrans sold in a sample of retail and nonretail outlets.

Results.—The FDA received 366 clinical dextran adverse event reports from 1969 to 2004, of which 90 (24.6%) were anaphylaxis/anaphylactoid events. The ratio of hospitalizations where clinical dextran was administered to hospitalizations where dextran 1 was administered was 28.4:1. The expected ratio would be 1:1 if all clinical dextran patients had received dextran 1 pretreatment. The ratio of clinical dextran doses sold to dextran 1 doses sold in the United States was 38.6:1.

Conclusions.—A high proportion of adverse event reports for clinical dextrans described anaphylaxis or anaphylactoid reactions. Hospital discharge and product sales data suggest that dextran 1 has not been used consistently before clinical dextran administration in recent years. To reduce the risk of anaphylactoid reactions, physicians should consider routine administration of dextran 1 before the infusion of a clinical dextran.

▶ One way to avoid anaphylactic reactions with the use of dextran is not to use dextran. With the availability and excellent safety profiles of low-molecular-weight heparin and clopidogrel, it seems silly to administer a dangerous drug if other, perhaps safer, alternatives are available. I haven't given a patient dextran in more than 10 years.

G. L. Moneta, MD

Thromboembolic Adverse Events After Use of Recombinant Human Coagulation Factor VIIa

O'Connell KA, Wood JJ, Wise RP, et al (Food and Drug Administration, Rockville, Md)
JAMA 295:293-298, 2006

Context.—The US Food and Drug Administration (FDA) licensed recombinant human coagulation factor VIIa (rFVIIa) on March 25, 1999, for bleeding in patients with hemophilia A or B and inhibitors to factors VIII or IX. Use in patients without hemophilia has been increasing since licensure.

Objective.—To review serious thromboembolic adverse events (AEs) reported to the FDA's Adverse Event Reporting System (AERS).

Design, Setting, and Patients.—The AERS database was reviewed from March 25, 1999, through December 31, 2004, for thromboembolic AE reports with rFVIIa. The AERS database includes US and non-US spontaneous AE reports from both approved (specific indications for patients with hemophilia) and unlabeled uses. It also includes serious AEs in patients enrolled in postlicensure clinical trials who received rFVIIa. Manufacturer reporting to FDA is mandatory, but primary notification from clinicians and others to FDA or manufacturers is voluntary for spontaneous reports; therefore, AERS underrepresents actual event occurrences.

Main Outcome Measure.—Reported thromboembolic events occurring in patients administered rFVIIa.

Results.—A total of 431 AE reports for rFVIIa were found, of which 168 reports described 185 thromboembolic events. Seventeen events occurred in patients with hemophilia and 59 occurred in patients enrolled in postlicensure trials. Unlabeled indications accounted for 151 of the reports, most with active bleeding (n = 115). Reported AEs were thromboembolic cerebrovascular accident (n = 39), acute myocardial infarction (n = 34), other arterial thromboses (n = 26), pulmonary embolism (n = 32), other venous thromboses (including deep vein thrombosis) (n = 42), and clotted devices (n = 10). In 36 (72%) of 50 reported deaths, the probable cause of death was the thromboembolic event. In 144 patients with timing information, 73 events (52%) occurred in the first 24 hours after the last dose (30 events within 2 hours). Sixty-four reports (38%) noted concomitant use of hemostatic agents. Most reports lacked sufficient information to evaluate potential dosage associations.

Conclusions.—Most reported thromboembolic AEs followed the use of rFVIIa for unlabeled indications and occurred in arterial and venous systems, often resulting in serious morbidity and mortality. Analysis of the relationship between AEs and rFVIIa is hindered by concomitant medications, preexisting medical conditions, confounding by indication, and inherent limitations of passive surveillance. Randomized controlled trials are needed to establish the safety and efficacy of rFVIIa in patients without hemophilia (Fig 4).

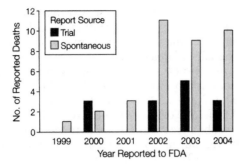

FIGURE 4.—Number of Reported Deaths Among Patients Administered Recombinant Human Coagulation Factor VIIa With a Thromboembolic Event by Year and Source. FDA indicates US Food and Drug Administration. (Courtesy of O'Connell KA, Wood JJ, Wise RP, et al. Thromboembolic adverse events after use of recombinant human coagulation factor VIIa. *JAMA.* 2006;295:293-298. Copyright 2006, American Medical Association.)

▶ Off-label use of recombinant activated factor VIIa is increasing.[1] All vascular surgeons are occasionally faced with a patient with a seemingly unrelenting coagulopathy. In such patients, the use of rFVIIa will likely be considered. Although the Food and Drug Administration adverse event reporting system does not allow for precise determination of the frequency of adverse events related to this drug, physicians should be aware that, if an adverse event occurs, it very well may be severe and result in death.

G. L. Moneta, MD

Reference

1. Ghorashian S, Hunt BJ. "Off-license" use of recombinant activated factor VII. *Blood Rev.* 2004;18:245-249.

Effects of Argatroban Therapy, Demographic Variables, and Platelet Count on Thrombotic Risks in Heparin-Induced Thrombocytopenia
Lewis BE, Wallis DE, Hursting MJ, et al (Loyola Univ, Maywood, Ill; Midwest Heart Specialists, Downers Grove, Ill; Clinical Science Consulting, Austin, Tex; et al)
Chest 129:1407-1416, 2006

Study Objectives.—We investigated the effects of the direct thrombin inhibitor argatroban, patient demographics, and the platelet count on thrombotic risks in heparin-induced thrombocytopenia (HIT), a serious thrombotic condition, to determine if argatroban provides effective antithrombotic therapy in patients with HIT without increasing bleeding.
Design.—We retrospectively analyzed thrombotic outcomes in 882 HIT patients (697 patients receiving mean argatroban doses of 1.7 to 2.0 µg/kg/min for 5 to 7 days, plus 185 historical control subjects) from previously reported prospective studies. Time-to-event analyses of our primary end point—a thrombotic composite of death due to thrombosis, amputation sec-

ondary to HIT-associated thrombosis, or new thrombosis within 37 days—and the individual components were conducted, with hazard ratios estimated for treatment with and without adjustments for patient age, gender, race, weight, and baseline platelet count.

Measurements and Results.—Argatroban, vs control, significantly reduced the thrombotic composite risk (HIT: hazard ratio, 0.33; 95% confidence interval [CI], 0.20 to 0.54, p < 0.001; HIT with thrombosis: hazard ratio, 0.39; 95% CI, 0.25 to 0.62, p < 0.001), regardless of covariate adjustments. More argatroban-treated patients than control subjects remained thrombotic event free during follow-up, regardless of whether baseline thrombosis was absent (91% vs 73%) or present (72% vs 50%). Argatroban significantly reduced new thrombosis (p < 0.001) and death due to thrombosis (p ≤ 0.001). Major bleeding was similar between groups (6 to 7%, p = 0.74). Thrombotic risks were 2 times greater in nonwhite than in white patients, 1.7 times greater in female than male patients with HIT and thrombosis, and increased with decreasing weight or platelet count.

Conclusions.—Argatroban, vs control, provides effective antithrombotic therapy in patients with HIT, without increasing bleeding. Patients at higher risk for HIT-associated thrombosis include women, nonwhites, and individuals with current HIT-associated thrombosis, lower body weight, or more severe thrombocytopenia.

▶ The study confirms the effectiveness of argatroban in treating heparin-associated thrombocytopenia (HIT). Note that HIT patients with lower body weight and more severe thrombocytopenia, as well as those who are not white, had greater HIT-associated thrombotic complications.

G. L. Moneta, MD

The Risk of Hemorrhage Among Patients With Warfarin-Associated Coagulopathy

Garcia DA, Regan S, Crowther M, et al (Univ of New Mexico, Albuquerque; Harvard Med School; McMaster Univ, Hamilton, Ont, Canada; et al)
J Am Coll Cardiol 47:804-808, 2006

Objectives.—Among warfarin-treated patients with international normalized ratio (INR) >5, we sought to determine the risk of major bleeding within 30 days.

Background.—For warfarin-treated patients, the risk of bleeding increases as the INR rises, particularly if the INR exceeds 4. The 30-day risk of hemorrhage among outpatients with excessively prolonged INR values is unknown.

Methods.—To assess anticoagulation care in the U.S., a cohort of 6,761 patients taking warfarin was prospectively assembled from 101 participating sites (43% were community-based cardiology practices). From this cohort, 1,104 patients were identified with a first episode of INR >5.

Results.—A total of 979 met eligibility criteria; complete follow-up information was available for 976 (99.7%). Ninety-six percent (n = 937) of patients had an INR value between 5 and 9; 80% of INR values were <7. Thirteen patients (1.3%) experienced major hemorrhage during the 30-day follow-up period; among patients whose INR was >5 and <9, 0.96% experienced major hemorrhage. None of the bleeding events was fatal. Intervention with vitamin K was uncommon (8.7%). Warfarin doses were withheld for the majority of patients. Fifty percent of patients who were managed conservatively and retested on day 4 or 5 had an INR of 2.0 or less.

Conclusions.—For warfarin-treated outpatients presenting with an INR >5 and <9, the 30-day risk of major bleeding is low (0.96%). Intervention with vitamin K among asymptomatic patients presenting with an INR <9 is not routine practice in the U.S.

▶ Warfarin coagulopathy is common but easily treated in the large majority of patients by simply withholding warfarin and rechecking the INR in a few days. Conservative treatment is indicated in patients with warfarin therapy who present with INRs that are elevated but less than 9.0. Reduction in the INR to an acceptable level can be expected within a few days with a minimal incidence of bleeding complications.

G. L. Moneta, MD

Prevalence of MRSA in Emergency and Elective Patients Admitted to a Vascular Surgical Unit: Implications for Antibiotic Prophylaxis
Muralidhar B, Anwar SM, Handa AI, et al (John Radcliffe Hosp, Oxford, England)
Eur J Vasc Endovasc Surg 32:402-407, 2006

Objectives.—

1. Audit adequacy of admission screening for MRSA in vascular surgery patients.
2. Establish the prevalence of MRSA carriage at the time of admission in emergency/transfer and elective patients.
3. Establish a threshold presence of MRSA that should trigger the use of prophylactic antibiotics active against MRSA.
4. Model some of the costs and efficacy of glycopeptides such as vancomycin, compared to aminoglycosides such as gentamicin, for the prevention of MRSA surgical site infections.

Materials and Methods.—200 consecutive emergency/transfer and 150 consecutive elective patients admitted between April 2004 and January 2005, were studied. Data was obtained from departmental Morbidity and Mortality records and the computerised laboratory medicine information system.

Results.—261 (75%) of the 350 patients were screened for MRSA on admission (target 100%). The proportions of emergency/transfer and elective patients screened were similar (78% and 72% respectively). The prevalence of MRSA carriage detected by admission screening in emergency/transfer patients 30/153 (20%), was significantly higher ($p<0.0001$) than in elective patients 2/108 (2%). A simple decision analysis model suggests that gentamicin should be used when the prevalence of MRSA reaches 10% and vancomycin when the prevalence reaches 50%.

Conclusions.—The high prevalence of MRSA colonisation in emergency/transfer patients has important implications for pre-operative antibiotic prophylaxis.

▶ An important concept is presented here. It is possible to identify certain types of vascular surgical patients who are at high risk for MRSA infection. A different regimen of prophylactic antibiotics should be considered in patients at high risk for MRSA if they must be operated on before their MRSA status can be confirmed. A better solution, of course, is to reduce the prevalence of MRSA colonization in hospitalized patients.[1]

G. L. Moneta, MD

Reference

1. Thompson M. An audit demonstrating a reduction in MRSA infection in a specialised vascular unit resulting from a change in infection control protocol. *Eur J Vasc Endovasc Surge.* 2006;31:609-615.

An Audit Demonstrating a Reduction in MRSA Infection in a Specialised Vascular Unit Resulting from a Change in Infection Control Protocol

Thompson M (St George's Hosp, London)
Eur J Vasc Endovasc Surg 31:609-615, 2006

Introduction.—In 2003, 18% of all admissions to our vascular ward were colonised by MRSA, with an MRSA infection rate of 10.6%. Standard practice was to segregate patients with proven MRSA from the rest of the patient pool. After a prospective audit, regression analysis was used to identify factors that could stratify patients into high and low risk for MRSA colonisation. A change in isolation policy was introduced that segregated patients according to their risk of MRSA acquisition, and isolated all patients undergoing prosthetic vascular reconstruction. Antibiotic policy was also altered. This audit reports the impact of these changes on MRSA colonisation and infection rates.

Methods.—The MRSA status of patients during 777 in-patient episodes was prospectively recorded during three time spans; period 1 (November 2002–April 2003) before the change in isolation and antibiotic policy and, periods 2 (August–December 2003) and 3 (October 2004–January 2005) after the change in policy.

Results.—Hospital acquired MRSA colonisation was reduced from 10.6% in period 1, to 1.1 and 1.4% in periods 2 and 3, respectively ($pM<0.001$). Similarly, MRSA infection rates fell from 10.6 to 2.9 and 0.9%

over the same time frame (*p*<0.001). The most dramatic changes in MRSA infection rates occurred in patients undergoing aneurysm repair (MRSA infection 30.1% in period 1 *vs*. 3.9 and 2.9% in periods 2 and 3) and lower limb revascularization (31 *vs*. 0 *vs*. 4.2%). Stepwise regression analysis revealed that the system of isolation was a significant factor reducing MRSA infection and colonisation rates (*p*<0.001).

Conclusions.—These data demonstrate that a change in infection control policy can significantly reduce MRSA infection in a vascular unit.

▶ This study was performed in a hospital where vascular surgical patients were housed in multipatient rooms. Therefore, it may not apply to many United States hospitals where most patients have individual rooms. Nevertheless, the idea of identifying patients at risk for MRSA infection and instituting infection control policies on the basis of risk rather than actual infection is interesting and indicates a proactive approach to this difficult problem. It is certainly possible that even in hospitals with individual patient rooms, a policy of increased contact precautions in patients at risk of MRSA infection may prove worthwhile.

G. D. Moneta, MD

Comparison of Two Fluid-Management Strategies in Acute Lung Injury
Wiedemann HP, for The National Heart, Lung, and Blood Institute Acute Respiratory Distress Syndrome (ARDS) Clinical Trials Network (Cleveland Clinic, Ohio; et al)
N Engl J Med 354:2564-2575, 2006

Background.—Optimal fluid management in patients with acute lung injury is unknown. Diuresis or fluid restriction may improve lung function but could jeopardize extrapulmonary-organ perfusion.

Methods.—In a randomized study, we compared a conservative and a liberal strategy of fluid management using explicit protocols applied for seven days in 1000 patients with acute lung injury. The primary end point was death at 60 days. Secondary end points included the number of ventilator-free days and organ-failure-free days and measures of lung physiology.

Results.—The rate of death at 60 days was 25.5 percent in the conservative-strategy group and 28.4 percent in the liberal-strategy group (P=0.30; 95 percent confidence interval for the difference, −2.6 to 8.4 percent). The mean (±SE) cumulative fluid balance during the first seven days was −136±491 ml in the conservative-strategy group and 6992±502 ml in the liberal-strategy group (P<0.001). As compared with the liberal strategy, the conservative strategy improved the oxygenation index ([mean airway pressure × the ratio of the fraction of inspired oxygen to the partial pressure of arterial oxygen]×100) and the lung injury score and increased the number of ventilator-free days (14.6±0.5 vs. 12.1±0.5, P<0.001) and days not spent in the intensive care unit (13.4±0.4 vs. 11.2±0.4, P<0.001) during the first 28 days but did not increase the incidence or prevalence of shock during

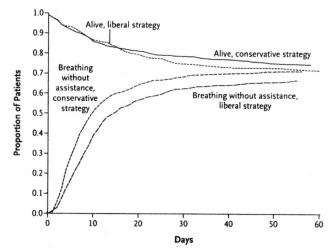

FIGURE 3.—Probability of Survival to Hospital Discharge and of Breathing without Assistance during the First 60 Days after Randomization. (Reprinted by permission of *The New England Journal of Medicine* from Wiedemann HP, for The National Heart, Lung, and Blood Institute Acute Respiratory Distress Syndrome [ARDS] Clinical Trials Network. Comparison of two fluid-management strategies in acute lung injury. *N Engl J Med.* 2006;354:2564-2575. Copyright ©2006, Massachusetts Medical Society. All rights reserved.)

the study or the use of dialysis during the first 60 days (10 percent vs. 14 percent, P=0.06).

Conclusions.—Although there was no significant difference in the primary outcome of 60-day mortality, the conservative strategy of fluid management improved lung function and shortened the duration of mechanical ventilation and intensive care without increasing nonpulmonary-organ failures. These results support the use of a conservative strategy of fluid management in patients with acute lung injury. (ClinicalTrials.gov number, NCT00281268 [ClinicalTrials.gov].) (Fig 3).

▶ A conservative fluid management strategy did not decrease death at 60 days versus a liberal fluid management strategy in patients with adult respiratory distress syndrome (ARDS). However, intensive care unit days were reduced and lung function was improved with a conservative fluid management posture. The results are consistent with other recent reports suggesting improved overall patient outcome with conservative fluid management of ARDS. The days of essentially drowning patients with acute lung injury to preserve distal organ perfusion should be over.

G. L. Moneta, MD

N-Acetylcysteine and Contrast-Induced Nephropathy in Primary Angioplasty

Marenzi G, Assanelli E, Marana I, et al (Univ of Milan, Italy)
N Engl J Med 354:2773-2782, 2006

Background.—Patients with acute myocardial infarction undergoing primary angioplasty are at high risk for contrast-medium–induced nephropathy because of hemodynamic instability, the need for a high volume of contrast medium, and the lack of effective prophylaxis. We investigated the antioxidant *N*-acetylcysteine for the prevention of contrast-medium–induced nephropathy in patients undergoing primary angioplasty.

Methods.—We randomly assigned 354 consecutive patients undergoing primary angioplasty to one of three groups: 116 patients were assigned to a standard dose of *N*-acetylcysteine (a 600-mg intravenous bolus before primary angioplasty and 600 mg orally twice daily for the 48 hours after angioplasty), 119 patients to a double dose of *N*-acetylcysteine (a 1200-mg intravenous bolus and 1200 mg orally twice daily for the 48 hours after intervention), and 119 patients to placebo.

Results.—The serum creatinine concentration increased 25 percent or more from baseline after primary angioplasty in 39 of the control patients (33 percent), 17 of the patients receiving standard-dose *N*-acetylcysteine (15 percent), and 10 patients receiving high-dose *N*-acetylcysteine (8 percent, $P<0.001$). Overall in-hospital mortality was higher in patients with contrast-medium–induced nephropathy than in those without such nephropathy (26 percent vs. 1 percent, $P<0.001$). Thirteen patients (11 percent) in the control group died, as did five (4 percent) in the standard-dose *N*-acetylcysteine group and three (3 percent) in the high-dose *N*-acetylcysteine group ($P=0.02$). The rate for the composite end point of death, acute renal failure requiring temporary renal-replacement therapy, or the need for mechanical ventilation was 21 (18 percent), 8 (7 percent), and 6 (5 percent) in the three groups, respectively ($P=0.002$).

Conclusions.—Intravenous and oral *N*-acetylcysteine may prevent contrast-medium-induced nephropathy with a dose-dependent effect in patients treated with primary angioplasty and may improve hospital outcome. (ClinicalTrials.gov number, NCT00237614[ClinicalTrials.gov]).

▶ This is obviously a study of urgent angiography and angioplasty in patients with coronary artery disease. However, it is likely the results can be extrapolated to patients with peripheral vascular disease. The importance of the article resides in the fact that it may be possible to prevent contrast nephropathy with *N*-acetylcysteine prophylaxis administrated at the time of the angiographic procedure rather than beginning the days before the procedure.

G. L. Moneta, MD

6 Grafts and Graft Complications

Engineered Living Blood Vessels: Functional Endothelia Generated From Human Umbilical Cord-Derived Progenitors
Schmidt D, Asmis LM, Odermatt B, et al (OBGYN Ctr Seefeld/Hirslanden Clinic Group Zurich, Switzerland; Univ Hosp Zurich, Switzerland; Swiss Federal Inst of Technology (ETH), Zurich, Switzerland)
Ann Thorac Surg 82:1465-1471, 2006

Background.—Tissue-engineered living blood vessels (TEBV) with growth capacity represent a promising new option for the repair of congenital malformations. We investigate the functionality of TEBV with endothelia generated from human umbilical cord blood–derived endothelial progenitor cells.

Methods.—Tissue-engineered living blood vessels were generated from human umbilical cord–derived myofibroblasts seeded on biodegradable vascular scaffolds, followed by endothelialization with differentiated cord blood–derived endothelial progenitor cells. During in vitro maturation the TEBV were exposed to physiologic conditioning in a flow bioreactor. For functional assessment, a subgroup of TEBV was stimulated with tumor necrosis factor-α. Control vessels endothelialized with standard vascular endothelial cells were treated in parallel. Analysis of the TEBV included histology, immunohistochemistry, biochemistry (extracellular matrix analysis, DNA), and biomechanical testing. Endothelia were analyzed by flow cytometry and immunohistochemistry (CD31, von Willebrand factor, thrombomodulin, tissue factor, endothelial nitric oxide synthase).

Results.—Histologically, a three-layered tissue organization of the TEBV analogous to native vessels was observed, and biochemistry revealed the major matrix constituents (collagen, proteoglycans) of blood vessels. Biomechanical properties (Young's modulus, 2.03 ± 0.65 MPa) showed profiles resembling those of native tissue. Endothelial progenitor cells expressed typical endothelial cell markers CD31, von Willebrand factor, and endothelial nitric oxide synthase comparable to standard vascular endothelial cells. Stimulation with tumor necrosis factor-α resulted in physiologic upregulation of tissue factor and downregulation of thrombomodulin expression.

Conclusions.—These results indicate that TEBV with tissue architecture and functional endothelia similar to native blood vessels can be successfully generated from human umbilical cord progenitor cells. Thus, blood-derived progenitor cells obtained before or at birth may enable the clinical realization of tissue engineering constructs for pediatric applications.

▶ This is a fascinating approach to achieve a functional bioactive endothelium in an arterial substitute. Obviously this work is in its early stages and clearly not perfect because some endothelial cells end up in the medial layer and the vessel is relatively thick walled. Nevertheless, the bioengineered blood vessel developed by the authors greatly approximates a normal vessel. Perhaps someday we will be storing umbilical cord blood to eventually serve as a basis for a late-in-life small-caliber arterial substitute.

G. L. Moneta, MD

Percutaneous transplantation of genetically-modified autologous fibroblasts in the rabbit femoral artery: a novel approach for cardiovascular gene therapy

Mazighi M, Tchétché D, Gouëffic Y, et al (Unité INSERM U698, Paris; Assistance Publique-Hôpitaux de Paris)
J Vasc Surg 44:1067-1075, 2006

Objective.—Arterial cell and gene therapies are promising strategies for the treatment of cardiovascular diseases; however, the optimal cell type and delivery technique for such treatment remain to be determined. The aim of the present study was to design a new approach for arterial cell and gene therapy in which genetically modified autologous skin fibroblasts are percutaneously delivered in stented rabbit femoral arteries in vivo.

Methods.—Autologous skin fibroblasts underwent in vitro transfection with the cationic lipid FuGene and plasmids expressing the human form of the tissue inhibitor of metalloproteinase (hTIMP-1) or nls-LacZ reporter genes.

Result.—Transfection efficiency was about 50% and there were high levels of hTIMP-1 secretion up to 14 days after gene transfer. We demonstrated the feasibility of in vivo percutaneous transplantation of fluorescent fibroblasts in the rabbit femoral artery. Results were confirmed by scanning electron microscopy. In vivo local delivery of hTIMP-1-expressing fibroblasts in stented femoral arteries also resulted in high-levels of hTIMP-1 secretion ex vivo for 7 days. Fibroblast transplantation resulted in a modest increase in intimal hyperplasia at the target site, which was reversed with hTIMP-1-transfected fibroblasts.

Conclusion.—Percutaneous transplantation of genetically modified autologous fibroblasts could be used as a cellular platform for locoregional secretion of therapeutic proteins to treat either specific arterial diseases or the diseased organ (eg, the heart) supplied by the target artery (Fig 2).

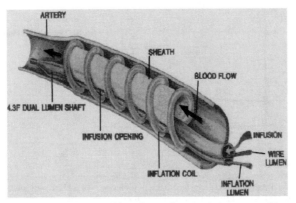

FIGURE 2.—The Dispatch catheter used for cell transplantation incorporates a 20-mm-long × 3-mm-diameter spiral inflation coil wrapped around a urethane sheath covered by a layer of 24 perforated channels, each with a single 100-μm infusion opening through which cells are delivered via an independent infusion lumen. (Reprinted by permission of the publisher from Mazighi M, Tchétché D, Gouëffic Y, et al. Percutaneous transplantation of genetically-modified autologous fibroblasts in the rabbit femoral artery: a novel approach for cardiovascular gene therapy. *J Vasc Surg*. 2006;44:1067-1075. Copyright 2006 by Elsevier.)

▶ Cell transplantation into arteries has been previously demonstrated using operative exposures that allow very controlled conditions and, therefore, potentially engraftment of a large percentage of cells. A percutaneous approach is obviously more desirable. The catheter used to deliver the cells in this study was also capable of retrieving nonengrafted cells, thus limiting distal cell dissemination. If this technology eventually achieves clinical importance, the percutaneous technique described here will certainly facilitate intravascular therapy.

G. L. Moneta, MD

Heparin immobilization reduces thrombogenicity of small-caliber expanded polytetrafluoroethylene grafts

Heyligers JMM, Verhagen HJM, Rotmans JI, et al (Univ Med Ctr, Utrecht, The Netherlands)
J Vasc Surg 43:587-591, 2006

Objective.—The patency of small-diameter expanded polytetrafluoroethylene (ePTFE) grafts for vascular reconstruction is impaired by acute thrombotic occlusion. Prosthetic materials are thrombogenic and cause platelet adhesion and activation of the coagulation cascade. Heparin is a potent anticoagulant drug widely used to prevent and treat thrombosis. A new ePTFE graft with long-term bonding of heparin is now commercially available in several European countries, but a basic analysis of its mechanism of action in humans has never been performed. This study was performed to evaluate the thrombogenicity of heparin-bonded ePTFE grafts compared with standard ePTFE in a newly developed human ex vivo model.

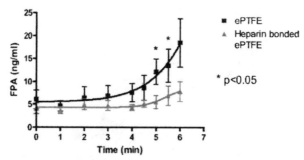

FIGURE 3.—Heparin immobilization reduces fibrin formation during ex vivo perfusion. Perfusions were performed in 10 volunteers by using both a noncoated and heparin-bonded graft in each volunteer. Serial samples were taken during perfusion, in which levels of fibrinopeptide A (*FPA*) were measured by enzyme-linked immunosorbent assay. Error bars indicate SEM. *ePTFE,* Expanded polytetrafluoroethylene. [Reprinted by permission of the publisher from Heyligers JMM, Verhagen HJM, Rotmans JI, et al. Heparin immobilization reduces thrombogenicity of small-caliber expanded polytetrafluoroethylene grafts. *J Vasc Surg.* 2006;43:587-591. Copyright 2006 by Elsevier.]

Methods.—Nonanticoagulated blood was drawn from antecubital veins of 10 healthy donors with a 19-gauge needle. The proximal end of a 60-cm ePTFE vascular graft with a diameter of 3 mm was connected to the needle while the distal end was connected to a syringe, which was placed in a syringe pump. Every volunteer served as his or her own control by using a heparin-bonded ePTFE graft on one arm and a standard ePTFE graft on the other arm. The perfusions were performed over 6 minutes with a flow rate of 20 mL/min, corresponding to a shear rate of 74/s. Serial samples were taken at the distal end of the graft for determination of prothrombin fragment 1 + 2, fibrinopeptide A, and P-selectin expression on perfused platelets. Fibrin deposition and platelet deposition were studied by using scanning electronic microscopy.

Results.—Fibrinopeptide A production over time was significantly reduced on the heparin-bonded ePTFE grafts compared with standard ePTFE grafts ($P < .05$). There was no increase in the production of prothrombin fragment 1 + 2 or P selectin over time on either type of graft. Scanning electronic microscopy scanning showed platelet deposition and fibrin formation on standard ePTFE grafts, whereas no platelets or fibrin were observed on heparin-bonded ePTFE grafts.

Conclusions.—Heparin immobilization substantially reduces the thrombogenicity of small-diameter ePTFE in a newly developed human ex vivo model. In this study, we provide evidence that the mechanism of action of the heparin bonding is due not only to anticoagulant but also to antiplatelet effects. Heparin bonding may be an important improvement of ePTFE, resulting in better patency rates for vascular reconstructions (Fig 3).

▶ The graft tested here is now available in the United States as well as in Europe. The heparin-bonded grafts reduced platelet adhesion to, basically, zero. It is interesting to speculate whether this will lead to decreased intimal anastomotic hyperplasia associated with these new grafts. However, I do remember when perioperative low-dose heparin was touted as a means of improving graft patency through decreased intimal hyperplasia.[1] We now know that this strategy was not effective. If the grafts described here really are advantageous over standard PTFE, my guess is it will not be through inhibition of intimal hyperplasia.

Reference

1. Taylor LM Jr, Troutman R, Feliciano P, Menashe V, Sunderland C, Porter JM. Late complications after femoral artery catheterization in children less than five years of age. *J Vasc Surg.* 1990;11:297-304.

G. L. Moneta, MD

PEG-hirudin/iloprost Coating of Small Diameter ePTFE Grafts Effectively Prevents Pseudointima and Intimal Hyperplasia Development
Heise M, Schmidmaier G, Husmann I, et al (Charité, Univ Medicine, Berlin; Charité, Campus Virchow Klinikum, Berlin)
Eur J Vasc Endovasc Surg 32:418-424, 2006

Objectives.—Small diameter PTFE grafts are prone to thrombosis and intimal hyperplasia development. Heparin graft coating has beneficial effects but also potential drawbacks. The purpose of this study was to evaluate the experimental efficacy of PEG-hirudin/iloprost coated small caliber PTFE grafts.

Methods.—Thirty-six femoro-popliteal ePTFE grafts (expanded polytetrafluoroethylene, diameter 4 mm) were inserted into 18 pigs. Grafts were randomised individually for each leg and grouped for 3 groups. Group I consisted of native ePTFE grafts, group II were grafts coated with a polylactide polymer (PLA) without drugs and group III grafts were coated with PLA containing a polyethylene glycol (PEG)-hirudin/iloprost combination. The follow-up period was 6 weeks. Patency rates were calculated and development of pseudointima inside the grafts was noted. Thickness of intimal hyperplasia at the distal anastomoses was measured using light microscopy.

Results.—Patency rates for group I were 6/9 (67%), for group II 9/10 (90%) and 12/12 (100%) for group III. In groups I and II there was a significant reduction of blood flow proximal to the graft at graft harvest, to 29 ± 12 and 28 ± 20 ml/min respectively (both $p < 0.01$ versus preoperative value), whilst in group III blood flow, 99 ± 21 ml/min, remained at the preoperative level. Subtotal stenosis due to development of pseudointima was noted in each of the native and PLA coated grafts but not in group III grafts. Intimal hyperplasia at the distal anastomosis was lowest in group III.

Conclusions.—The PEG-hirudin/iloprost coating of ePTFE prostheses effectively reduced pseudointima and intimal hyperplasia development and led to superior graft patency (Fig 2).

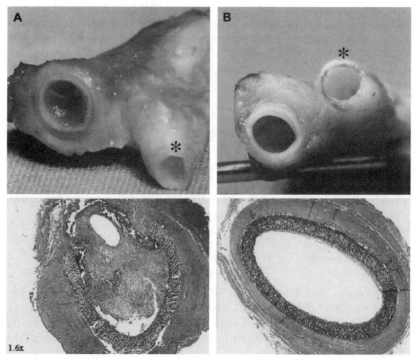

FIGURE 2.—Comparison of the distal anastomoses of an uncoated (A) versus a PEG-hirudin/iloprost coated (B) ePTFE graft. A marked pseudointima, resulting in a subtotal stenosis, developed in all uncoated/PLA coated prostheses (n = 19), while only a thin layer was seen in antithrombotic coated grafts (n = 12). *denotes distal femoral/popliteal artery ePTFE-expanded polytetrafluoroethylene. (Verhoeff van Giesson stain, original magnification ×1.6). (Reprinted from Heise M, Schmidmaier G, Husmann I, et al. PEG-hirudin/iloprost coating of small diameter ePTFE grafts effectively prevents pseudointima and intimal hyperplasia development. *Eur J Vasc Endovasc Surg.* 2006;32:418-424, by permission of the publisher.)

▶ Another approach to potentially inhibiting intimal hyperplasia associated with PTFE grafts (Heparin immobilization reduces thrombogenicity of small-caliber expanded polytetrafluoroethylene grafts). However, the conclusion of this abstract is a bit misleading because intimal hyperplasia was not statistically different in the hirudin/iloprost-coated grafts except at one site, and there was no statistical correction performed for multiple comparisons. The principal mechanism of improved patency is likely to be reduced pseudointima rather than decreased intimal hyperplasia.

G. L. Moneta, MD

In Vivo Behavior of Decellularized Vein Allograft

Martin ND, Schaner PJ, Tulenko TN, et al (Thomas Jefferson Univ, Philadelphia)
J Surg Res 129:17-23, 2005

Background.—We are investigating decellularized vein allograft as a scaffold to engineer a non-synthetic, small-diameter vascular graft. This study examines the in vivo behavior of this scaffolding after implantation into the arterial circulation.

Materials and Methods.—Canine animals underwent bilateral carotid interposition grafting using jugular vein implanted as either: 1) fresh autograft, 2) fresh allograft, or 3) decellularized allograft. Decellularization was achieved using sodium dodecyl sulfate. Grafts were examined with duplex ultrasound biweekly to determine luminal diameter, thrombosis, stenosis, or anastomotic breakdown. After perfusion fixation at 2 or 8 weeks, grafts underwent histological, morphometric, and immunohistochemical examination.

Results.—All animals survived without neurological or hemorrhagic complication. No deterioration of graft integrity (rupture, aneurysm) was observed in any group. Luminal narrowing was observed in both allograft groups, but secondary to different pathology. Fresh allografts had significant mononuclear cell infiltrate, intimal hyperplasia, and intramural hemorrhage consistent with rejection. Conversely, decellularized allografts had minimal evidence of rejection but instead had a compact fibrin layer formed along their lumen. This fibrin layer was absent in the peri-anastomotic regions where endothelium had migrated from the native artery. By 8 weeks, decellularized grafts had repopulated with cells staining positive for smooth muscle α-actin.

Conclusions.—After 8 weeks of arterial flow, decellularized vein allograft exhibits satisfactory strength, reduced antigenicity compared to fresh allograft, and supports cellular repopulation. These characteristics make it satisfactory for further tissue engineering; combined with luminal vascular cell seeding, it may prove useful as a small-diameter arterial bypass graft.

▶ These guys remove the luminal cells from cadaver veins and hope that when the resulting matrix is repopulated with vascular cells that it will be in time to prevent degeneration of the matrix with preservation of the lumen of the graft. At 8 weeks everything seems okay. Measurements of endothelial function and vasoreactivity are needed to demonstrate that the grafts not only maintain a lumen, but also a functional luminal surface.

G. L. Moneta, MD

Endovascular Repair for Aorto-enteric Fistula: A Bridge Too Far or a Bridge to Surgery?

Danneels MIL, Verhagen HJM, Teijink JAW, et al (Ghent Univ, Gent, Belgium; Univ Med Ctr Utrecht, The Netherlands; Atrium Med Ctr Heerlen, The Netherlands; et al)

Eur J Vasc Endovasc Surg 32:27-33, 2006

Purpose.—To review our experience of endovascular treatment of aorto-enteric fistula (AEF).

Methods.—Between March 1999 and March 2005, 15 patients in five university and teaching hospitals in Belgium and The Netherlands were treated for AEF by endovascular repair. Twelve (80%) were male. The mean age was 67 years. Thirteen (87%) had had previous aortic or iliac surgery, 1.7–307 months before. All patients showed clinical or biochemical signs of bleeding. Eight (53%) were in shock, five (33%) had systemic signs of infection. Eight (53%) patients were treated in an emergency setting. Ten (67%) were treated with an aortouniiliac device, three (20%) with an aortobiiliac device, one with a tube graft and one with occluders only. All patients received antibiotics postoperatively for a prolonged period of time.

Results.—All AEF were successfully sealed, the 30-days mortality was nil. Mean hospital stay was 20 (2–81) days. One patient died 2.7 months later of postoperative complications, one died of lung cancer. Until now, there are no signs of reinfection in four (27%) patients (mean follow-up 15.7 (1–44) months). However, reinfection or recurrent AEF occurred in nine (60%) patients after 9.5 (0.61–31) months. Seven patients were reoperated successfully, two patients died after reintervention.

Conclusion.—Endovascular sealing of AEF is a promising technique, which provides time to treat shock, local and systemic infection, and co-morbidity. This creates a better situation to perform open repair in the future with possibly better outcome. Danger of reinfection remains high. Endovascular sealing of AEF should, therefore, be seen as a bridge to open surgery when possible.

▶ Placement of an aortic stent graft for definitive treatment of an aorto-enteric fistula seems like a silly idea. It violates virtually every known surgical principle. Nevertheless, it does not seem unreasonable to use an aortic endograft in patients with aortic enteric fistula as a temporizing measure. This can convert an emergency to a more elective situation and may make a high-risk operation a bit safer.

G. L. Moneta, MD

Neoaortic Reconstruction for Aortic Graft Infection: Need for Endovascular Adjunctive Therapies?

Faulk J, Dattilo JB, Guzman RJ, et al (Vanderbilt Univ, Nashville, Tenn; VA Hosp, Nashville, Tenn)
Ann Vasc Surg 19:774-781, 2005

Neoaortic reconstruction using an autogenous conduit is an increasingly accepted option for the management of aortic graft infections. However, this approach is not without technical challenges and potential graft-related problems, some of which can be solved with endovascular techniques. All patients who underwent neoaortic reconstruction with femoral-popliteal vein for aortic graft infection over a 6-year period were identified from the operative registry. Those patients requiring endovascular adjunctive therapies form the basis of this report. Of 17 cases of neoaortic reconstruction for aortic graft infection, five (29%) required endovascular adjunctive procedures. These included stent placement for graft stenosis ($n = 3$), stent graft placement for proximal anastomotic stenosis ($n = 1$), and stent graft placement for anastomotic disruption ($n = 1$). While two of these procedures occurred within 30 days of the original neoaortic reconstruction, three were required during late follow-up. Although there were no direct complications related to the endovascular procedures, the patient with anastomotic disruption died within 30 days of causes unrelated to the endovascular procedure. Primary patency of neoaortic reconstruction was 87% at 30 days and 61% at 3 years, with assisted primary patency increasing to 100% at 3 years after endovascular adjunctive intervention. While neoaortic reconstruction using an autogenous conduit for aortic graft infection has proven durability, it is not without potential early and late graft complications. When graft problems occur, endovascular options are an attractive alternative to reoperative open aortic procedures, especially in the setting of a vastly altered surgical field.

▶ This article provides a hint that neoaortic reconstructions with femoral vein are not immortal and may be subject to the same problems as smaller-caliber vein grafts. Indeed, the primary patency of the neoaortic reconstructions in this series at 3 years was somewhat disappointing at 61%. This is not terribly unlike that reported by others.[1] We need to pay attention to the fine print when choosing one type of procedure over another for treatment of aortic graft infection. The choice is seldom as clear cut as might be suggested by enthusiasts of various procedures.

G. L. Moneta, MD

Reference

1. Gordon LL, Hagino RT, Jackson MR, Modrall JG, Valentine RJ, Clagett GP. Complex aortofemoral prosthetic infections: the role of autogenous superficial femoropopliteal vein reconstruction. *Arch Surg.* 1999;134:615-621.

Treatment of Femoral Pseudoaneurysms with Endograft in High-risk Patients

Derom A, Nout E (Ziekenhuis Zeeuws-Vlaanderen, Terneuzen, The Netherlands)
Eur J Vasc Endovasc Surg 30:644-647, 2005

Introduction.—Anastomotic aneurysms are a late complication after arterial reconstruction. Current treatment usually consists of open repair but we describe our experience with endovascular repair of femoral pseudoaneurysms.

Report.—Six patients with seven femoral pseudoaneurysms were treated with percutaneously inserted endografts. Control angiography confirmed immediate technical success in all cases. Exclusion of the para-anastomotic aneurysm was obtained in all cases. No major complications or postoperative mortality were observed. No occlusions of the endografts occurred and no endoleaks were noticed.

Discussion.—Endovascular exclusion of femoral pseudoaneurysms is feasible and reliable. Long-term follow-up will demonstrate if this approach in selected patients is justified.

▶ With the development of more flexible endovascular prostheses, the groin is no longer "no man's land" for endograft enthusiasts. Longer follow-up is required to see whether the approach described here is durable. Obviously, there should be no sign of primary graft infection when treating a pseudoaneurysm with an endograft. In addition, because femoral pseudoaneurysm repair with open techniques is not all that complicated, I would hope those wishing to treat a femoral pseudoaneurysm with an endograft will not fail, and thus sacrifice, the profunda femoris artery.

G. L. Moneta, MD

7 Aortic Aneurysm

Cost-effectiveness of screening women for abdominal aortic aneurysm
Wanhainen A, Lundkvist J, Bergqvist D, et al (Uppsala Univ, Sweden; Karolinska Inst, Uppsala, Sweden)
J Vasc Surg 43:908-914, 2006

Background.—Women are usually not considered for abdominal aortic aneurysm (AAA) screening because of their lower prevalence of disease. This position may, however, be questioned given the higher risk of rupture and the longer life expectancy among women. The purpose of this study was to assess the cost-effectiveness of screening 65-year-old women for AAA.

Methods.—A systematic review of the literature was conducted to obtain data of importance to evaluate the effectiveness of screening women for AAA. Data were entered into a Markov simulation cohort model.

Results.—The review suggested some main assumptions for women with AAA. Prevalence is 1.1%. In 6.8%, the AAA is of a size that merits surgery, and the patients are fit for a procedure. For patients with an AAA, the yearly risk for elective surgery and the rupture incidence was 3.1% and 2.4%, respectively, in the invited group and 1.1% and 5.7% in the noninvited group. The operative mortality for elective surgery was 3.5%, and the total mortality for ruptured AAA was 86.3%. The long-term mortality for AAA patients was 3.6 times higher than for an age-matched healthy population. Screening reduced the AAA rupture incidence by 33% and the AAA-related death rate by 35%. The cost per life year gained was estimated at $5911.

Conclusion.—The incremental cost-effectiveness ratio was similar to that found for screening men, which reflects the fact that the lower AAA prevalence in women is balanced by a higher rupture rate. Screening women for AAA may be cost-effective, and future evaluations on screening for AAA should include women.

▶ Many assumptions are required for Markov simulations, and those who enjoy this type of mathematical exercise have to admit they are at the mercy of the quality of the data available to them. It is important to keep in mind that recommendations not supporting AAA screening in women are primarily based on lack of data on the subject and not on negative data. Therefore, although imperfect, articles such as this should at least raise the possibility among regulatory agencies and payers that screening for AAA in women may actually be indicated and cost-effective.

G. L. Moneta, MD

Influence of sex on expansion rate of abdominal aortic aneurysms
Mofidi R, Goldie VJ, Kelman J, et al (Royal Infirmary of Edinburgh, Scotland)
Br J Surg 94:310-314, 2007

Background.—The UK Small Aneurysm Trial suggested that female sex is an independent risk factor for rupture of abdominal aortic aneurysm (AAA). This study assessed the effect of sex on the growth rate of AAA.

Methods.—Between January 1985 and August 2005 all patients who were referred to the Royal Infirmary of Edinburgh with an AAA who were not considered for early aneurysm repair were assessed by serial abdominal ultrasonography. Maximum anteroposterior and transverse diameters of the AAAs were measured.

Results.—A total of 1255 patients (824 men and 431 women) were followed up for a median of 30 (range 6-185) months. A median of six examinations (range 2-37) was performed for each patient. Median diameter on initial examination was 41 (range 25-83) mm. Median growth rate overall was 2·79 (range − 4·80-37·02) mm per year. Median growth rate of AAA was significantly greater in women than men (3·67 (range − 1·2-37·02) *versus* 2·03 (range − 4·80-21·00) mm per year; $P < 0·01$). Weighted linear regression analysis revealed that large initial anteroposterior AAA diameter and female sex were significant predictors of faster aneurysm growth rate ($P < 0·001$ and $P = 0·006$ respectively).

Conclusion.—The growth rate of AAA was significantly greater in women than in men. This may have implications for the frequency of follow-up and timing of repair of AAA in women.

▶ In the UK Small Aneurysm Trial, female sex was an independent risk factor for AAA rupture. Despite smaller initial anteroposterior diameters, the rupture rate in women was 3 times higher than that of men. Longitudinal studies suggest ruptures are more common in aneurysms that expand at higher rates.[1] These previous data and the current article argue for increased frequency of follow-up in women with AAA, and repair of the aneurysm at a smaller diameter than is generally recommended for men.

G. L. Moneta, MD

Reference

1. Brown PM, Zelt DT, Sobolev B. The risk of rupture in untreated aneurysms: the impact of size, gender, and expansion rate. *J Vasc Surg.* 2003;37:280-284.

Growth Rate and Associated Factors in Small Abdominal Aortic Aneurysms

Vega de Céniga M, Gómez R, Estallo L, et al (Hosp de Galdakao, Bizkaia, Spain)
Eur J Vasc Endovasc Surg 31:231-236, 2006

Objective.—To study the growth rate and factors influencing progression of small infrarenal abdominal aortic aneurysms (AAA).

Design.—Observational, longitudinal, prospective study.

Patients and Methods.—We followed patients with AAA <5 cm in diameter in two groups. Group I (AAA 3–3.9 cm, $n = 246$) underwent annual ultrasound scans. Group II (AAA 4–4.9 cm, $n = 106$) underwent 6-monthly CT scans.

Results.—We included 352 patients (333 men and 19 women) followed for a mean of 55.2±37.4 months (6.3–199.8). The mean growth rate was significantly greater in group II (4.72±5.93 *vs.* 2.07±3.23 mm/year; $p<0.0001$). Group II had a greater percentage of patients with rapid aneurysm expansion (>4 mm/year) (36.8 vs. 13.8%; $p<0.0001$). The classical cardiovascular risk factors did not influence the AAA growth rate in group I. Chronic limb ischemia was associated with slower expansion ($\leq$4 mm/year) (OR 0.47; CI 95% 0.22–0.99; $p = 0.045$). Diabetic patients in group

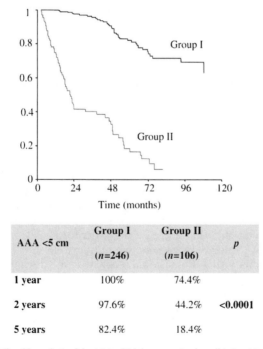

AAA <5 cm	Group I (n=246)	Group II (n=106)	p
1 year	100%	74.4%	
2 years	97.6%	44.2%	<0.0001
5 years	82.4%	18.4%	

FIGURE 2.—Life-table analysis of the AAA which have remained small (<5 cm) in groups I and II (statistical analysis: univariate Cox regression). (Reprinted by permission of the publisher from Vega de Céniga M, Gómez R, Estallo L, Rodríguez M, Baquer M, Barba A. Growth rate and associated factors in small abdominal aortic aneurysms. *Eur J Vasc Endovasc Surg.* 2006;31:231-236.)

II had a significantly smaller mean AAA growth rate than non-diabetics (1.69±3.51 vs. 5.22±6.11 mm/year; p = 0.032).

Conclusions.—The expansion rate of small AAA increases with the AAA size. AAA with a diameter of 3–3.9 cm expand slowly, and they are very unlikely to require surgical repair in 5 years. Many 4–4.9 cm AAA can be expected to reach a surgical size in the first 2 years of follow-up. Chronic limb ischemia and diabetes are associated with reduced aneurysm growth rates (Fig 2).

▶ The differential effects of cardiovascular risk factors and growth rates of aneurysms, although known, are not widely appreciated. In the UK Small Aneurysm Trial, there were decreased growth rates of aneurysms in patients with peripheral arterial disease, diabetes, or both.[1] The observation in this study that peripheral arterial disease and diabetes are associated with a lower growth rate of an AAA is, therefore, unlikely to be the result of chance. Perhaps there are changes in the collagen versus elastin content of the aortic wall in patients with diabetes, or in those whose atherosclerotic risk factors have produced both occlusive as well as aneurysm disease.

G. L. Moneta, MD

Reference

1. Brady AR, on behalf of the UK Small Aneurysm Trial Participants. Abdominal aortic aneurysm expansion. Risk factors and time intervals for surveillance. *Circulation.* 2004;110:16-21.

Surveillance of small aortic aneurysms does not alter anatomic suitability for endovascular repair
Yau FS, Rosero EB, Clagett GP, et al (Univ of Texas, Dallas; Dallas Veterans Affairs Med Ctr)
J Vasc Surg 45:96-100, 2007

Objective.—Small abdominal aortic aneurysms (AAAs; 4-5.4 cm) are more likely to be suitable for endovascular aneurysm repair (EVAR) than large aortic aneurysms (>5.5 cm). The purpose of this study was to determine whether small AAA growth is associated with the development of morphologic characteristics that decrease eligibility for EVAR.

Methods.—We studied 54 patients who underwent 2 or more computed tomography scans with 3-dimensional reconstruction during surveillance of small AAAs. Morphologic aortic aneurysm features and changes were measured according to Society for Vascular Surgery reporting standards. Suitability for EVAR was determined by neck anatomy (diameter, length, and angulations), iliac artery morphology, and total aortic aneurysm angulation and tortuosity.

Results.—The median age of the study cohort was 73 years (interquartile range [IQR], 65-77 years). The median follow-up period was 24 months (IQR, 15-36 months). The median small AAA diameter increased from 44.5

mm (IQR, 41-48 mm) to 48.9 mm (IQR, 45.7-52.0 mm). The median aortic neck diameter increased from 23.0 to 24.0 mm ($P = .002$), whereas median neck length decreased from 26.5 to 20.0 mm ($P = .001$). Aortic aneurysm median tortuosity index increased from 1.09 to 1.11 ($P = .05$). No significant changes in iliac artery morphology occurred. Overall, the anatomic suitability for endovascular repair did not significantly change during the study period (74% vs 69%; McNemar test; $P = .25$).

Conclusions.—Changes in aortic morphology are frequently associated with small AAA growth at mid-term follow-up, but such changes are minor and do not affect overall anatomic suitability for EVAR. These data reveal that continued surveillance of small AAAs does not threaten the window of opportunity for EVAR.

▶ There is currently great interest in treating small AAAs (4-5 cm) with aortic endografts. One of the arguments is that if you treat the aneurysm early, you will be able to treat it with an endograft, whereas if the aneurysm is allowed to progress in size it may not remain suitable for an aortic endograft. Obviously, this article argues against this sort of logic. The current push to treat small AAAs with endografts may have a lot more to do with industry profit motive and surgeon ego than the natural history of aortic aneurysm disease.

G. L. Moneta, MD

Age stratified, perioperative, and one-year mortality after abdominal aortic aneurysm repair: A statewide experience

Rigberg DA, Zingmond DS, McGory ML, et al (Univ of California, Los Angeles; West Los Angeles VA Med Ctr)
J Vasc Surg 43:224-229, 2006

Objective.—The purpose of this study was to determine the in-hospital, 30-day, and 365-day mortality for the open repair of abdominal aortic aneurysms (AAAs), when stratified by age, in the general population. Age stratification could provide clinicians with information more applicable to an individual patient than overall mortality figures.

Methods.—In a retrospective analysis, data were obtained from the California Office of Statewide Health Planning and Development (OSHPD) for the years 1995 to 1999. Out-of-hospital mortality was determined via linkage to the state death registry. All patients undergoing AAA repair as coded by International Classification of Diseases, 9th Revision (ICD-9) procedure code 38.44 and diagnosis codes 441.4 (intact) and 441.3/441.5 (ruptured) in California were identified. Patients <50 years of age were excluded. We determined in-hospital, 30-day, and 365-day mortality, and stratified our findings by patient age. Multivariate logistic regression was used to determine predictors of mortality in the intact and ruptured AAA cohorts.

Results.—We identified 12,406 patients (9,778 intact, 2,628 ruptured). Mean patient age was 72.4 ± 7.2 years (intact) and 73.9 ± 8.2 (ruptured). Men comprised 80.9% of patients, and 90.8% of patients were white. Overall, intact AAA patient mortality was 3.8% in-hospital, 4% at 30 days, and 8.5% at 365 days. There was a steep increase in mortality with increasing age, such that 365-day mortality increased from 2.9% for patients 51 to 60 years old to 15% for patients 81 to 90 years old. Mortality from day 31 to 365 was greater than both in-hospital and 30-day mortality for all but the youngest intact AAA patients. Perioperative (in-hospital and 30-day) mortality for ruptured cases was 45%, and mortality at 1 year was 54%.

Conclusions.—There is continued mortality after the open repair of AAAs during postoperative days 31 to 365 that, for many patients, is greater than the perioperative death rate. This mortality increases dramatically with age for both intact and ruptured AAA repair.

▶ Well, I guess repair of an AAA does not convey immortality, and older people die at a greater rate than younger people. Also, the sun rises in the east, and none of us get out of this alive. In other words, there is not much unexpected in this article. The article, however, does serve to remind us to look beyond the perioperative period when determining whether a patient is an appropriate candidate for a prophylactic procedure of any sort.

G. L. Moneta, MD

N-Acetylcysteine for the Prevention of Kidney Injury in Abdominal Aortic Surgery: A Randomized, Double-Blind, Placebo-Controlled Trial
Hynninen MS, Niemi TT, Pöyhiä R, et al (Helsinki Univ, Finland)
Anesth Analg 102:1638-1645, 2006

In this prospective, randomized, placebo-controlled, double-blind trial we studied the effects of IV N-acetylcysteine for prevention of renal injury in patients undergoing abdominal aortic surgery. Seventy patients without previously documented renal dysfunction were randomly allocated to receive either N-acetylcysteine (150 mg/kg mixed in 250 mL of 5% dextrose infused in 20 min, followed by an infusion of 150 mg/kg in 250 mL of 5% dextrose over 24 h) or placebo. The infusion was started after the induction of anesthesia. The primary outcome measure was renal injury as measured by the increases in urinary N-acetyl-β-D-glucosaminidase (NAG)/creatinine ratio (indicator of renal tubular injury) and urinary albumin/creatinine ratio (indicator of glomerular injury). Renal function was assessed by measuring plasma creatinine and serum cystatin C concentrations. The urinary NAG/creatinine ratio increased significantly from baseline to before crossclamp and remained increased on day 5 in both groups. The urinary albumin/creatinine ratio increased significantly from baseline to 6 h after declamping in the N-acetylcysteine group. However, the changes in the NAG/creatinine ratio and the albumin/creatinine ratio were not significantly different between the two groups. Plasma creatinine and serum cystatin C values remained unchanged during the study period in both groups. In conclusion, N-acetylcysteine did not offer any significant protection from renal injury during elective aortic operation in patients with normal preoperative renal function, and some degree of tubular injury seems to occur before aortic crossclamp.

▶ It is known that infrarenal and suprarenal aortic cross-clamping can induce renal dysfunction. However, it would seem more likely that suprarenal aortic clamping may produce changes in renal function of greater magnitude than infrarenal aortic clamping. It would be interesting to repeat this study in centers with a high volume of thoracoabdominal aneurysm repair and/or centers in which there are relatively large numbers of open abdominal aortic aneurysm repairs requiring suprarenal aortic clamps. There were only 2 patients with suprarenal aortic clamps in this study.

G. L. Moneta, MD

Replanting the inferior mesentery artery during infrarenal aortic aneurysm repair: Influence on postoperative colon ischemia
Senekowitsch C, Assadian A, Assadian O, et al (Wilhelminenspital, Vienna; Med Univ Vienna)
J Vasc Surg 43:689-694, 2006

Background.—Replanting the inferior mesentery artery (IMA) to prevent ischemic colitis (IC) has been discussed for many years; yet, to our knowledge, no prospective studies have been conducted to compare the incidence of histologically proven IC in patients with and without IMA revascularization. The aim of this prospective study, with histologic evaluation of the sigmoid colon mucosa, was to assess the influence of replanting the IMA on IC and mortality.

Methods.—From January 1999 to December 2003, 160 consecutive patients who were operated on for a symptomatic (n = 21) or asymptomatic (n = 139) infrarenal aortic aneurysm were prospectively assessed and randomly assigned either to replanting or ligating the IMA. Sigmoidoscopy with biopsy was performed on day 4 or 5 after surgery; an autopsy was performed on patients not surviving to day 5 after surgery. All patients gave written informed consent.

Results.—Of the 160 randomized patients, 128 had a confirmed patent IMA and formed the basis of this study. Their age was 70 ± 8 years (men, 70 ± 8 years; women, 73 ± 7 years). The IMA was replanted in 67 patients (52%) and ligated in 61 (48%) intraoperatively. IC developed in six patients with a replanted IMA and in 10 with a ligated IMA (relative risk [RR], 0.55; 95% confidence interval [CI], 0.21 to 1.41; χ^2 = 1.62; P = .203). Blood loss in the two cohorts did not differ significantly (P = .788); however, patients with IC had a significantly higher blood loss compared with the cohort without IC (P = .012) and were older (P = .017). Age, sex distribution, clamping time, the use of tube or bifurcated grafts, and intraoperative hypotension did not differ between patients with ligated or replanted IMA.

Conclusion.—Although replanting the IMA did not confer a statistically significant reduction of perioperative morbidity or mortality in this study, it appears that older patients and patients with increased intraoperative blood loss might benefit from IMA replantation, because this maneuver does not increase perioperative morbidity or substantially increase operation time.

▶ The conclusion of this article should be that routine reimplantation of the IMA does not influence all degrees of colon ischemia after abdominal aortic aneurysm repair. The authors admit that their study was underpowered to truly detect a difference for routine IMA reimplantation. It is also most certainly underpowered to detect a difference in patients at higher risk for colon ischemia, such as those with patent, large IMAs and bilateral hypogastric disease. Do not use this article to talk yourself out of reimplanting the IMA in a patient at high risk for postoperative colon ischemia.

G. L. Moneta, MD

Factors affecting outcomes of open surgical repair of pararenal aortic aneurysms: A 10-year experience
West CA, Noel AA, Bower TC, et al (Mayo Clinic, Rochester, Minn)
J Vasc Surg 43:921-928, 2006

Purpose.—Few large series document surgical outcomes for patients with pararenal abdominal aortic aneurysms (PAAAs), defined as aneurysms including the juxtarenal aorta or renal artery origins that require suprarenal aortic clamping. No standard endovascular alternatives presently exist; however, future endovascular branch graft repairs ultimately must be compared with the gold standard of open repair. To this end, we present a 10-year experience.

Methods.—Between 1993 and 2003, 3058 AAAs were repaired. Perioperative variables, morbidity, and mortality were retrospectively assessed. Renal insufficiency was defined as a rise in the concentration of serum creatinine by ≥ 0.5 mg/dL. Factors predicting complications were identified by multivariate analyses. Morbidity and 30-day mortality were evaluated with multiple logistic regression analysis.

Results.—Of a total of 3058 AAA repairs performed, 247 were PAAAs (8%). Mean renal ischemia time was 23 minutes (range, 5 to 60 minutes). Cardiac complications occurred in 32 patients (13%), pulmonary complications in 38 (16%), and renal insufficiency in 54 (22%). Multivariate analysis associated myocardial infarction with advanced age ($P = .01$) and abnormal preoperative serum creatinine (>1.5 mg/dL) ($P = .08$). Pulmonary complications were associated with advanced age ($P = .03$), renal artery bypass ($P = .02$), increased mesenteric ischemic time ($P = .01$), suprarenal aneurysm repair ($P < .0008$), and left renal vein division ($P = .01$). Renal insufficiency was associated with increased mesenteric ischemic time ($P = .001$), supravisceral clamping ($P = .04$), left renal vein division ($P = .04$), and renal artery bypass ($P = .0002$), but not renal artery reimplantation or endarterectomy. New dialysis was required in 3.7% (9/242). Abnormal preoperative serum creatinine (>1.5 mg/dL) was predictive of the need for postoperative dialysis (10% vs 2%; $P = .04$). Patients with normal preoperative renal function had improved recovery (93% vs 36%; $P = .0002$). The 30-day surgical mortality was 2.5% (6/247) but was not predicted by any factors, and in-hospital mortality was 2.8% (7/247). Median intensive care and hospital stays were 3 and 9 days, respectively, and longer stays were associated with age at surgery ($P = .007$ and $P = .0002$, respectively) and any postoperative complication.

Conclusions.—PAAA repair can be performed with low mortality. Renal insufficiency is the most frequent complication, but avoiding renal artery bypass, prolonged mesenteric ischemia time, or left renal vein transection may improve results.

▶ The authors utilized a transperitoneal approach to the aorta in most cases. While it is certainly possible to repair pararenal aneurysms transperitoneally, as evidenced by the excellent early results presented here, a retroperitoneal approach seems preferable in most cases of pararenal aneurysms. With the retroperitoneal approach there is no need to divide the renal vein or shift between retractor setups to clamp above the celiac artery. Initial exposure is a bit more of a hassle, but aortic clamping, a key part of any aortic procedure, is facilitated by the retroperitoneal approach for pararenal aneurysms.

G. L. Moneta, MD

Preoperative and Intraoperative Determinants of Incisional Bulge following Retroperitoneal Aortic Repair
Matsen SL, Krosnick TA, Roseborough GS, et al (Johns Hopkins Univ, Baltimore, Md)
Ann Vasc Surg 20:183-187, 2006

Although the left flank retroperitoneal incision is a useful approach for many patients undergoing major aortic reconstruction for aneurysmal and occlusive disease, it has been associated with weakening of the flank muscles, resulting in bulges varying from slight asymmetry to huge hernias. The purpose of this study was to determine if the incidence of this complication correlated with identifiable preoperative or intraoperative factors. Fifty consecutive patients undergoing aortic reconstruction via the retroperitoneal approach were followed for 1 year postoperatively for evidence of disfiguring bulges. Bulges were scored as follows: normal/mild, <1-inch protrusion; moderate, protrusion 1-2 inches; severe, protrusion >2 inches and/or pain or true herniation. Preoperatively, patients were administered a questionnaire to elicit demographic and comorbidity data. Fifty-six percent of patients developed a bulge at 1 year. In 43% of these, the bulge was deemed mild and in 54% moderate. One patient developed a severe bulge. Among preoperative comorbidities, no statistically significant correlations were found on bivariate analysis. However, likelihood ratios for bulge development of 5.5 for renal disease and 3.1 for cancer were demonstrated. Conversely, peripheral vascular disease had a likelihood ratio of 0.21 for bulge formation and emphysema, 0.28. On logistic analysis, incision >15 cm and body mass index (BMI) >23 mg/kg^2 were found to correlate strongly with bulge formation (p = 0.003, odds ratio = 9.1, and p = 0.018, odds ratio = 16.9, respectively). Together, these yielded a pseudo r^2 of 0.32. BMI >23 mg/ kg^{2}was found to yield the greatest explanatory power. These same two variables were found to correlate with severity of bulge: p = 0.02 for incision >15 cm and p = 0.006 for BMI >23. Of note, gender, age, and extension of the incision into the interspace were not significant on logistic analysis. Preoperatively, surgeons should warn obese patients and those requiring large incisions for extensive disease of their increased risk for poor healing. Intraoperatively, surgeons should aim to minimize incision length.

▶ An old-fashioned analysis where only the doctor's perception of a problem was addressed. We perform most open aortic surgery through flank incisions. Hernias are very uncommon, bulges of some sort frequent, and patient complaints very unusual, but perhaps that is because we don't ask the patient whether their incisions interfere with their quality of life.

G. L. Moneta, MD

Retroperitoneal Aortic Aneurysm Repair: Long-Term Follow-Up Regarding Wound Complications and Erectile Dysfunction
Ballard JL, Abou-Zamzam AM Jr, Teruya TH, et al (Univ of California, Irvine, Orange; Loma Linda Univ, Calif; Univ of Hawaii, Honolulu; et al)
Ann Vasc Surg 20:195-199, 2006

The long-term impact of retroperitoneal aortic exposure regarding wound complications in all patients and erectile dysfunction in men was studied in a consecutive group of 107 patients (81 males and 26 females). Postoperative wound complications were classified into the following groups: none, flank bulge, hernia, and chronic pain. Patient demographic features including body mass index (BMI) were statistically analyzed in relation to the incidence of long-term wound problems. Information regarding erectile dysfunction was obtained before surgery in all men and stratified into three groups after surgery: no change, inability to consistently obtain an erection, and retrograde ejaculation. Mean patient follow-up was 2.9 years (range 1-4.36, median 2.8). Flank bulge was the only long-term wound complication, and this was noted in nine patients (8%). The incidence of true hernia and chronic pain was 0%. BMI >28 was the only factor that positively impacted the incidence of wound complications (p < 0.0001). Erectile dysfunction prior to surgery was noted in 37 men (46%), while 44 (54%) reported normal erectile function. Erectile function improved after surgery in one patient but remained unchanged in the rest. Postoperative retrograde ejaculation occurred with a frequency of 9% (four of 45 patients). Retroperitoneal abdominal aortic aneurysm (rAAA) exposure with incision based on the twelfth rib tip and rectus abdominis muscle sparing results in an overall low incidence of long-term wound complications. Postoperative flank bulge is associated with patient BMI >28. In addition, erectile function is not worsened by infrarenal autonomic nerve sparing rAAA exposure. However, a small percentage of potent men will experience postoperative retrograde ejaculation.

▶ Similar to an article by Matsen et al,[1] BMI was associated with an increased incidence of postoperative flank bulge. There is no reason to suspect that rAAA repair ought to have any greater or lesser incidence of erectile dysfunction than open AAA repair. It also must be remembered that older men with AAAs have an increasing prevalence of erectile dysfunction with age regardless of whether the AAA is repaired.

G. L. Moneta, MD

Reference

1. Matsen SL, Krosnick TA, Roseborough GS, et al. Preoperative and intraoperative determinants of incisional bulge following retroperitoneal aortic repair. *Ann Vasc Surge.* 2006;20:183-187.

Angiotensin-converting enzyme inhibitors and aortic rupture: a population-based case-control study
Hackam DG, Thiruchelvam D, Redelmeier DA (Univ of Toronto)
Lancet 368:659-665, 2006

Background.—Angiotensin-converting enzyme (ACE) inhibitors prevent the expansion and rupture of aortic aneurysms in animals. We investigated the association between ACE inhibitors and rupture in patients with abdominal aortic aneurysms.

Methods.—We did a population-based case-control study of linked administrative databases in Ontario, Canada. The sample included consecutive patients older than 65 (n=15 326) admitted to hospital with a primary diagnosis of ruptured or intact abdominal aortic aneurysm between April 1, 1992, and April 1, 2002.

Findings.—Patients who received ACE inhibitors before admission were significantly less likely to present with ruptured aneurysm (odds ratio [OR] 0.82, 95% CI 0·74–0·90) than those who did not receive ACE inhibitors. Adjustment for demographic characteristics, risk factors for rupture, comorbidities, contraindications to ACE inhibitors, measures of health-care use, and aneurysm screening yielded similar results (0·83, 0·73–0·95). Consistent findings were noted in subgroups at high risk of rupture, including patients older than 75 years and those with a history of hypertension. Conversely, such protective associations were not observed for β blockers (1·02, 0·89–1·17), calcium channel blockers (1·01, 0·89–1·14), α blockers (1·15,

0·86–1·54), angiotensin receptor blockers (1·24, 0·71–2·18), or thiazide diuretics (0·91, 0·78–1·07).

Interpretation.—ACE inhibitors are associated with a reduced risk of ruptured abdominal aortic aneurysm, unlike other antihypertensive agents. Randomised trials of ACE inhibitors for prevention of aortic rupture might be warranted.

▶ This study has several important limitations. Healthier patients, perhaps with a lower risk of rupture, may have been more likely to receive ACE inhibitors. Most importantly, the authors did not control for AAA size, and certainly diameters are a significant predictor of AAA rupture. In addition, AAAs grow over a long period, and there was no analysis for the length of time the patients were on ACE inhibitors. The data are interesting but insufficient to recommend routine treatment of AAA patients with ACE inhibitors at this time.

G. L. Moneta, MD

Outcomes after Ruptured Abdominal Aortic Aneurysms: The "Halo Effect" of Trauma Center Designation
Utter GH, Maier RV, Rivara FP, et al (Harborview Med Ctr, Seattle; Univ of Washington, Seattle)
J Am Coll Surg 203:498-505, 2006

Background.—Trauma centers have an array of services available around the clock that help reduce mortality in injured patients. Having such services available can benefit patients other than those who are injured. We set out to determine whether patients hospitalized with ruptured abdominal aortic aneurysms experience lower morbidity and mortality at regional trauma centers than at other acute care hospitals.

Study Design.—We conducted a retrospective cohort study with the exposure being care at a trauma center and outcomes either mortality or organ failure. We evaluated all patients 40 to 84 years of age with a diagnosis of a ruptured abdominal aortic aneurysm who underwent operation during 2001 in 20 US states with organized systems of trauma care. We determined the relative risk of either death or organ failure at regional trauma centers compared with nondesignated centers.

Results.—Of 2,450 patients hospitalized for ruptured abdominal aortic aneurysm, 867 (35%) hospitalizations occurred at regional trauma centers. At trauma centers, 41.4% of patients died before hospital discharge, compared with 45.2% of patients at nondesignated hospitals (odds ratio [OR], 0.85; 95% CI, 0.71–1.02). After adjusting for payor, hospital beds, annual hospital admissions, annual inpatient operations, affiliation with a vascular surgery fellowship, and comorbid illnesses, the likelihood of death or organ failure was lower at trauma centers (OR, 0.72; 95% CI, 0.55–0.93).

Conclusions.—Care at regional trauma centers after operative repair of ruptured abdominal aortic aneurysm is associated with improved outcomes.

We postulate that these benefits reflect the ability of both vascular and general surgeons to immediately mobilize resources for care of the patient requiring urgent operative intervention. The beneficial effects of trauma center designation might extend beyond caring for the critically injured.

▶ The data suggest that patients with a ruptured abdominal aortic aneurysm have improved outcomes when cared for in trauma centers versus nondesignated centers. The ability to mobilize massive resources, the ready availability of emergent operative care, and the intense dedication to surgical intensive care at designated trauma centers all likely combine to result in improved outcomes for patients with a ruptured abdominal aortic aneurysm.

G. L. Moneta, MD

Outcome of common iliac arteries after straight aortic tube-graft placement during elective repair of infrarenal abdominal aortic aneurysms
Hassen-Khodja R, for the University Association for Research in Vascular Surgery (Univ Hosp of Nice, France; et al)
J Vasc Surg 44:943-948, 2006

Purpose.—To determine the relative rates of common iliac artery (CIA) expansion after elective straight aortic tube-graft replacement of infrarenal abdominal aortic aneurysms (AAA).

Methods.—Five participating centers in this 2004 study entered patients they had managed by an aortoaortic tube graft for elective AAA repair. The procedures took place between January 1995 and December 2003. Postoperative computed tomography (CT) scans were obtained for all patients in 2004 to assess changes in CIA diameter. Measurements on preoperative and postoperative CT scans were all made at the same level using the same technique.

Results.—Entered in the study were 147 patients (138 men, 9 women) with a mean age of 68 years. Mean follow-up from aortic surgery to verification of CIA diameter on the postoperative CT scan was 4.8 years. Mean preoperative CIA diameter was 13.6 mm vs 15.2 mm postoperatively. No patient developed occlusive iliac artery disease during follow-up. Three patients (2%) required repeat surgery during follow-up for a CIA aneurysm. The 147 patients were divided into three groups based on preoperative CIA diameter shown in CT scan: group A (n = 59, 40.1%), both CIA were of normal diameter; group B (n = 53, 36.1%), ectasia (diameter between 12 and 18 mm) of at least one CIA; group C (n = 35, 23.8%), an aneurysm (diameter >18 mm) of at least one CIA. CIA diameter increased by a mean of 1 mm (9.4%) over 5.5 years in group A vs 1.7 mm (12.1%) over 4.3 years in group B and 2.3 mm (12.7%) over 4.2 years in group C. The three patients who required repeat surgery for a CIA aneurysm during follow-up were all in group C (Fig 2). Four variables were associated with aneurysmal change in CIA: initial CIA diameter, celiac aorta diameter on the preoperative CT scan, a coexisting aneurysm site, and the follow-up duration.

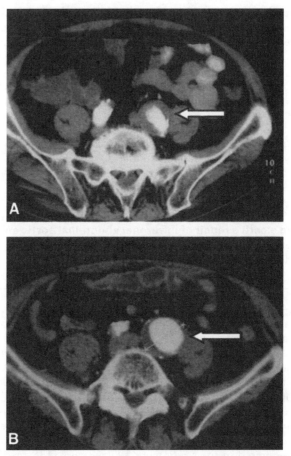

FIGURE 2.—**A,** Left common iliac artery aneurysm (*arrow*) measuring 30 mm on the preoperative computed tomography scan. **B,** Four years after aortic tube-graft placement, the left common iliac artery aneurysm (*arrow*) measures 45 mm in diameter on the postoperative computed tomography scan. (Courtesy of Hassen-Khodja R, for the University Association for Research in Vascular Surgery. Outcome of common iliac arteries after straight aortic tube-graft placement during elective repair of infrarenal abdominal aortic aneurysms. *J Vasc Surg.* 2006;44:943-948. Copyright 2006 by Elsevier. Reprinted by permission.)

Conclusions.—Tube-graft placement during AAA surgery is justified even for moderate CIA dilatation (<18 mm). CIA aneurysms with a preoperative diameter ≥25 mm enlarge more rapidly and warrant insertion of a bifurcated graft during the same surgical session as AAA repair. The evolutive potential of CIA between 18 mm and 25 mm in diameter justifies a bifurcated graft when the celiac aorta diameter is >25 mm or the patient's life expectancy is ≥8 years.

▶ Essentially, this article confirms conventional wisdom but suggests quantitative guidelines for open tube versus bifurcated repairs of AAAs. Quantitative guidelines are generally better than ego-based guidelines. The information in this article is, however, less useful than it would have been in the past, as most aneurysms are now managed with endovascular techniques. Nevertheless, open repairs are still common, and marginally sized iliac arteries are also common. Tube-graft repair of AAA is a good operation, and preferential use of tube grafts for open repair seems justified. When the CIA is greater than 25 mm and the patient seems reasonably healthy, a bifurcated graft does, however, seem reasonable based on these data.

G. L. Moneta, MD

Increased psychiatric morbidity after abdominal aortic surgery: Risk factors for stress-related disorders
Liberzon I, Abelson JL, Amdur RL, et al (Univ of Michigan, Ann Arbor; Cleveland Clinic Found, Ohio)
J Vasc Surg 43:929-934, 2006

Objective.—Research on surgical outcomes has focused on technical results and physical morbidity. However, postoperative psychiatric complications are common and can undermine functional results. High rates of posttraumatic stress disorder and major depressive disorder have been documented after cardiac events or surgery. These complications are also expected after abdominal aortic surgery, but their incidence and relevant risk factors in this population have not been documented.

Methods.—We examined the development of posttraumatic stress and depressive symptoms in patients with aortic aneurysms or occlusive disease, comparing surgical with nonsurgical patients and predicting that surgery and a prolonged intensive care stay would contribute to the development of psychiatric morbidity. A consecutive sample of vascular surgery patients (n = 109) was recruited 6 months to 2 years after surgery. Data were analyzed by using group comparisons, regression, and path analyses.

Results.—Rates of objectively determined postoperative psychiatric morbidity were extremely high (32%). Surgical patients were more than four times more likely to develop psychiatric disorders (odds ratio, 4.8; P = .02). Being younger, having increased preoperative blood pressure, and being intubated at the end of surgery were linked to greater rates of psychiatric morbidity (P < .05), but a longer intensive care stay was not.

Conclusions.—New-onset psychiatric symptoms are common after abdominal aortic surgery, and preoperative and surgical factors were more predictive than postoperative complications and stress, as reflected in intensive care unit stays. Prospective examination of vulnerability in this model could identify risk factors for stress-related psychiatric morbidity and help improve surgical outcomes.

▶ There are several interesting findings in this article. First and foremost, significant psychologic stress after abdominal aortic aneurysm repair is very common, and patients and families should know about this preoperatively. Second, younger patients suffer greater stress than older patients and, perhaps most interesting, prolonged ICU stays were not associated with greater stress levels. I suspect the latter is due to assiduous attention to patient sedation by nursing staff in the ICU. It would be interesting to know how stress levels after abdominal aortic aneurysm repair influence a patient's future utilization of the health care system.

G. L. Moneta, MD

8 Abdominal Aortic Endografting

Long-term Outcomes After Endovascular Abdominal Aortic Aneurysm Repair: The First Decade
Brewster DC, Jones JE, Chung TK, et al (Massachusetts Gen Hosp, Boston)
Ann Surg 244:426-438, 2006

Objective.—The proper role of endovascular abdominal aortic aneurysm repair (EVAR) remains controversial, largely due to uncertain late results. We reviewed a 12-year experience with EVAR to document late outcomes.

Methods.—During the interval January 7, 1994 through December 31, 2005, 873 patients underwent EVAR utilizing 10 different stent graft devices. Primary outcomes examined included operative mortality, aneurysm rupture, aneurysm-related mortality, open surgical conversion, and late survival rates. The incidence of endoleak, migration, aneurysm enlargement, and graft patency was also determined. Finally, the need for reintervention and success of such secondary procedures were evaluated. Kaplan-Meier and multivariate methodology were used for analysis.

Results.—Mean patient age was 75.7 years (range, 49–99 years); 81.4% were male. Mean follow-up was 27 months; 39.3% of patients had 2 or more major comorbidities, and 19.5% would be categorized as unfit for open repair. On an intent-to-treat basis, device deployment was successful in 99.3%. Thirty-day mortality was 1.8%. By Kaplan-Meier analysis, freedom from AAA rupture was 97.6% at 5 years and 94% at 9 years. Significant risk factors for late AAA rupture included female gender (odds ratio OR, 6.9; $P = 0.004$) and device-related endoleak (OR, 16.06; $P = 0.009$). Aneurysm-related death was avoided in 96.1% of patients, with the need for any reintervention (OR, 5.7 $P = 0.006$), family history of aneurysmal disease (OR, 9.5; $P = 0.075$), and renal insufficiency (OR, 7.1; $P = 0.003$) among its most important predictors. 87 (10%) patients required reintervention, with 92% of such procedures being catheter-based and a success rate of 84%. Significant predictors of reintervention included use of first-generation devices (OR, 1.2; $P < 0.01$) and late onset endoleak (OR, 64; $P < 0.001$). Current generation stent grafts correlated with significantly improved outcomes. Cumulative freedom from conversion to open repair was 93.3% at 5 through 9

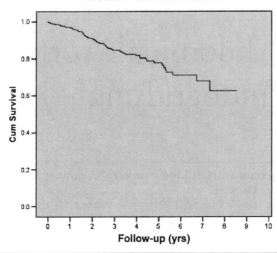

Freedom From Reintervention

Time (yrs)	1	2	3	4	5	6	7	8	9
No. Entering Interval	851	569	358	215	134	73	37	19	3
No. of Events	20	30	20	6	5	5	1	1	0
Cum. Proportion Surviving	97.2%	91.1%	85.0%	82.1%	78.2%	71.4%	68.9%	62.9%	62.9%
SE	0.6%	1.2%	1.7%	2.0%	2.6%	3.7%	4.4%	7.0%	7.0%

FIGURE 5.—Kaplan-Meier freedom from reintervention. (Courtesy of Brewster DC, Jones JE, Chung TK, et al. Long-term outcomes after endovascular abdominal aortic aneurysm repair: The first decade. *Ann Surg.* 2006;244:426-438.)

years, with the need for prior reintervention (OR, 16.7; $P = 0.001$) its most important predictor. Cumulative survival was 52% at 5 years.

Conclusions.—EVAR using contemporary devices is a safe, effective, and durable method to prevent AAA rupture and aneurysm-related death. Assuming suitable AAA anatomy, these data justify a broad application of EVAR across a wide spectrum of patients (Fig 5).

▶ This article emphasizes the durability of EVAR with modern devices and makes a case, at least indirectly, for EVAR as the preferred technique for AAA repair. All modern devices may not be equal, and there is some hint that devices with hooked fixation are less subject to late migration and, therefore, development of late type I endoleak. Given the results here, modern hook devices, and a commitment to the use of endografts within the specification of the manufacturer, it would appear appropriate to offer endografts as preferred therapy. If one pushes the indications, all bets are off. Please see the report by Sicard et al.[1]

G. L. Moneta, MD

Reference

1. Sicard GA, Zwolak RM, Sidawy AN, White RA, Siami FS; Society for Vascular Surgery Outcomes Committee. Endovascular abdominal aortic aneurysm repair: long-term outcome measures in patients at high-risk for open surgery. *J Vasc Surg.* 2006;44:229-236.

Endovascular abdominal aortic aneurysm repair: Long-term outcome measures in patients at high-risk for open surgery
Sicard GA, Zwolak RM, Sidawy AN, et al (Washington Univ, St Louis; Dartmouth-Hitchcock Med Ctr, Lebanon, NH; Washington VA Med Ctr, Washington, DC; et al)
J Vasc Surg 44:229-236, 2006

Purpose.—The study was conducted to determine the outcome in the United States after endovascular repair (EVAR) of infrarenal abdominal aortic aneurysms (AAAs) in patients at high-risk for open surgery by using independently audited, high-compliance, chart-verified data sets, and to compare those results with open surgery.

Methods.—High-risk was defined to match a recent European trial (EVAR2) and included age of $\geq$60 years with aneurysm size of $\geq$5.5 cm, plus at least one cardiac, pulmonary, or renal comorbidity. Data from five multicenter investigational device exemption clinical trials leading to Food and Drug Administration (FDA) approval were analyzed. Of 2216 EVAR patients, 565 met the high-risk criteria. Of 342 surgical controls (OPEN), 61 met high-risk criteria. Primary outcome comparisons included AAA-related death, all-cause death, and aneurysm rupture. Secondary measures were endoleak, AAA sac enlargement, and migration.

Results.—Average age of the high-risk EVAR subset was 76 ± 7 years vs 74 ± 6 years OPEN ($P = 0.07$), mean EVAR AAA size was 6.4 ± 0.8 cm vs 6.6 ± 1.0 cm OPEN ($P = .33$), and average EVAR follow-up was 2.7 years vs 2.5 years OPEN. The 30-day operative mortality was 2.9% in EVAR vs 5.1% in OPEN ($P = .32$). The AAA-related death rate after EVAR was 3.0% at 1 year and 4.2% at 4 years compared with 5.1% at both time points after OPEN ($P = .58$). Overall survival at 4 years after EVAR was 56% vs 66% in OPEN ($P = .23$). After treatment, EVAR successfully prevented rupture in 99.5% at 1 year and in 97.2% at 4 years.

Conclusions.—Endovascular repair of large infrarenal AAAs in anatomically suited high-surgical-risk patients using FDA-approved devices in the United States is safe and provides lasting protection from AAA-related mortality. EVAR mortality remained comparable with OPEN up to 4 years. The decision to treat AAAs in patients with advanced age and significant comorbidities must be individualized and carefully considered, but repair provides excellent protection from AAA-related death.

▶ The definition of "high risk" appears a bit liberal in this article. Patients only had to be aged 60 years or older with one comorbidity to be classified as high risk. That is really not my picture of the "high-risk" aneurysm patient. Overall survival in the high-risk patients was 56% at 5 years in this article. This is better than the 52% described in the report by Brewster et al,[1] which did not report to be operating only on high-risk patients! This article was basically a response to the EVAR2 report.[2] But, likely the patients in EVAR2 were substantially less fit than those analyzed here. If you are going to use this article to help your decision for surgery in "high-risk" aneurysm patients, make sure your "high-risk" patients are not all that high of a risk! I suggest reading the commentary by Dr Buth that accompanies this article.

G. L. Moneta, MD

Reference

1. Brewster DC, Jones JE, Chung TK, et al. Long-term outcomes after endovascular abdominal aortic aneurysm repair: the first decade. *Ann Surg.* 2006;244:426-438.
2. EVAR Trial Participants. Endovscular aneurysm repair and outcome in patients unfit for open repair of abdominal aortic aneurysm (EVAR Trial 2): randomized controlled trial. *Lancet.* 2005;365:2187-2192.

Factors Affecting Long-term Mortality After Endovascular Repair of Abdominal Aortic Aneurysms
de Virgilio C, Tran J, Lewis R, et al (Harbor-UCLA Med Ctr, Torrance, Calif)
Arch Surg 141:905-910, 2006

Hypothesis.—Endovascular repair of abdominal aortic aneurysms has made considerable advancements with respect to perioperative mortality. However, fewer data are available regarding factors affecting long-term mortality, including the impact of adverse perioperative cardiac events. Perioperative clinical cardiac risk factors are significant predictors of long-term mortality.

Design, Setting, and Patients.—Retrospective review of a prospective database of 468 patients who underwent endovascular abdominal aortic aneurysm repair from June 3, 1996, to January 31, 2005.

Main Outcome Measures.—Preoperative, intraoperative, and postoperative factors were analyzed using multivariate Cox proportional hazards models to identify statistically significant independent predictors of long-term survival (beyond 30 days and after discharge from the hospital).

Results.—The mean age was 74 years, and 90% of the patients were male. Median follow-up was 2.57 years (interquartile range, 0.92-4.06 years). The leading cause of death was cardiac in nature. On multivariate analysis, the number of preoperative clinical cardiac risk factors ($P<.001$) (Fig 1), spending 2 or more days in the intensive care unit ($P<.001$), and having an ST-segment elevation myocardial infarction ($P<.001$) were predictors of decreased long-term survival. Of note, having a perioperative non-ST-segment elevation myocardial infarction was not predictive of decreased survival ($P=.09$).

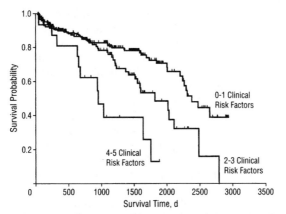

FIGURE 1.—Long-term survival by number of clinical cardiac risk factors. (Courtesy of de Virgilio C, Tran J, Lewis R, et al. Factors affecting long-term mortality after endovascular repair of abdominal aortic aneurysms. *Arch Surg.* 2006;141:905-910. Copyright 2006, American Medical Association.)

Conclusions.—Adverse cardiac events are the leading cause of long-term mortality following endovascular repair of abdominal aortic aneurysms. Preoperative clinical cardiac risk factors are significant predictors of long-term mortality, as are a prolonged intensive care unit stay and a perioperative ST-segment elevation myocardial infarction. A perioperative non-ST-segment elevation myocardial infarction did not influence long-term outcome.

▶ No surprises here; patients with vascular disease tend to die of cardiac causes. We already know that, and that this sort of information applies to patients with abdominal aortic aneurysm as well. Treating an aneurysm with an endograft would not be expected to change this. It has already been shown that there is no long-term survival advantage to treatment of an abdominal aortic aneurysm with an endograft versus open repair. Predicting late cardiac death by perioperative cardiac events is also not very useful. It makes for an article, but there is no "undo" key in life.

G. L. Moneta, MD

Open Versus Endovascular Abdominal Aortic Aneurysm Repair in VA Hospitals
Bush RL, Johnson ML, Collins TC, et al (Michael E DeBakey Veterans Affairs Med Ctr, Houston; Baylor College of Medicine; Univ of Colorado, Denver; et al)
J Am Coll Surg 202:577-587, 2006

Background.—Endovascular abdominal aortic aneurysm repair (EVAR), when compared with conventional open surgical repair, has been shown to reduce perioperative morbidity and mortality. We performed a retrospective cohort study with prospectively collected data from the Department of Veterans Affairs to examine outcomes after elective aneurysm repair.

Study Design.—We studied 30-day mortality, 1-year survival, and postoperative complications in 1,904 patients who underwent elective abdominal aortic aneurysm repair (EVAR n=717 [37.7%]; open n=1,187 [62.3%]) at 123 Department of Veterans Affairs hospitals between May 1, 2001 and September 30, 2003. We investigated the influence of patient, operative, and hospital variables on outcomes.

Results.—Patients undergoing EVAR had significantly lower 30-day (3.1% versus 5.6%, p = 0.01) and 1- year mortality rates (8.7% versus 12.1%, p = 0.018) than patients having open repair. EVAR was associated with a decrease in 30-day postoperative mortality (adjusted odds ratio[OR] = 0.59; 95% CI = 0.36, 0.99; p = 0.04). The risk of perioperative complications was much less after EVAR (15.5% versus 27.7%; p < 0.001; unadjusted OR 0.48; 95% CI = 0.38, 0.61; p < 0.001). Patients operated on at low volume hospitals (25% of entire cohort) were more likely to have had open repair (31.3% compared with 15.9% EVAR; p < 0.001) and a nearly two-fold increase in adjusted 30-day mortality risk (OR = 1.9; 95% CI = 1.19, 2.98; p = 0.006).

Conclusions.—In routine daily practice, veterans who undergo elective EVAR have substantially lower perioperative mortality and morbidity rates compared with patients having open repair. The benefits of a minimally invasive approach were readily apparent in this cohort, but we recommend using caution in choosing EVAR for all elective abdominal aortic aneurysm repairs until longer-term data on device durability are available.

▶ The VA surgeons do a good job, but the data suggest things could be better if the patients were uniformly treated in high-volume hospitals. Someone in Central Office should notice these data. It is hard not to be impressed with a 100% increase in mortality related to aneurysm repair in low-volume versus high-volume VA hospitals. The private sector has difficulty mandating regionalization of care, but the VA system can do it if it wishes to.

G. L. Moneta, MD

Influence of anesthesia type on outcome after endovascular aortic aneurysm repair: An analysis based on EUROSTAR data

Ruppert V, Leurs LJ, Steckmeier B, et al (Univ Munich; Catharina Hosp, Eindhoven, The Netherlands; Klinikum der Universitat Munchen, Munich; et al)
J Vasc Surg 44:16-21, 2006

Background.—Local and regional anesthesia was used in endovascular aortic aneurysm repair (EVAR) shortly after its introduction, and the feasibility has been documented several times. Nevertheless, locoregional anesthesia has not become accepted on a large scale, probably owing to a traditional surgical attitude preferring general anesthesia. This study compared various anesthesia techniques in patients treated with EVAR for infrarenal aortic aneurysms.

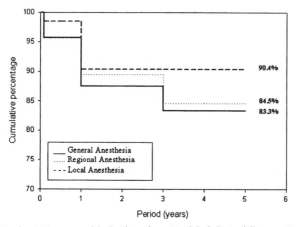

FIGURE.—Kaplan-Meier curves of the freedom of type II endoleak during follow-up. (Reprinted by permission of the publisher from Ruppert V, Leurs LJ, Steckmeier B, et al. Influence of anesthesia type on outcome after endovascular aortic aneurysm repair: An analysis based on EUROSTAR data. *J Vasc Surg.* 2006;44:16-21. Copyright 2006 by Elsevier.)

Methods.—From July 1997 to August 2004, 5557 patients who underwent EVAR repair in 164 centers were enrolled in the EUROSTAR registry. Data were compared among three groups: a general anesthesia group (GA-G) of 3848 patients (69%), a regional anesthesia group (RA-G) of 1399 patients (25%), and the local anesthesia group (LA-G) of 310 patients (6%). Differences in preoperative and operative details among the three study groups were analyzed using the χ^2 test for discrete variables and the Kruskal-Wallis test for continuous variables. Multivariate logistic regression analysis was performed on early complications.

Results.—The duration of the operation was reduced in the LA-G (115.7 ± 42.2 minutes) compared with the RA-G (127.6 ± 52.8 min, $P < .0009$) and GA-G (133.3 ± 59.1 minutes, $P < .0001$). Admission to the intensive care unit was significantly less for LA-G patients (2%) than RA-G (8.3%, $P = .0004$) and GA-G (16.2%, $P < .0001$), but RA-G still had a distinct advantage ($P < .0001$) over GA-G. Hospital stay was significantly shorter in LA-G (3.7 ± 3.1 days [$P < .0001$] vs GA-G [$P = .007$] vs RA-G), but RA-G (5.1 ± 7.5 days) still had an advantage ($P < .0001$) vs GA-G (6.2 ± 8.5 days). In EUROSTAR, systemic complications were significantly lower both for LA-G (6.6%, $P = .0015$) and RA-G (9.5%, $P = .0007$) than for GA-G (13.0%).

Conclusion.—The EUROSTAR data indicate that patients appeared to benefit when a locoregional anesthetic technique was used for EVAR. Locoregional techniques should be used more often to enhance the perioperative advantage of EVAR in treating infrarenal aneurysms of the abdominal aorta (Fig).

▶ The conclusion of this article should be that local or regional anesthesia can be an acceptable alternative to general anesthesia during EVAR. The patients in the local anesthesia group are not the same as those in the general anesthesia group, as the general anesthesia patients had more complex aneurysms, more additional procedures, and, as a result, longer operative times. In addition, well over 50% of the local anesthesia patients came from a single high-volume center, making it difficult to eliminate both surgeon and institutional experience as contributing to a potential benefit of local anesthesia. This article should not be used to justify blanket use of local or regional anesthesia for EVAR. It tells you such techniques can be used; it does not tell you on whom they should be used.

G. L. Moneta, MD

Outcome after hypogastric artery bypass and embolization during endovascular aneurysm repair
Lee WA, Nelson PR, Berceli SA, et al (Univ of Florida, Gainesville; Malcom Randall Veterans Affairs Med Ctr, Gainesville, Fla)
J Vasc Surg 44:1162-1169, 2006

Background.—Multiple strategies have been devised to extend the applicability of endovascular aneurysm repair (EVAR) in patients with common iliac artery (CIA) aneurysms. This study was designed to examine outcome in patients undergoing EVAR with either hypogastric artery embolization or common iliac artery bifurcation advancement by hypogastric bypass.

Methods.—A retrospective review of all patients undergoing EVAR since the inception of our program (1997-2006) was performed. Data were prospectively collected in an EVAR registry. Patients with large common iliac artery aneurysms ($\geq$20 mm) and patent hypogastric arteries not amenable to a cuff or "bell bottom" technique were treated with coil embolization (EMBO) and/or hypogastric revascularization (BYPASS) (Fig 1). The perioperative and mid-term outcomes were compared with the larger group of patients undergoing EVAR that did not require either treatment (CTRL). Bilateral common iliac artery aneurysms were treated with unilateral coil embolization and contralateral bypass.

Results.—Common iliac artery aneurysms were present in 137 (31%) of the 444 patients undergoing EVAR, but only 57 (42%) of 137 required direct management. This included hypogastric artery embolization alone (EMBO) in 31 or hypogastric artery revascularization (BYPASS) in 26, with and without contralateral embolization (both revascularization/embolization in 46%). The procedure length (CTRL, 159 ± 72 minutes; EMBO, 153 ± 39 minutes; BYPASS, 283 ± 75 minutes) and estimated blood loss (CTRL, 251 ± 313 mL; EMBO, 233 ± 158 mL; BYPASS, 400 ± 287 mL) were significantly greater ($P < .05$) in the BYPASS group. The incidence of any postoperative complication (CTRL, 26%; EMBO, 68%; BYPASS, 54%), any ischemic complication (CTRL, 6%; EMBO, 55%; BYPASS, 27%), and new-onset buttock claudication (CTRL, 3%; EMBO, 39%; BYPASS, 27%) were all significantly greater in the BYPASS and EMBO group relative to the control (CTRL) group (n = 387). The incidence of new-onset buttock claudication ipsilateral to the hypogastric bypass was 4%; the balance of

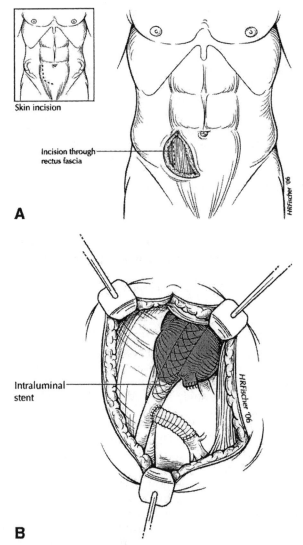

Skin incision

Incision through
rectus fascia

A

Intraluminal
stent

B

FIGURE 1.—A, A curvilinear skin incision was made halfway between the umbilicus and symphysis pubis (*inset*), and the anterior rectus sheath was incised along its lateral border. **B,** The completed repair is shown with the endoluminal stent and hypogastric bypass. (Courtesy of Lee WA, Nelson PR, Berceli SA, Seeger JM, Huber TS. Outcome after hypogastric artery bypass and embolization during endovascular aneurysm repair. *J Vasc Surg.* 2006;44:1162-1169. Copyright 2006 by Elsevier. Reprinted by permission.)

the new onset claudication in the BYPASS group was due to the contralateral embolization. The primary hypogastric artery bypass patency was 91 ± 11% (SE) at 36 months by life-table analysis.

Conclusions.—Despite its increased complexity, hypogastric artery bypass is an excellent alternative to embolization in terms of patency and freedom from ischemic symptoms for patients with large common iliac artery aneurysms undergoing EVAR.

▶ Dr Lee is a founding member of the Hypogastric Artery Preservation Society. It does make sense to preserve major arteries when possible, and in good-risk, active patients who are likely to be significantly bothered by buttock claudication, hypogastric bypass in the course of EVAR seems reasonable. However, there are clearly many endograft abdominal aortic aneurysm patients who are not likely to be significantly affected by hypogastric coverage or embolization. Hypogastric artery bypass adds time, complexity, and complications to EVAR. Its use should be selective, as life-threatening complications of hypogastric embolization or coverage are quite rare. Please see the comments from Dr Veith and Dr Turnipseed that accompany the original article.

G. L. Moneta, MD

Preservation of pelvic circulation with hypogastric artery bypass in endovascular repair of abdominal aortic aneurysm with bilateral iliac artery aneurysms
Unno N, Inuzuka K, Yamamoto N, et al (Hamamatsu Univ, Shizuoka, Japan)
J Vasc Surg 44:1170-1175, 2006

Purpose.—The endovascular repair (EVAR) of an abdominal aortic aneurysm (AAA) with a bilateral common iliac artery aneurysm (CIAA) often requires exclusion of the bilateral hypogastric artery (HA), which can be associated with pelvic ischemic complications such as erectile dysfunction and buttock claudication. This study assessed the effect of HA bypass on improving pelvic circulation.

Methods.—Five patients who underwent endovascular repair with HA bypass for an AAA with bilateral CIAA were evaluated. In all patients, the patency of the inferior mesenteric artery and bilateral HAs arteries was confirmed with preoperative computed tomography (CT) scans and angiography. During EVAR, penile blood flow was monitored with pulse-volume plethysmography measuring the penile brachial pressure index (PBI), and bilateral buttock blood flow was monitored with near-infrared spectroscopy measuring the gluteal tissue oxygenation index (TOI). An aortouni-external iliac artery stent graft with a crossover bypass was performed after embolization of the contralateral HA. HA bypass was performed between the crossover bypass graft and the ipsilateral HA via a retroperitoneal incision.

Results.—Unilateral coil embolization of the contralateral side HA trunk slightly decreased blood flow to the contralateral side buttock but did not cause significant changes in penile blood flow. At the completion of EVAR, the levels of both PBI and the contralateral side TOI were significantly lower than the baseline levels. After ipsilateral side HA revascularization with HA bypass, both PBI and bilateral gluteal flow returned almost to the baseline levels. Postoperative angiography and CT scans demonstrated the patency of all HA bypasses and no endoleaks. None of the patients experienced new onset of erectile dysfunction or buttock claudication 1 month after surgery.

Conclusion.—Bilateral HA interruption during EVAR for AAA with bilateral CIAA was associated with significant depletion of both penile and gluteal blood flow. Intraoperative monitoring of PBI and TOI at the bilateral buttocks showed significant improvement of both parameters after HA bypass. HA bypass is an excellent procedure to improve pelvic circulation despite its increased surgical complexity.

▶ There is also a Japanese chapter of the Hypogastric Artery Preservation Society. This is a small series (n = 5) that focused on erectile dysfunction and penile blood flow and its preservation with a type of hypogastric bypass accompanying EVAR. However, keep in mind that erectile dysfunction occurs over time frequently in patients treated for AAA for reasons that are independent of the original operation. Hypogastric preservation to preserve erectile function is an issue, but long-term development of erectile dysfunction will still likely occur in many of these patients.

G. L. Moneta, MD

Effect of challenging neck anatomy on mid-term migration rates in AneuRx endografts

Fulton JJ, Farber MA, Sanchez LA, et al (Univ of North Carolina, Chapel Hill; Washington Univ, St Louis)
J Vasc Surg 44:932-937, 2006

Objective.—To establish the effect of challenging neck anatomy on the mid- and long-term incidence of migration with the AneuRx bifurcated device in patients treated after Food and Drug Administration approval and to identify the predictive factors for device migration.

Methods.—Prospectively maintained databases at the University of North Carolina (UNC) and Washington University (WU) were used to identify 595 patients (UNC, n = 230; WU, n = 365) who underwent endovascular repair of an infrarenal abdominal aortic aneurysm with the AneuRx bifurcated stent graft. Those patients with at least 30 months of follow-up were identified and underwent further assessment of migration (UNC, n = 25; WU, n = 59) by use of multiplanar reconstructed computed tomographic scans.

Results.—Eighty-four patients with a mean follow-up time of 40.3 months (range, 30-55 months) were studied. Seventy percent of the patients (n = 59) met all inclusion criteria for neck anatomy (length, angle, diameter, and quality) as defined by the revised instructions for use guidelines and are referred to as those with favorable neck anatomy (FNA). The remaining 25 patients retrospectively fell outside of the revised instructions for use guidelines and are referred to as those with unfavorable neck anatomy (UFNA). Life-table analysis for FNA patients at 2 and 4 years revealed a migration rate of 0% and 6.1%, respectively (Fig 1). For UFNA patients, it was 24.0%

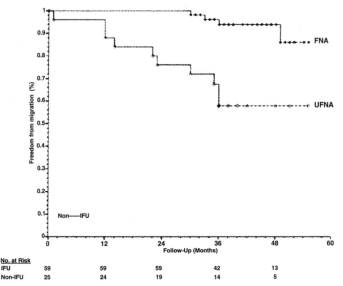

FIGURE 1.—Freedom from migration by Kaplan-Meier analysis for those with favorable neck anatomy (*FNA*) and unfavorable neck anatomy (*UFNA*). (Reprinted by permission of the publisher from Fulton JJ, Farber MA, Sanchez LA, et al. Effect of challenging neck anatomy on mid-term migration rates in AneuRx endografts. *J Vasc Surg.* 2006;44:932-937. Copyright 2006 by Elsevier.)

and 42.1% at 2 and 4 years, respectively ($P < .0001$). The overall (FNA and UFNA) migration rate was 7.1% and 17.1% at 2 and 4 years, respectively. Overall, late graft-related complications occurred in 38% of patients (FNA, 27%; UFNA, 64%; $P = .003$; relative risk, 1.7). There was no incidence of late rupture or open conversion. The relative risk of migration for UFNA patients was 2.5 compared with FNA patients ($P = .0003$). A larger neck angle and a longer initial graft to renal artery distance were predictors of migration, whereas shorter neck length approached but did not reach statistical significance.

Conclusions.—Patients who have unfavorable aneurysm neck anatomy experience significantly higher migration, device-related complication, and secondary intervention rates. However, there was no incidence of open conversion, rupture, or abdominal aortic aneurysm–related death, thereby supporting the AneuRx device as a feasible alternative to open repair even in patients with challenging neck characteristics. Enhanced surveillance should be used in these high-risk patients.

▶ The conclusion of this article does not make much sense to me. Patients with UFNA had a migration rate of 42% at 4 years! Even though there were no ruptures, this is clearly an unacceptable number. With sufficient time, there will be a need for more interventions and conversions, and there will be ruptures. This device does appear acceptable and reasonable when used according to the manufacturer's recommendations. With alternative devices available it makes no sense to place this device under conditions where it is not capable of doing well.

G. L. Moneta, MD

Secondary interventions following endovascular abdominal aortic aneurysm repair using current endografts. A EUROSTAR report
Hobo R, for the EUROSTAR collaborators (Catharina Hosp, Eindhoven, The Netherlands)
J Vasc Surg 43:896-902, 2006

Objective.—The purpose of this study was to evaluate the need for secondary interventions after endovascular abdominal aortic aneurysm repair with current stent-grafts.

Methods.—Studied were data from 2846 patients treated from December 1999 until December 2004. The data were recorded from the EUROSTAR registry. The only patients studied were those with a follow-up of at least 12 months or until they had a secondary intervention within the first 12 months. The cumulative incidences of secondary transabdominal, extra-anatomic, and transfemoral interventions during follow-up (after the first postoperative month) were investigated.

Results.—A secondary intervention was performed in 247 patients (8.7%) at a mean of 12 months after the initial procedure within a follow-up period of a mean of 23 ± 12 months. Of these, 57 (23%) transabdominal, 43 (16%) involved an extra-anatomic bypass, and 147 (60%) were by transfemoral approach. The cumulative incidence of secondary interventions was 6.0%, 8.7%, 12%, and 14% at 1, 2, 3, and 4 years, respectively. This corresponded with an annual rate of secondary interventions of 4.6%, which was remarkably lower than in a previously published EUROSTAR study of patients treated before 1999. Type I endoleaks (33% of procedures), migration (16%), and rupture (8.8%) were the most frequent reasons for secondary transabdominal interventions. Graft limb thrombosis was the indication for extra-anatomic bypass (60%). Type I endoleak (17%), type II endoleak (23%), device limb stenosis (14%), thrombosis (23%), and device migration (14%) were the most frequent reasons for secondary transfemoral interventions. Operative mortality was higher after secondary transabdominal interventions (12.3%, *P* = .007) compared with transfemoral interventions (2.7%). Overall survival was lower in patients with secondary transabdominal (*P* = .016) and extra-anatomic interventions (*P* < .0001) compared with patients without a secondary intervention.

Conclusion.—Although the incidence of secondary interventions after endovascular aneurysm repair has substantially decreased in recent years, continuing need for surveillance for device-related complications remains necessary.

▶ Fewer secondary interventions are being performed with modern abdominal aortic aneurysm stent grafts. Devices have gotten better, and we have gotten smarter about what are the best indications for a secondary intervention. At some point the rate of secondary interventions will plateau, but it will never be zero, and we will have to know whether these secondary interventions actually save lives and prevent rupture. We also need to figure out who needs to be followed up closely and who needs less intensive follow-up. In addition to identifying factors associated with secondary interventions, we need to identify factors that are not associated with secondary intervention and combinations of variables that predict no need for secondary intervention.

G. L. Moneta, MD

An 8-year experience with type II endoleaks: Natural history suggests selective intervention is a safe approach
Silverberg D, Baril DT, Ellozy SH, et al (Mount Sinai School of Medicine, New York)
J Vasc Surg 44:453-459, 2006

Objective.—The treatment of type II endoleaks remains controversial because little is known about their long-term natural history and impact on changes in aneurysm morphology. This study reviews type II endoleaks occurring in patients after endovascular abdominal aortic aneurysm repair (EVAR) at a single-institution over an 8-year period.

Methods.—All patients undergoing EVAR who had type II endoleaks documented on follow-up imaging studies at our institution between January 1997 and March 2005 were reviewed. Data regarding patient demographics in addition to aneurysm size, device type, operative complications, and secondary interventions were reviewed. Outcomes evaluated included the rate of spontaneous sealing, freedom from secondary intervention, and aneurysm enlargement, rupture, or conversion.

Results.—Type II endoleaks were present in 154 of 965 patients (16.0%) undergoing EVAR. Mean follow-up time was 22.0 months (range, 1 to 72 months). Fifty-five patients (35.7%) with type II endoleaks sealed spontaneously in a mean time of 14.5 months. According to Kaplan-Meier analysis, approximately 75% of type II endoleaks sealed spontaneously within a 5-year period (Fig 2). Nineteen patients (12.3%) with type II endoleaks were treated at a mean time of 19.9 months at the operating surgeon's discretion, including 13 with sac enlargement >5 mm. Kaplan-Meier analysis estimated that approximately 65% of the patients remained free of intervention after a period of 4 years. Thirteen patients (8.4%) experienced aneurysm sac enlargement >5 mm. Kaplan-Meier analysis estimated that approximately 80% of patients with type II endoleaks remained free of sac enlargement >5 mm over a 4-year period. No patients with type II endoleaks experienced rupture or required conversion to open repair during their follow-up. Cox regression analysis showed that cancer, coronary artery disease, and chronic obstructive pulmonary disease were associated with earlier spontaneous closure of the type II endoleaks ($P < .05$).

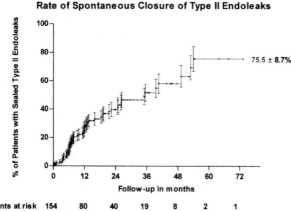

FIGURE 2.—Kaplan-Meier analysis demonstrates the rate of spontaneous closure of type II endoleaks. (Reprinted by permission of the publisher from Silverberg D, Baril DT, Ellozy SH, et al. An 8-year experience with type II endoleaks: natural history suggests selective intervention is a safe approach. *J Vasc Surg.* 2006;44:453-459. Copyright 2006 by Elsevier.)

Conclusions.—We observed that type II endoleaks have a relatively benign course, and in the absence of sac expansion, can be followed for a prolonged course of time without the need for intervention. The rate of spontaneous seal continues to increase with time and, therefore, close follow-up of patients with type II endoleaks who show no signs of aneurysm expansion is a safe approach. For patients in whom the exact etiology of their endoleak is in question, dynamic imaging should be used to exclude the presence of a type I endoleak.

▶ There is a lot of good quantitative information in this article regarding the natural history of type II endoleaks. The main points are that a large percentage will seal spontaneously, and very few are associated with aneurysm sac expansion. Also, unfortunately, about one third of patients who undergo successful treatment of a type II endoleak continue to have sac expansion, suggesting the presence of an additional undetected type II or even a type I endoleak. I predict in the future the emphasis will shift from documenting the presence of endoleak to documenting a lack of sac expansion during follow-up. This has huge implications for what imaging will be needed to follow-up abdominal aortic aneurysms treated with stent grafts.

G. L. Moneta, MD

Intraoperative Colon Mucosal Oxygen Saturation During Aortic Surgery

Lee ES, Bass A, Arko FR, et al (Univ of California, Davis; Saklar School of Medicine, Tel Aviv, Israel; UT Southwestern Med Ctr at Dallas; et al)
J Surg Res 136:19-24, 2006

Background.—Colonic ischemia after aortic reconstruction is a devastating complication with high mortality rates. This study evaluates whether Colon Mucosal Oxygen Saturation (CMOS) correlates with colon ischemia during aortic surgery.

Materials and Methods.—Aortic reconstruction was performed in 25 patients, using a spectrophotometer probe that was inserted in each patient's rectum before the surgical procedure. Continuous CMOS, buccal mucosal oxygen saturation, systemic mean arterial pressure, heart rate, pulse oximetry, and pivotal intra-operative events were collected.

Results.—Endovascular aneurysm repair (EVAR) was performed in 20 and open repair in 5 patients with a mean age of 75 ± 10 (SE) years. CMOS reliably decreased in EVAR from a baseline of 56% ± 8% to 26 ± 17% ($P <$ 0.0001) during infrarenal aortic balloon occlusion and femoral arterial sheath placement. CMOS similarly decreased during open repair from 56% ± 9% to 15 ± 19% ($P <$ 0.0001) when the infrarenal aorta and iliac arteries were clamped. When aortic circulation was restored in both EVAR and open surgery, CMOS returned to baseline values 56.5 ± 10% ($P = 0.81$). Mean recovery time in CMOS after an aortic intervention was 6.4 ± 3.3 min. Simultaneous buccal mucosal oxygen saturation was stable (82% ± 6%) during aortic manipulation but would fall significantly during active bleeding. There were no device related CMOS measurement complications.

Conclusions.—Intra-operative CMOS is a sensitive measure of colon ischemia where intraoperative events correlated well with changes in mucosal oxygen saturation. Transient changes demonstrate no problem. However, persistently low CMOS suggests colon ischemia, thus providing an opportunity to revascularize the inferior mesenteric artery or hypogastric arteries to prevent colon infarction.

▶ The technique offers a potential method of monitoring colonic perfusion intraoperatively. Obviously, a number of details still need to be determined, such as what is the lowest level of CMOS that will sustain colonic viability. In addition, the potential ability of this technique to monitor for postoperative colon ischemia seems like an interesting line of inquiry.

G. L. Moneta, MD

Acute Abdominal Aortic Aneurysms: Cost Analysis of Endovascular Repair and Open Surgery in Hemodynamically Stable Patients with 1-year Follow-up
Visser JJ, van Sambeek MRHM, Hunink MGM, et al (Erasmus Med Ctr, Rotterdam, The Netherlands; Harvard School of Public Health, Boston; Erasmus Univ Rotterdam, The Netherlands; et al)
Radiology 240:681-689, 2006

Purpose.—To retrospectively assess the in-hospital and 1-year follow-up costs of endovascular aneurysm repair and conventional open surgery in patients with acute infrarenal abdominal aortic aneurysm (AAA) by using a resource-use approach.

Materials and Methods.—Institutional Review Board approval was obtained, and informed consent was waived. In-hospital costs for all consecutive patients (61 men, six women; mean age, 72.0 years) who underwent endovascular repair ($n = 32$) or open surgery ($n = 35$) for acute infrarenal AAA from January 1, 2001, to December 31, 2004, were assessed by using a resource-use approach. Patients who did not undergo computed tomography before the procedure were excluded from analysis. One-year follow-up costs were complete for 30 patients who underwent endovascular repair and for 34 patients who underwent open surgery. Costs were assessed from a health care perspective. Mean costs were calculated for each treatment group and were compared by using the Mann-Whitney U test ($\alpha = .05$). The influence of clinical variables on the total in-hospital cost was investigated by using univariate and multivariate analyses. Costs were expressed in euros for the year 2003.

Results.—Sex, age, and comorbidity did not differ between treatment groups ($P > .05$). The mean total in-hospital costs were lower for patients who underwent endovascular repair than for those who underwent open surgery (€20 767 vs €35 470, respectively; $P = .004$). The total costs, including those for 1-year follow-up, were €23 588 for patients who underwent endovascular repair and €36 448 for those who underwent open surgery ($P = .05$). The results of multivariate analysis indicated that complications had a significant influence on total in-hospital cost; patients who had complications incurred total in-hospital costs that were 2.27 times higher than those for patients who had no complications.

Conclusion.—Total in-hospital costs and total overall costs, which included 1-year follow-up costs, were lower in patients with acute AAA who underwent endovascular repair than in those who underwent open surgery.

▶ I hate misleading articles like this. It is a bit of a bait-and-switch between the abstract and the discussion. Nowhere in the abstract does it tell you that 71% of the open repair group had a ruptured AAA, and only 44% of the endovascular group had a ruptured AAA ($P = .02$). The abstract also does not mention 33 patients with symptomatic or ruptured juxtarenal aneurysms who were excluded. These facts make the conclusions derived by the authors totally unreliable and a bit irresponsible. Must have been a slow month for submissions to *Radiology*.

G. L. Moneta, MD

Endovascular treatment of iliac artery aneurysms with a tubular stent-graft: Mid-term results
Tielliu IFJ, Verhoeven ELG, Zeebregts CJ, et al (Univ Med Ctr Groningen, The Netherlands)
J Vasc Surg 43:440-445, 2006

Objective.—To report the mid term results of a prospective cohort of iliac artery aneurysms (IAAs) treated with endovascular tubular stent-grafts.

Methods.—All IAAs referred to the University Medical Center Groningen between June 1998 and June 2005 were evaluated for endovascular repair. Criteria for repair were a diameter of ≥30 mm for anastomotic aneurysms and ≥35 mm for true aneurysms. Preferentially, tubular grafts were used. Follow-up included both radiographs of the abdomen and duplex examination.

Results.—In 35 patients, 40 IAAs were treated endovascularly with a tubular stent-graft. Elective repair was performed in 30 patients (86%) and emergent repair in five patients (14%). Aneurysms were false in 26 cases (65%) and true in 14 cases (35%). Local anesthesia was used in 74% of the cases. The stent-grafts that were used included the Excluder contralateral limb (n = 28, 70%), Passager (n = 9, 22.5%), Hemobahn (n = 2, 5%), and Wallgraft (n = 1, 2.5%). The mean operation time was 83 ± 28 minutes (range, 50 to 150 minutes). Mean hospital stay was 3.3 ± 2.3 days (range, 1 to 12 days). There was no 30-day mortality. Patients were followed up for a mean of 31.2 ± 20.7 months (range, 3 to 83 months). Complications occurred in two patients during follow-up, including migration with a proximal type I endoleak in one, and occlusion of the stent-graft in the other. The internal iliac artery was intentionally sacrificed in 28 patients (70%), and this led to gluteal claudication in three patients.

Conclusion.—Endovascular repair of iliac artery aneurysms with flexible stent-grafts is a minimally invasive technique and is associated with low mortality and morbidity. Follow-up results up to 5 years suggest that the technique is durable. It should be regarded as a first choice treatment option for suitable aneurysms.

▶ I think stent-grafts are a clear winner for treatment of iliac artery pseudoaneurysms. Tube stent-grafts for isolated, native common iliac artery (CIA) aneurysms may be a different story, as these patients are at risk for abdominal aortic aneurysm as well. There are only 6 isolated, native CIA aneurysms treated in this study. The remainder of the CIA aneurysms occurred distal to an aortic tube-graft. The small number of native artery aneurysms and short follow-up do not allow one to conclude that tubular stent-grafts are a good treatment for an isolated CIA aneurysm. Data and personal experience with CIA pseudoaneurysms again suggest that stent-grafts are the preferred mode of treatment for this problem, even if it requires coverage of the hypogastric artery.

G. L. Moneta, MD

9 Visceral and Renal Artery Disease

Progression of atherosclerotic renovascular disease: a prospective population-based study
Pearce JD, Craven BL, Craven TE, et al (Wake Forest Univ, Winston-Salem, NC)
J Vasc Surg 44:955-963, 2006

Objective.—Previous reports from select hypertensive patients suggest that atherosclerotic renovascular disease (RVD) is rapidly progressive and associated with a decline in kidney size and kidney function. This prospective, population-based study estimates the incidence of new RVD and progression of established RVD among elderly, free-living participants in the Cardiovascular Health Study (CHS).

Method.—The CHS is a multicenter, longitudinal cohort study of cardiovascular risk factors, morbidity, and mortality among men and women aged >65 years old. From 1995 through 1996, 834 participants underwent renal duplex sonography (RDS) to define the presence or absence of significant RVD. Between 2002 and 2005, a second RDS study was performed in 119 participants (mean study interval, 8.0 ± 0.8 years). Significant RVD was defined as hemodynamically significant stenosis (renal artery peak systolic velocity [RA-PSV] exceeding 1.8 m/s) or renal artery occlusion. Prevalent RVD was significant RVD at the first RDS, and incident disease was defined as new significant RVD at the second RDS. Significant change of RVD was defined as a change in RA-PSV of greater than two times the standard deviation of expected change over time, regardless of hemodynamic significance or progression to renal artery occlusion.

Results.—The second RDS study cohort included 119 CHS participants with 235 kidneys (35% men; mean age, 82.8 ± 3.4). On follow-up, no prevalent RVD (n = 13 kidneys; 6.0%) progressed to occlusion. Twenty-nine kidneys without RVD at the first RDS demonstrated significant change in PSV at the second RDS; including nine kidneys with new significant RVD (8 new stenoses; 1 new occlusion). Controlling for within-subject correlation, the overall estimated change in RVD among all 235 kidneys was 14.0% (95% confidence interval [CI], 9.2% to 21.4%), with progression to significant RVD in 4.0% (95% CI, 1.9% to 8.2%). Longitudinal increase in diastolic blood pressure and decrease in renal length were significantly associated with progression to new (ie, incident) significant RVD but not prevalent RVD.

Conclusions.—This is the first prospective, population-based estimate of incident RVD and progression of prevalent RVD among free-living elderly Americans. In contrast to previous reports among select hypertensive patients, CHS participants with a low rate of clinical hypertension demonstrated a significant change of RVD in only 14.0% of kidneys on follow-up of 8 years (annualized rate, 1.3% per year). Progression to significant RVD was observed in only 4.0% (annualized rate, 0.5% per year), and no prevalent RVD progressed to occlusion.

▶ The results of this study indicate that the rate of progression of RVD in the elderly population is low. I am inclined to look favorably upon this article because its conclusions support my bias that renal artery stenoses found incidentally should be left alone and that "drive-by" renal intervention is not justified. Unfortunately, the low rate of patient follow-up (14%) significantly limits my ability to offer this study as proof of my position. As noted in the invited commentary, only well-designed multicenter studies can provide the solid data on which we can base clinical judgments related to the treatment of RVD. We are still waiting for such data.

G. L. Moneta, MD

The management of renal artery atherosclerosis for renal salvage: Does stenting help?
Kashyap VS, Sepulveda RN, Bena JF, et al (Cleveland Clinic Found, Ohio)
J Vasc Surg 45:101-109, 2007

Objective.—The use of endovascular techniques to treat renal artery stenosis (RAS) has increased in recent years but remains controversial. The purpose of this study was to review the outcomes and durability of percutaneous transluminal angioplasty and stenting (PTA/S) for patients with RAS and decreasing renal function.

Methods.—Between 1999 and 2004, 125 consecutive patients underwent angiography and intervention for renal salvage and formed the basis of this study. Inclusion criteria for this study included serum creatinine greater than 1.5 mg/dL, ischemic nephropathy, and high-grade RAS perfusing a single functioning kidney. Patients undergoing PTA/S for renovascular hypertension or fibromuscular dysplasia or in conjunction with endovascular stent grafting for aneurysm repair were excluded. The original angiographic imaging was evaluated for lesion grade and parenchymal kidney size. All medical records and noninvasive testing were reviewed. Preoperative and postoperative patient data were standardized and analyzed by using χ^2 tests for nominal values and t tests for continuous variables. The Modification of Diet in Renal Disease equation was used to estimate glomerular filtration rate (GFR), and univariate analysis was performed.

Results.—Preoperative variables included the presence of coronary artery disease (93%), diabetes (44%), tobacco use (48%), and hypercholesterolemia (70%). RAS was suspected on the basis of preoperative duplex imaging or magnetic resonance angiography. Aortography and PTA/S were performed in 125 patients (mean age, 71 years; 59% male) with a mean baseline creatinine level of 2.2 mg/dL. There were two mortalities (1.6%) in the 30-day postoperative period, but there was no case of acute renal loss. Blood pressure decreased after PTA/S (151/79 mm Hg before vs 139/72 mm Hg after 1 month; $P < .03$). For all patients, the estimated GFR went from 33 ± 12 mL · min^{-1} · 1.73 m^{-2} (mean $\pm$ SD) to 37 ± 19 mL · min^{-1} · 1.73 m^{-2} at 6 months ($P = .10$). Sixty-seven percent of treated patients had improvement (>10% increase in GFR) or stabilization of renal function. A rapid decline in GFR before intervention was correlated with improvement after PTA/S. Responders after PTA/S had a 27% decrease in GFR before intervention (44 ± 13 mL · min^{-1} · 1.73 m^{-2} to 32 ± 13 mL · min^{-1} · 1.73 m^{-2}; $P < .001$) with a negative to positive slope change in GFR values. Ten patients underwent reintervention for in-stent restenosis. Cases without improvement in GFR after PTA/S were associated with eventual dialysis need ($P = .01$; mean follow-up, 19 months). Survival at 3 years was 76%, and dialysis-free survival was 63% as estimated by Kaplan-Meier analyses.

Conclusions.—Renal artery stenoses causing renal dysfunction can be safely treated via endovascular means. Rapidly decreasing renal function is associated with the response to renal artery angioplasty/stenting and helps identify patients for renal salvage.

▶ Clearly there are patients with renal insufficiency due to RAS who will benefit from renal angioplasty and stenting. The challenge is to differentiate those patients who will benefit from the procedure from those who won't. Retrospective studies such as this that broadly define inclusion criteria, that do not have a standardized pre- or postprocedure clinical evaluation routine, and that have inconsistent follow-up cannot provide us with any meaningful information from which we can base treatment decisions. Consequently, this study is a valiant but ultimately fruitless effort.

G. L. Moneta, MD

Iliorenal Bypass: Indications and Outcomes following 41 Reconstructions
Grigoryants V, Henke PK, Watson NC, et al (Univ of Michigan, Ann Arbor)
Ann Vasc Surg 21:1-9, 2007

Iliorenal bypass is a nonanatomic means of renal revascularization usually performed in high-risk patients. Its efficacy was assessed in this review of 35 patients (17 males and 18 females, two children and 33 adults) ranging in age 8–84 years, who were subjected to 41 iliorenal bypasses at the University of Michigan Hospital during 1975–2003. Renal artery lesions included arteriosclerosis ($n = 20$), developmental narrowing ($n = 10$), arterial fibrodysplasia ($n = 3$), penetrating trauma ($n = 1$), and aortorenal dissection associated with Marfan disease ($n = 1$). All patients had hypertension attributed to their renal artery disease. Twenty patients exhibited renal insufficiency (serum creatinine >1.8 mg/dL). Primary reasons for selecting an iliorenal reconstruction over a more conventional open revascularization included advanced aortic arteriosclerosis ($n = 9$); prior aortoaortic, aortoiliac, or aortofemoral reconstruction ($n = 7$); a small aortic aneurysm not justifying aortic surgery ($n = 6$); prior aortorenal surgery ($n = 6$); congenital abdominal aortic coarctation ($n = 4$); a hostile retroperitoneum ($n = 2$); or compromised cardiac status ($n = 1$). Eleven patients had prior ipsilateral renal artery interventions. Iliorenal bypasses were to the right kidney ($n = 20$), the left kidney ($n = 9$), and bilateral ($n = 12$). Conduits were saphenous veins ($n = 29$), synthetic prostheses ($n = 11$), or direct renal artery-iliac artery reimplantation ($n = 1$). Initial bypass patency was 93%. Follow-up averaged 7.5 years. Three early and six late graft complications resulted in eight secondary operations. The mean preoperative and postoperative serum creatinine of all 35 patients did not vary (1.9 vs. 1.8 mg/dL), although on an individual basis renal function improved in eight, remained stable in 21, and deteriorated in six patients. The series' mean preoperative blood pressure of 180/97 mm Hg decreased postoperatively to 140/78 mm Hg ($P < 0.001$). Hypertension was cured in three patients, improved in 27, and became worse in four. Antihypertensive medication numbers decreased postoperatively, from a median of three to two ($P < 0.0001$). Surgical mortality was limited to one patient succumbing from perioperative intestinal infarction. Iliorenal bypass is an effective means of renal revascularization in patients not amenable to more conventional open or transluminal procedures.

▶ Secondary graft interventions were required in about 20% of cases in this series. This seemingly high rate of graft interventions is probably due in part to the length of bypass needed to reach from the iliac to the renal artery. I will place this procedure in my list of alternatives for renal revascularization; however, considering that I only have 15 to 20 years left to practice, it is unlikely I will ever have to use it.

G. L. Moneta, MD

Distal embolic protection during renal artery angioplasty and stenting
Edwards MS, Craven BL, Stafford J, et al (Wake Forest Univ, Winston-Salem, NC)
J Vasc Surg 44:128-135, 2006

Background.—Percutaneous renal artery angioplasty and/or stenting (RA-PTAS) is increasingly being used as an alternative to surgery for renal artery revascularization. Unfortunately, renal function responses after RA-PTAS appear to be inferior to those observed after surgical revascularization both in terms of improving and preventing deterioration of renal function postintervention. Atheroembolism during RA-PTAS has been postulated as a potential cause for the disparate results. Strategies to limit the occurrence of atheroembolism, such as the use of distal embolic protection (DEP) systems, may result in improved outcomes after RA-PTAS.

Methods.—All RA-PTAS procedures performed with DEP (using a commercially available temporary balloon occlusion and aspiration catheter) between October 2003 and July 2005 were reviewed (Fig 2). Glomerular filtration rate (eGFR) was estimated preintervention and 4 to 6 weeks postintervention using the abbreviated Modification of Diet in Renal Disease formula. Renal function and hypertension response rates as well as procedural data were classified and reported according to American Heart Association guidelines. Renal function improvement and deterioration were defined as a 20% increase and decrease in eGFR, respectively, compared with preoperative values. Continuous and categoric data were analyzed using paired t tests and repeated measures linear models.

Results.—DEP was used in 32 RA-PTAS procedures in 15 women and 11 men with a mean age of 71 years. All patients were hypertensive, 24 (92%) had renal insufficiency, and the mean preintervention degree of renal artery stenosis was 79%. Immediate technical success was achieved in 100% of RA-PTAS cases. Mean pre- and postintervention serum creatinine and eGFR values were 1.9 vs 1.6 mg/dL ($P < .001$) and 37 vs 43 mL/min/1.73 m² ($P < .001$), respectively. Renal function was defined as improved after 17 (53%) of 32 procedures and worsened in none (0%).

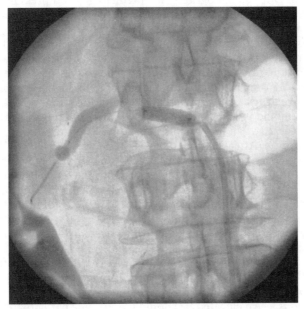

FIGURE 2.—Hand injection angiogram demonstrates complete renal artery occlusion using the distal embolic protection system before stent placement. (Courtesy of Edwards MS, Craven BL, Stafford J, et al. Distal embolic protection during renal artery angioplasty and stenting. *J Vasc Surg.* 2006;44:128-135. Copyright 2006 by Elsevier. Reprinted by permission.)

Conclusions.—RA-PTAS using DEP resulted in 4- to 6-week postintervention renal function results approximating those of surgical revascularization. These data suggest that DEP use may prevent renal function harm during RA-PTAS as a result of atheroembolism and warrant further investigation.

▶ This provocative study suggests that the renal functional deterioration that often occurs after renal artery angioplasty in some cases might be caused by parenchymal injury from atheromatous embolization sustained during the procedure. The results of this small case series showed no deterioration in renal function after renal artery angioplasty in the early postprocedure period with the use of a DEP device. This study will have important clinical implications if its results are borne out in larger controlled clinical trials.

G. L. Moneta, MD

Value of Doppler Sonography for Predicting Clinical Outcome After Renal Artery Revascularization in Atherosclerotic Renal Artery Stenosis
Garcia-Criado A, Gilabert R, Nicolau C, et al (Hosp Clinic of Barcelona)
J Ultrasound Med 24:1641-1647, 2005

Objective.—The purpose of this study was to prospectively evaluate the usefulness of Doppler sonography for predicting blood pressure and renal function improvement after percutaneous renal angioplasty in patients with unilateral atherosclerotic renal artery stenosis.

Methods.—Thirty-six patients with successfully revascularized unilateral atherosclerotic renal artery stenosis were included. Patients were evaluated by Doppler sonography before treatment, with the resistive index (RI) and acceleration being measured in both kidneys. Blood pressure, number of antihypertensive drugs, and serum creatinine concentration were assessed before treatment and thereafter during a 23 ± 15-month (mean $\pm$ SD) period.

Results.—In 20 of the 36 patients (55%), the RI was less than 0.80 before revascularization. After treatment, blood pressure improved in 17 (85%) of those 20 patients and improved in 8 (50%) of 16 patients with an RI of greater than 0.80 ($P < .05$). Twenty-five patients had renal insufficiency pretreatment, and 11 (44%) had a baseline RI of less than 0.80. Improvement in renal function after angioplasty was shown in 5 (45%) of these 11 patients and in 4 (28.5%) of 14 in the group with high RI ($P > .05$, not significant). On analysis of acceleration, blood pressure improved in 9 (69%) of 13 patients with acceleration of greater than 3 m/s^2 and in 16 (69.5%) of 23 with acceleration of less than 3 m/s^2 ($P > .05$). In patients with renal insufficiency, 5 (50%) of 10 cases with normal baseline acceleration and 4 (27%) of 15 with low acceleration showed improvement in renal function ($P > .05$).

Conclusions.—An elevated RI should not exclude patients from a revascularization procedure because, although renal RI does correlate with blood pressure response to revascularization, it is not a useful parameter in predicting renal function outcome. Acceleration has no prognostic value.

▶ In the presence of a good contralateral kidney, improvement in renal function would not usually be expected after unilateral treatment of renal artery stenosis. The number of patients here is too few with such limited information on the contralateral kidney, that any conclusions by the authors are somewhat tenuous. The χ^2 analysis used by the authors was too simplistic. A multivariable analysis would have added strength to the authors' conclusions. The article is not convincing enough to dismiss RI as a predictor of response to unilateral renal artery angioplasty.

G. L. Moneta, MD

Endovascular Versus Open Mesenteric Revascularization: Immediate Benefits Do Not Equate with Short-Term Functional Outcomes
Sivamurthy N, Rhodes JM, Lee D, et al (Univ of Rochester, NY)
J Am Coll Surg 202:859-867, 2006

Background.—Percutaneous therapy for symptomatic visceral occlusive disease is rapidly gaining popularity in many centers. This study evaluates the anatomic and functional outcomes of open and endovascular therapy for chronic mesenteric ischemia at an academic medical center.

Study design.—We performed a retrospective review of patients who underwent endovascular or open mesenteric arterial revascularization for chronic mesenteric ischemia between January 1989 and September 2003. Indications for revascularization included postprandial abdominal pain (92%) or weight loss (54%). All had atherosclerotic visceral occlusive disease with a median of 2 vessels with more than 50% stenosis or occlusion on angiography. Sixty patients (44 women, mean age 66 years) underwent 67 interventions (43 vessels bypassed, 23 vessel endarterectomies, 22 vessel angioplasty and stents). The median numbers of vessels revascularized were two in the open group and one in the endovascular group.

Results.—Thirty-day mortality and cumulative survival at 3 years were similar (open, 15% and 62% ± 9%; endovascular, 21% and 63% ± 14%, respectively; p = NS). Cumulative patencies at 6 months were 83% ± 7% and 68% ± 14% in the open and endovascular groups, respectively (p = NS). Major morbidity, median postoperative length of stay, and cumulative freedom from recurrent symptoms at 6 months were significantly greater in the open group (open, 46%, 23 days, and 71% ± 7%, respectively; endovascular, 19%, 1 day, and 34% ± 10%, respectively; p < 0.01).

Conclusions.—Endovascular revascularization is attractive because it carries equivalent patency to open revascularization. Symptomatic benefit of endovascular revascularization is not achieved, probably as a result of incomplete revascularization. Despite incomplete revascularization, endovascular therapy has equivalent survival and lower morbidity compared with open revascularization. Complete endovascular revascularization needs further evaluation to determine if it is superior to open revascularization. In the interim, endovascular therapy should be reserved for the patient unable to undergo open revascularization.

▶ It is a little unclear what to make of these data, as it is very likely a significant number of the patients actually did not have classic mesenteric ischemia. Only 64% of the open group had 2 or more diseased vessels with significant stenosis. Significant stenosis was defined as greater than 50%, a very liberal definition of a critical stenosis in the mesenteric circulation. Less than half of the endovascular group had 2 or more vessels with greater than 50% stenosis, and weight loss was uncommon in the endovascular group. I wonder how many of these patients in the endovascular group were victims of the ocular stenotic reflex?

G. L. Moneta, MD

Clinical significance of splanchnic artery stenosis
Mensink PBF, van Petersen AS, Geelkerken RH, et al (Medisch Spectrum Twente, Enschede, The Netherlands)
Br J Surg 93:1377-1382, 2006

Background.—The clinical relevance of splanchnic artery stenosis is often unclear. Gastric exercise tonometry enables the identification of patients with actual gastrointestinal ischaemia. A large group of patients with splanchnic artery stenosis was studied using standard investigations, including tonometry.

Methods.—Patients referred with possible intestinal ischaemia were analysed prospectively, using duplex imaging, conventional abdominal angiography and tonometry. All results were discussed within a multidisciplinary team.

Results.—Splanchnic stenoses were found in 157 (49.7 percent) of 316 patients; 95 patients (60.5 percent) had one-vessel, 54 (34.4 percent) two-vessel and eight (5.1 percent) had three-vessel disease. Chronic splanchnic syndrome was diagnosed in 107 patients (68.2 percent), 54 (57 percent) with single-vessel, 45 (83 percent) with two-vessel and all eight with three-vessel stenoses. Treatment was undertaken in 95 patients, 62 by surgery and 33 by endovascular techniques. After a median follow-up of 43 months, 84 percent of patients were symptom free.

Conclusion.—Gastric exercise tonometry proved crucial in the evaluation of possible intestinal ischaemia. Comparing patients with single- and multiple-vessel stenoses, there were significant differences in clinical presentation and mortality rates.

▶ Many, if not most, of the patients in this study would not be considered to have intestinal ischemia using the classic definition of postprandial abdominal pain, food fear, and weight loss. These degrees of symptoms, however, are obviously extreme and indicate advanced disease. It makes sense that there may be patients with milder degrees of intestinal ischemia who do not have classic symptoms. The authors' technique is extremely interesting and potentially may help guide revascularization strategies in patients with visceral artery stenosis but less than classic symptoms of intestinal ischemia.

G. L. Moneta, MD

Splenic artery aneurysms: postembolization syndrome and surgical complications
Piffaretti G, Tozzi M, Lomazzi C, et al (Univ of Insubria-Varese, Italy)
Am J Surg 193:166-170, 2007

Background.—This study assessed the endovascular embolization of splenic artery aneurysms and false aneurysms with special consideration given to postoperative complications.

Methods.—Fifteen patients (11 women; mean age, 56 y; range, 39–80 y) with splenic artery aneurysm (n = 13) or false aneurysm (n = 2) were treated with coil embolization. The lesion was asymptomatic in 9 patients, symptomatic in 5 patients, and ruptured in 1 patient. The mean aneurysm diameter was 33 ± 23 mm (range, 15–80 mm). Postoperative follow-up evaluation included a clinical visit and spiral computed tomography at 1, 4, and 12 months, and yearly thereafter.

Results.—Endovascular treatment was possible in 14 patients (93%) (1 failure: neck cannulation). Perioperative mortality was not observed. Morbidity included postembolization syndrome in 5 patients (30%). Neither pancreatitis nor spleen abscess occurred (Fig 2). The mean follow-up period was 36 months (range, 3–60 mo). During follow-up evaluation we detected 1 sac reperfusion that was sealed successfully with additional coils. Surgical conversion or open repair were never required.

Conclusions.—At our institute, endovascular treatment represents the first-line treatment for splenic artery aneurysms. Postembolization syndrome and infarcts are common events but generally resolve without sequelae.

▶ Coil embolization of splenic artery aneurysms is generally safe and effective but apparently not applicable to all patients with splenic artery aneurysms. After embolization, a few patients will have significant symptoms and splenic infarcts. Hospitalization can be prolonged in these patients, and perhaps with the availability of laparoscopic splenectomy, splenectomy should be considered in those patients with massive splenic infarcts after coil embolization of a splenic artery aneurysm.

G. L. Moneta, MD

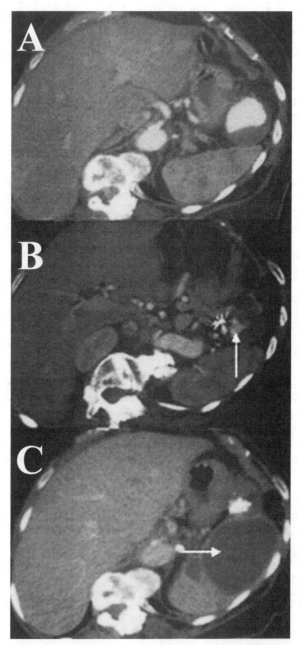

FIGURE 2.—(A) Preoperative CT angiography of a 7-cm aneurysm of the distal portion of the splenic artery. At 4 months the CT control revealed a (B) mild reperfusion (*arrow*) of the sac that was totally excluded with (C) adjunctive coil (*arrow*) embolization. (Courtesy of Piffaretti G, Tozzi M, Lomazzi C, et al. Splenic artery aneurysms: postembolization syndrome and surgical complications. *Am J Surg.* 2007;193:166-170. Copyright 2007, with permission from Excerpta Medica Inc.)

Management of aneurysms involving branches of the celiac and superior mesenteric arteries: A comparison of surgical and endovascular therapy

Sachdev U, Baril DT, Ellozy SH, et al (Mount Sinai Med Ctr, New York)
J Vasc Surg 44:718-724, 2006

Objective.—Aneurysms involving branches of the superior mesenteric and celiac arteries are uncommon and require proper management to prevent rupture and death. This study compares surgical and endovascular treatment of these aneurysms and analyzes outcome.

Methods.—Patients at the Mount Sinai Medical Center in New York who were treated for aneurysms in the branches of the celiac artery and superior mesenteric artery were identified through a search of the institution's medical records and endovascular database. Patient demographics, history, clini-

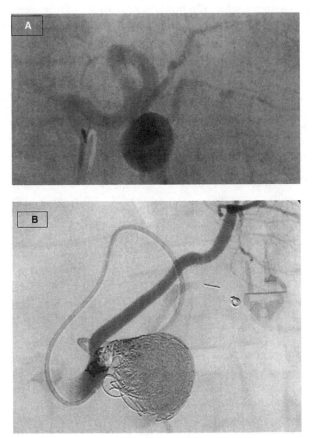

FIGURE 2.—A, Angiogram of splenic artery aneurysm before coil embolization. B, Angiogram of splenic artery aneurysm after coil embolization. (Courtesy of Sachdev U, Baril DT, Ellozy SH, et al. Management of aneurysms involving branches of the celiac and superior mesenteric arteries: a comparison of surgical and endovascular therapy. *J Vasc Surg.* 2006;44:718-724. Copyright 2006 by Elsevier. Reprinted with permission from Excerpta Medica, Inc.)

cal presentation, aneurysm characteristics, treatments, and follow-up outcome were retrospectively recorded. Significant differences between patients treated by surgical or endovascular therapy were determined by using Student's t test and χ^2 analysis.

Results.—Between January 1, 1991, and July 1, 2005, 59 patients with 61 aneurysms were treated at a single institution. Twenty-four patients had surgical repair, and 35 underwent endovascular treatment, which included coil embolization and stent-graft therapy. Splenic (28) and hepatic (22) artery aneurysms predominated (Fig 2). Eighty-nine percent of splenic artery aneurysms were true aneurysms and were treated by endovascular and surgical procedures in near equal numbers (14 and 11, respectively). Pseudoaneurysms were significantly more likely to be treated by endovascular means ($P < .01$). The technical success rate of endovascular treatment for aneurysms was 89%, and failures were successfully treated by repeat coil embolization in all patients who presented for retreatment. Patients treated by endovascular techniques had a significantly higher incidence of malignancy than patients treated with open surgical techniques ($P = .03$). Furthermore, patients treated by endovascular means had a shorter in-hospital length of stay (2.4 vs 6.6 days, $P < .001$).

Conclusion.—Endovascular management of visceral aneurysms is an effective means of treating aneurysms involving branches of the celiac and superior mesenteric arteries and is particularly useful in patients with comorbidities, including cancer. It is associated with a decreased length of stay in the elective setting, and failure of primary treatment can often be successfully managed percutaneously.

▶ These types of articles that examine a relatively rare condition treated in many ways by many surgeons over many years never really help that much, except to indicate a relatively rare condition can be treated by many techniques over many years by many surgeons, and most of the time the outcome will be favorable. This article should receive the Mayo Clinic stamp of approval!

G. L. Moneta, MD

10 Thoracic Aorta

Familial Thoracic Aortic Aneurysms and Dissections—Incidence, Modes of Inheritance, and Phenotypic Patterns
Albornoz G, Coady MA, Roberts M, et al (Yale Univ, New Haven, Conn)
Ann Thorac Surg 82:1400-1406, 2006

Background.—We examined the genetic nature and phenotypic features of thoracic aortic aneurysms (TAAs) and dissections in a large cohort of patients.

Methods.—Interviews were conducted with 520 patients with TAAs and their pedigrees were compiled to identify family members with aneurysms. Study patients were divided into three groups: 101 non-Marfan patients, in 88 pedigrees, had a family pattern for TAA (familial group), 369 had no family pattern (sporadic group), and 50 had Marfan syndrome (MFS). We de-

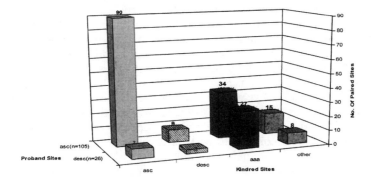

Proband sites		Kindred sites				Total paired sites
		asc	desc	AAA	other	
asc	105	90	9	34	15	148
desc	26	7	3	27	8	45
						193

FIGURE 4.—Distribution of sites of arterial aneurysms and dissections in kindred of familial probands. *AAA* = abdominal aortic aneurysm; *asc* = ascending; *desc* = descending. (Courtesy of Albornoz G, Coady MA, Roberts M, et al. Familial thoracic aortic aneurysms and dissections: incidence, modes of inheritance, and phenotypic patterns. *Ann Thorac Surg.* 2006;82:1400-1406. Reprinted with permission from the Society of Thoracic Surgeons.)

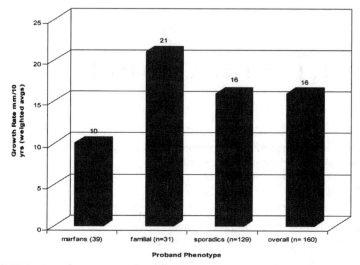

FIGURE 2.—Rate of aneurysm growth in different groups. (Courtesy of Albornoz G, Coady MA, Roberts M, et al. Familial thoracic aortic aneurysms and dissections: incidence, modes of inheritance, and phenotypic patterns. *Ann Thorac Surg.* 2006;82:1400-1406. Reprinted with permission from the Society of Thoracic Surgeons.)

termined incidence of familial clustering, age at presentation, rate of aneurysm growth, incidence of hypertension, correlation of aneurysm sites among kindred, and pedigree inheritance patterns.

Results.—An inherited pattern for TAA was present in 21.5% of non-MFS patients. The predominant inheritance pattern was autosomal dominant (76.9%), with varying degrees of penetrance and expressivity. The familial TAA group was significantly younger than the sporadic group ($p < 0.0001$), but not as young as the MFS group ($p < 0.0001$) (mean ages, 58.2 versus 65.7 versus 27.4 years). Among all 197 probands and kindred with aneurysm, 131 (66.5%) had TAA, 49 (24.9%) had abdominal aortic aneurysm (AAA), and 17 (8.6%) had cerebral or other aneurysms. Ascending aneurysm paired most commonly with ascending, and descending with abdominal (Fig 4). Abdominal aortic aneurysms (AAAs) and hypertension were more often associated with descending than with ascending TAAs ($p < 0.001$). Aortic growth rate was highest for the familial group (0.21 cm/y), intermediate for the sporadic group (0.16 cm/y), and lowest for the Marfan group (0.1 cm/y; $p < 0.01$) (Fig 2).

Conclusions.—TAAs are frequently familial diseases. The predominant mode of inheritance is autosomal dominant. Familial TAAs have a relatively early age of onset. Aneurysms in relatives may be seen in the thoracic aorta, the abdominal aorta, or the cerebral circulation. Screening of first-order relatives of probands with TAA is essential. Familial TAAs tend to grow at a higher rate, exemplifying a more aggressive clinical entity.

▶ A familial pattern of AAA has long been recognized. Surprisingly, there have been relatively few studies examining familial predisposition to TAA and thoracic aortic dissection. The important points of this article are that many TAAs and dissections are familial (20% of non-MFS patients). In addition, patients with a familial pattern of TAA have a higher rate of aneurysm growth than those with sporadic disease. The data suggest screening for aneurysm disease in first-order relatives and probands of patients with TAA.

G. L. Moneta, MD

Novel Measurement of Relative Aortic Size Predicts Rupture of Thoracic Aortic Aneurysms
Davies RR, Gallo A, Coady MA, et al (Yale Univ, New Haven, Conn)
Ann Thorac Surg 81:169-177, 2006

Background.—Optimal operative decision making in thoracic aortic aneurysms requires accurate information on the risk of complications during expectant management. Cumulative and yearly risks of rupture, dissection, and death before operative repair increase with increasing aortic size, but previous work has not addressed the impact of relative aortic size on complication rates.

Methods.—Our institutional database contains data on 805 patients followed up serially with thoracic aortic aneurysms. Body surface area information was obtained on 410 patients (257 male, 153 female). We calculated a new measure of relative aortic size, the "aortic size index," and examined its ability to predict complications in these patients.

Results.—Increasing aortic size index was a significant predictor of increasing rates of rupture ($p = 0.0014$) as well as the combined endpoint of rupture, death, or dissection ($p < 0.0001$). Using aortic size index, patients were stratified into three risk groups: less than 2.75 cm/m^2 are at low risk (approximately 4% per year), 2.75 to 4.24 cm/m^2 are at moderate risk (approximately 8% per year), and those above 4.25 cm/m^2 are at high risk (approximately 20% per year).

Conclusions.—This study confirms that (1) thoracic aortic aneurysm is a lethal disease, (2) relative aortic size is more important than absolute aortic size in predicting complications, and (3) a novel measurement of relative aortic size allows for the stratification of patients into three levels of risk, enabling appropriate surgical decision-making.

▶ This may be an advance over simple measurement of transverse or anterior-posterior diameter as a measure of potential rupture risk. It is, however, still relatively unsophisticated. The work of Fillinger et al, in which stress patterns of the abdominal aortic wall in abdominal aortic aneurysms are mapped, is a quantum leap beyond the approach in this article. That approach also needs to be applied to thoracic aneurysms and compared with the technique described here.

G. L. Moneta, MD

Long-Term Survival in Patients Presenting With Type B Acute Aortic Dissection: Insights From the International Registry of Acute Aortic Dissection

Tsai TT, for the International Registry of Acute Aortic Dissection (IRAD) (Univ of Michigan, Ann Arbor; et al)
Circulation 114:2226-2231, 2006

Background.—Follow-up survival studies in patients with acute type B aortic dissection have been restricted to a small number of patients in single centers. We used data from a contemporary registry of acute type B aortic dissection to better understand factors associated with adverse long-term survival.

Method and Results.—We examined 242 consecutive patients discharged alive with acute type B aortic dissection enrolled in the International Registry of Acute Aortic Dissection (IRAD) between 1996 and 2003. Kaplan-Meier survival curves were constructed, and Cox proportional hazards analysis was performed to identify independent predictors of follow-up mortality. Three-year survival for patients treated medically, surgically, or with endovascular therapy was 77.6±6.6%, 82.8±18.9%, and 76.2±25.2%, respectively (median follow-up 2.3 years, log-rank $P=0.61$). Independent predictors of follow-up mortality included female gender (hazard ratio [HR],1.99; 95% confidence interval [CI], 1.07 to 3.71; $P=0.03$), a history of prior aortic aneurysm (HR, 2.17; 95% CI, 1.03 to 4.59; $P=0.04$), a history of atherosclerosis (HR, 2.48; 95% CI, 1.32 to 4.66; $P<0.01$), in-hospital renal failure (HR, 2.55; 95% CI, 1.15 to 5.63; $P=0.02$), pleural effusion on chest radiograph (HR, 2.56; 95% CI, 1.18 to 5.58; $P=0.02$), and in-hospital hypotension/shock (HR, 12.5; 95% CI, 3.24 to 48.21; $P<0.01$).

Conclusions.—Contemporary follow-up mortality in patients who survive to hospital discharge with acute type B aortic dissection is high, approaching 1 in every 4 patients at 3 years. Current treatment and follow-up surveillance require further study to better understand and optimize care for patients with this complex disease.

▶ There were no differences in survival between medically managed, surgically managed, and endovascularly managed patients in this registry. However, since this was not a randomized study, it is possible that patients treated with surgical or endovascular techniques had additional risk factors for long-term mortality. Patients with acute type B aortic dissection to be treated by endografts will need to be stratified for additional risk factors. There are two other articles relating closely to this body of work: Mukherjee et al has produced an article on the implications of periaortic hematoma in patients with acute aortic dissection, [1] and Winnerkvist et al published an article studying medically treated acute type B aortic dissection.[2]

G. L. Moneta, MD

References

1. Mukherjee D, Evangelista A, Nienaber CA, et al. Implications of periaortic hematoma in patients with acute aortic dissection (from the International Registry of Acute Aortic Dissection). *Am J Cardiol.* 2005;96:1734-1738.
2. Winnerkvist A, Lockowandt U, Rasmussen E, Rådegran K. A prospective study of medically treated acute type B aortic dissection. *Eur J Vasc Endovasc Surg.* 2006;32:349-355.

Implications of Periaortic Hematoma in Patients With Acute Aortic Dissection (from the International Registry of Acute Aortic Dissection)

Mukherjee D, Evangelista A, Nienaber CA, et al (Univ of Kentucky, Lexington; Hosp Gen Universitari Vall d'Hebron, Barcelona; Univ of Rostock, Germany; et al)
Am J Cardiol 96:1734-1738, 2005

The clinical profiles, presentation, and outcomes of patients with acute aortic dissections and associated periaortic hematomas on aortic imaging have not been described in a large cohort. This study sought to assess the prognostic implications of periaortic hematomas in patients with aortic dissections and to identify factors associated with in-hospital mortality in patients with periaortic hematomas. The study population was 971 patients with acute aortic dissections enrolled in the International Registry of Acute Aortic Dissection with available imaging data on presentation with the presence or absence of periaortic hematomas. Patients with periaortic hematomas (n = 227, 23.4%) were more likely to be women, to have a history of hypertension and atherosclerosis, and to present early to the hospital. At presentation, they had greater frequencies of shock, cardiac tamponade, coma, and/or altered consciousness. Clinical outcomes were significantly worse in patients with periaortic hematomas, including significantly greater mortality (33% vs 20.3%, p <0.001). A multivariate model demonstrated periaortic hematomas to be an independent predictor of mortality in patients with aortic dissections (odds ratio 1.71, 95% confidence interval 1.15 to 2.54, p = 0.007). In conclusion, this study provides insight into the profiles, presentation, and outcomes of patients with periaortic hematomas and acute aortic dissections. The early identification and aggressive management of patients with periaortic hematomas may potentially improve clinical outcomes.

▶ The study shows that patients with acute aortic dissection and periaortic hematomas have many of the factors that logically predict poor outcome with aortic dissection. Periaortic hematomas may, in some cases, actually be better described as contained ruptures of the aorta with an expected adverse natural history. The article argues for more aggressive management of aortic dissection complicated by periaortic hematoma. Perhaps these are the patients with type B dissection who really should be acutely managed with a thoracic endograft.

G. L. Moneta, MD

A Prospective Study of Medically Treated Acute Type B Aortic Dissection
Winnerkvist A, Lockowandt U, Rasmussen E, et al (Karolinska Univ, Stockholm; Karolinska Institutet, Stockholm)
Eur J Vasc Endovasc Surg 32:349-355, 2006

Objective.—To study prospectively aneurysm formation, need of surgery, incidence of rupture and mortality in patients with conservatively treated acute type B aortic dissection.

Methods.—All patients referred to us with acute type B dissection between January 1990 and December 2001 were candidates for this prospective treatment and follow-up study. Patients deemed not to be in need of acute surgical repair were included after aggressive antihypertensive treatment. The follow-up protocol included close blood pressure control, clinic visits with physical examination, chest x-ray and spiral CT or MRI at 3 and 6 months and annually thereafter.

Results.—Sixty-six patients were followed for a mean of 79 months (range 22–179). The actuarial survival rate was 82% at 5 years and 69% at 10 years (Fig 1). Eighty-five percent remained free from dissection-related death at 5 years and 82% at 10 years. Ten patients (15%) developed aneurysm (>6 cm) of the dissected aorta. Three of these 10 patients died from aortic rupture and 2 underwent elective surgical repair. Of the 56 patients without aneurysm, one died from rupture and one died suddenly for causes unknown. One patient was treated with endovascular stent-graft. Five patients sustained a new type A aortic dissection which in all but one were fatal.

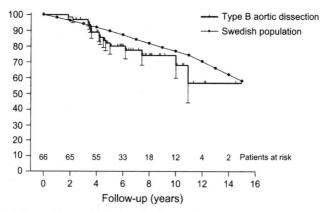

FIGURE 1.—Actuarial survival percentages for 66 patients followed after acute type B aortic dissection. The survival percentage for the entire age- and gender-matched Swedish population for each year of follow-up is plotted for comparison. Numbers above X-axis show patients at risk left in follow-up. (Reprinted by permission of the publisher from Winnerkvist A, Lockowandt U, Rasmussen E, Rådegran K. A prospective study of medically treated acute type B aortic dissection. *Eur J Vasc Endovasc Surg.* 2006;32:349-355.)

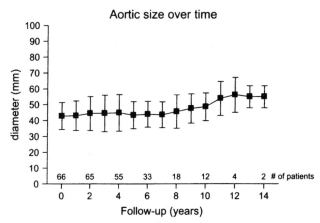

FIGURE 3.—The mean (±SD) maximal diameter of the dissected aorta for each year of follow-up. Numbers above the X-axis show number of patients available for analysis. (Reprinted by permission of the publisher from Winnerkvist A, Lockowandt U, Rasmussen E, Rådegran K. A prospective study of medically treated acute type B aortic dissection. *Eur J Vasc Endovasc Surg.* 2006;32:349-355.)

In 26 patients the initial dissection was categorized as intramural hematoma. Twelve of these patients had, in addition to the hematoma, areas with localized dissection/ulcer-like projection. The latter was found to be a predictor of aortic event (dissection-related death, rupture, new type A aortic dissection, aneurysm formation) during follow-up, as was an initial diameter of >4.0 cm at first CT-scan during the acute event.

Conclusions.—Conservatively treated acute type B dissection has a low incidence of aneurysm formation and rupture during the chronic phase. These results must be matched or improved upon before endovascular stent-grafting or early aortic surgical repair can be regarded as the primary treatment of choice (Fig 3).

▶ This article also suggests that while most patients with type B acute aortic dissection do well, some do not. Not all type B aortic dissections are the same, and some appear to have an adverse natural history. This is the type of information that will allow more intelligent selection of patients with type B dissection for primary endograft repair. Mukherjee et al also wrote a very important article on this topic.[1]

G. L. Moneta, MD

Reference

1. Mukherjee D, Evangelista A, Nienaber CA, et al. Implications of periaortic hematoma in patients with acute aortic dissection (from the International Registry of Acute Aortic Dissection). *Am J Cardiol.* 2005;96:1734-1738.

Acute limb ischemia associated with type B aortic dissection: Clinical relevance and therapy

Henke PK, Williams DM, Upchurch GR Jr, et al (Univ of Michigan, Ann Arbor)
Surgery 140:532-540, 2006

Background.—The goal of the current study is to characterize the presentation, therapy, and outcomes of acute limb ischemia (ALI) associated with type B aortic dissection (AoD).

Methods.—The prospective/retrospective International Registry for Acute Aortic Dissection (IRAD) database and a single institutional database were queried for all patients with type B AoD from 1996 to 2002. Univariate and multivariate statistics were used to delineate factors associated with morbidity and mortality outcomes.

Results.—According to the IRAD data (n = 458), the mean age of patients was 64 years, and 70% were men. The overall mortality was 12%; of these, 6% had ALI. Pulse (3-fold) and neurologic deficits (5-fold) were more common in those with ALI ($P < .001$). Endovascular, but not surgical therapy, was more commonly performed in patients with ALI compared with those without ALI (31% vs 10%, $P = .004$). No difference in age, race, gender, or origin of dissection was observed. ALI was associated with acute renal failure (odds ratio [OR] = 2.7; 95% confidence interval [CI] 1.1-7.1; $P = .048$) and acute mesenteric ischemia/infarction (OR = 6.9; 95% CI 2.5-20; $P < .001$). Adjusting for patient characteristics, ALI was associated with death (3.5; 95% CI 1.1-10; $P = .02$). The single institution analysis revealed similar patient demographics and mortality in 93 AoD patients, of whom 28 had ALI. Aortic fenestration or aorto-iliac stenting was the primary therapy in 93%; surgical bypass was used in 7%. Limb salvage was 93% in those with ALI at a mean of 18 months follow-up. The number of organ systems with malperfusion was 2-fold higher at aortography than suspected preprocedure ($P = .002$). By stepwise regression modeling, mortality was greater in those not taking a β-blocker (OR = 19; 95% CI 3.1-111; $P = .001$).

Conclusions.—ALI secondary to AoD is predictive of death and visceral ischemia. Endovascular therapy confers excellent limb salvage and allows diagnosis of unsuspected visceral ischemia.

▶ The main points to be taken from this article are that endovascular therapy works well for treatment of ALI in patients with type B AoD. In addition, other unsuspected areas of hypoperfusion will be discovered at the time of aortography.

G. L. Moneta, MD

Endograft exclusion of acute and chronic descending thoracic aortic dissections

Song TK, Donayre CE, Walot I, et al (Harbor-UCLA Med Ctr, Torrance, Calif)
J Vasc Surg 43:247-258, 2006

Objectives.—To analyze the results of endograft exclusion of acute and chronic descending thoracic aortic dissections (Stanford type B) with the AneuRx (n = 5) and Talent (n = 37) thoracic devices and to compare postoperative outcomes of endograft placement acutely (<2 weeks) and for chronic interventions.

Methods.—Patients treated for acute or chronic thoracic aortic dissections (Stanford type B) with endografts were included in this study. All patients (n = 42) were enrolled in investigational device exemption protocols from August 1999 to March 2005. Three-dimensional computed tomography reconstructions were analyzed for quantitative volume regression of the false lumen and changes in the true lumen over time (complete >95%, partial >30%).

Results.—Forty-two patients, all of whom had American Society of Anesthesiologists (ASA) risk stratification ≥III and 71% with ASA ≥IV, were treated for Stanford type B dissections (acute = 25, chronic = 17), with 42 primary and 18 secondary procedures. All proximal entry sites were identified intraoperatively by intravascular ultrasound (IVUS). The procedural stroke rate was 6.7% (4/60), with three posterior circulation strokes. Procedural mortality was 6.7% (4/60). The left subclavian artery was occluded in 11 patients (26%) with no complaints of arm ischemia, but there was an association with posterior circulation strokes (2/11) (18%). No postoperative paraplegia was observed after primary or secondary intervention. Complete

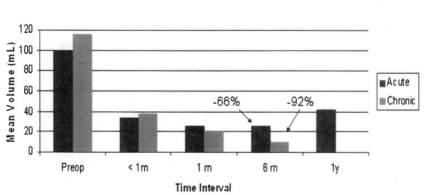

Acute vs Chronic:
False Lumen Blood Flow

FIGURE 4.—False lumen volume regression of acute and chronic dissections related to time. At the 6-month follow-up, there was a 66% decrease in false lumen (contrast) volume in the acute dissections and a 92% decrease in the chronic dissections compared with preoperative values. (Reprinted by permission of the publisher from Song TK, Donayre CE, Walot I, et al. Endograft exclusion of acute and chronic descending thoracic aortic dissections. *J Vasc Surg.* 2006;43:247-258. Copyright 2006 by Elsevier.)

thrombosis of the false lumen at the level of endograft coverage occurred in 25 (61%) of 41 patients ≤1 month and 15 (88%) of 17 patients at 12 months. Volume regression of the false lumen was 66.4% (acute) and 91.9% (chronic) at 6 months (Fig 4). Lack of true lumen volume (contrast) increase and increasing false lumen volume (contrast) suggests continued false lumen pressurization and the need for secondary reintervention. Thirteen patients (31%) required 18 secondary interventions for proximal endoleaks in 6, junctional leaks in 3, continued perfusion of the false lumen from distal re-entry sites in 3, and surgical conversion in 4 for retrograde dissection.

Conclusions.—Preliminary experience with endografts to treat acute and chronic dissections is associated with a reduced risk of paraplegia and lower mortality compared with open surgical treatment, the results of medical treatment alone, or a combination.

▶ The patients treated in this series comprise a selected group of thoracic dissections with either symptoms or specific indications for treatment, and do not represent all patients presenting with a type B dissection. Intravascular US was used extensively in this series of patients to aid in the evaluation and plan treatment. Its importance cannot be overstressed. Adjuvant procedures are rarely if ever needed to maintain visceral perfusion after thoracic endovascular aortic repair (TEVAR). Despite extensive coverage of the aorta, the incidence of paraplegia is also extremely low, and as with other published studies, stroke is the most common major complication. Retrograde dissection can occur with open or endovascular repair, and currently, its underlying cause in TEVAR (device configuration, timing of procedure, etc) has not been determined.

G. L. Moneta, MD

Thoracic Aortic Endografting Is the Treatment of Choice for Elderly Patients With Thoracic Aortic Disease

Kern JA, Matsumoto AH, Tribble CG, et al (Univ of Virginia, Charlottesville)
Ann Surg 243:815-823, 2006

Objective.—To assess the effect of age on outcomes following thoracic aortic endografting.

Summary Background Data.—Endograft therapy for thoracic aortic disease is rapidly evolving. This therapy is less invasive, and elderly patients with significant medical comorbidities are more frequently referred for endografting. We hypothesized that elderly patients over the age of 75 have worse outcomes after thoracic endografting than patients under the age of 75.

Methods.—We retrospectively reviewed the charts of the first 42 patients who underwent endografting for thoracic aortic pathology. Charts were reviewed for demographics, comorbid conditions, perioperative complications and death, endoleaks, and results at 3, 6, and 12 months. Preexisting medical conditions were also evaluated to determine if any patient characteristics were associated with adverse outcomes. Perioperative morbidity included cardiac, pulmonary, renal, hemorrhagic, and neurologic (stroke and spinal cord injury) complications.

Results.—Twenty-four patients were under the age of 75, and 18 patients were 75 or older. Baseline demographics and comorbidities were similar between the 2 groups. There were no differences in operative time, length of stay, perioperative mortality, or the incidence of significant complications between the 2 age groups. Gender, however, was associated with a statistically significant difference between the occurrence of complications, with more women experiencing complications than men ($P = 0.026$, relative risk = 2.36). One patient (age >75 years) in the entire cohort of 42 (2.4%) suffered a spinal cord injury. At 3 months, endoleaks were more common in the older age group ($P = 0.059$).

Conclusion.—Endograft therapy for thoracic aortic disease can be performed safely in elderly patients with no significant increase in perioperative morbidity or mortality compared with younger patients. Female gender is associated with a higher likelihood of perioperative complications, regardless of age. The overall incidence of spinal cord injury is very low. Endograft therapy, when anatomically possible, is the treatment of choice for thoracic aortic disease in elderly patients.

▶ While multiple references exist demonstrating poorer outcomes in elderly patients undergoing open thoracic aortic repairs, data are lacking with thoracic endovascular aortic repair. While this article concluded that there are no differences based on age, statistical analysis and study design are not ideal. Statistical evaluation for procedural aspects such as disease type, conduit use, and exclusion of patients from clinical trials with renal insufficiency was not conducted and may alter results. One thing is for sure—patient selection has always impacted outcomes.

G. L. Moneta, MD

Thirty-day mortality statistics underestimate the risk of repair of thoracoabdominal aortic aneurysms: A statewide experience
Rigberg DA, McGory ML, Zingmond DS, et al (UCLA, Los Angeles)
J Vasc Surg 43:217-223, 2006

Objective.—The purpose of this study was to determine the 30-day and 365-day mortality for the repair of thoracoabdominal aortic aneurysms (TAA), when stratified by age, in the general population. These data provide clinicians with information more applicable to an individual patient than mortality figures from a single institutional series.

Methods.—Data were obtained from the California Office of Statewide Health Planning and Development (OSHPD) for the years 1991 to 2002. These data were linked to the state death certificate file, allowing for continued information on the status of the patients after hospital discharge. All patients undergoing elective and ruptured TAA repair as coded by International Classification of Diseases, 9th Clinical Modification (ICD-9, CM) in

California were identified. Patients aged <50 or >90 years old were excluded. We determined 30- and 365-day mortality and stratified our findings by decade of patient age (eg, 50 to 59). Demographics of elective and ruptured cases were also compared.

Results.—We identified 1010 patients (797 elective, 213 ruptured) who underwent TAA repair. Mean patient ages were 70.0 (elective) and 72.1 years (ruptured). Men comprised 62% of elective and 68% of ruptured aneurysm patients, and 80% (elective) and 74% (ruptured) were white. Overall elective patient mortality was 19% at 30 days and 31% at 365 days. There was a steep increase in mortality with increasing age, such that elective 365-day mortality increased from about 18% for patients 50 to 59 years old to 40% for patients 80 to 89 years old. The elective case 31-day to 365-day mortality ranged from 7.8% for the youngest patients to 13.5%. Mortality for ruptured cases was 48.4% at 30 days and 61.5% at 365 days, and these rates also increased with age.

Conclusions.—Our observed 30-day mortality for TAA repairs is consistent with previous reports; however, mortality at 1 year demonstrates a significant risk beyond the initial perioperative period, and this risk increases with age. These data reflect surgical mortality for TAA repair in the general population and may provide more useful data for surgeons and patients contemplating TAA surgery.

▶ This is a sobering analysis. As pointed out by Dr Huber in the invited commentary accompanying this report, it is very unlikely that the 1-year rupture rate for this cohort of patients would have exceeded the 1-year mortality after repair. This is not a good thing for a prophylactic operation. If open TAA repair is really something we should be doing, it needs to be done in regionalized centers where it may be possible for the surgical outcome to "beat" the natural history of the disease and the natural history of the patient population with the disease.

G. L. Moneta, MD

Beyond the aortic bifurcation: Branched endovascular grafts for thoraco-abdominal and aortoiliac aneurysms
Greenberg RK, West K, Pfaff K, et al (Cleveland Clinic Found, Ohio)
J Vasc Surg 43:879-886, 2006

Objectives.—To evaluate the use of novel technology to treat complex aortic aneurysms involving branches that provide critical end-organ blood supply.

Methods.—A prospective study was conducted in patients with thoracoabdominal, suprarenal, or common iliac aneurysms (TAA, SRA, or CIA) at high risk for open surgical repair. An endovascular graft using the Zenith platform was customized to fit patient anatomy (TAA or SRA) and combined with Jomed balloon-expandable stent-grafts. Prefabricated hypogastric branches were used with a Zenith abdominal aortic aneurysm (AAA) or

Fluency self-expanding fenestrated device in conjunction with a self-expanding stent-graft. Analyses were conducted in accordance with the endovascular aneurysm reporting standards document. Follow-up studies occurred at discharge, 1, 6, and 12 months, and included computed tomography and duplex ultrasound scans, and flat plate radiography.

Results.—Fifty patients were treated (9 TAA, 20 SRA, 21 CIA). The mean aneurysm size was 7.6 cm (TAA), 7.2 cm (SRA), and 6.1 cm AAA size associated with a mean CIA size of 3.8 cm. Bilateral CIA aneurysms were present in 86% (18/21) of patients with CIA aneurysms. Perioperative mortality was 2% (1/50) and resulted from a myocardial infarction after a planned conduit and iliac endarterectomy required for device access. Five late deaths occurred (2 TAA, 2 SRA, 1 CIA), three of which (2 TAA, 1 SRA) were aneurysm related. Failure to access internal iliac arteries occurred in three cases, and two late hypogastric branch thromboses occurred. No visceral branches were lost acutely or occluded during follow-up. Sac shrinkage (>5 mm) was noted in 65% of patients at 6 months and in all patients (10/10) by 12 months. There were no ruptures or conversions, but nine patients required secondary interventions.

Conclusions.—Branch vessel technology has made it technically feasible to preserve critical end-organ perfusion in the setting of CIA, SRA, and TAA aneurysms. The relatively low acute mortality rate and lack of short-term branch vessel loss are encouraging and merit further investigation. These advances have the potential to markedly diminish the complications associated with conventional management of complex aneurysms.

▶ Early reports of outcomes using branched and fenestrated devices are beginning to accumulate. Technical success and branch graft patency are extremely high. Secondary procedures are not infrequent, however, and patients need close observation. These procedures are extremely complex and labor intensive. Modification of the current device and techniques will be required if this technique is to be disseminated beyond the expert interventionalist. Lastly, despite an increased number of publications for TAA and iliac branched configurations, great vessels branched/fenestrated "off-the-shelf" devices are currently not available and are not likely to be widely available anytime soon.

G. L. Moneta, MD

Mid-term results of endovascular aneurysm repair with branched and fenestrated endografts
Muhs BE, Verhoeven ELG, Zeebregts CJ, et al (Univ Med Ctr Groningen, The Netherlands; Univ Med Ctr Utrecht, The Netherlands)
J Vasc Surg 44:9-15, 2006

Purpose.—The technique of fenestrated and branched endovascular aneurysm repair (EVAR) has been used for the treatment of a variety of aortic aneurysms. Although technically successful, longer-term results have been

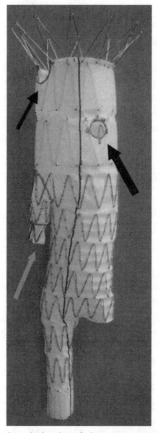

FIGURE 1.—Photograph of a branched endograft demonstrates a small fenestration (*thick arrow*), a scallop (*thin arrow*), and a premade branch (*gray arrow*). (Courtesy of Muhs BE, Verhoeven ELG, Zeebregts CJ, et al. Mid-term results of endovascular aneurysm repair with branched and fenestrated endografts. *J Vasc Surg.* 2006;44:9-15. Copyright 2006 by Elsevier. Reprinted by permission.)

lacking. This article reports on the mid-term results of aneurysm repair with fenestrated and branched endografts from a European center with a large endovascular experience.

Methods.—Between 2001 and 2005, 38 patients were prospectively enrolled in a single institution, investigational device protocol database. Indications for fenestrated or branched EVAR included unfavorable anatomy for traditional EVAR and an abdominal aortic aneurysm >5.5 cm in maximum diameter. Customized stent-grafts were either fenestrated or branched and based on the Zenith system (Fig 1). Data were analyzed on an intention-to-treat basis. Differences between groups were determined using analysis of variance with $P < .05$ considered significant.

Results.—The mean (SD) follow-up was 25.8 ± 12.7 months (median, 25.0 months; range, 9 to 46 months), and no patients were lost to follow-up. All cause mortality was 13% (5/38), with all deaths occurring within the first postoperative year; 30-day mortality was 2.6%. No patient died during the operation. Completion angiography demonstrated successful sealing in 37 of 38 patients and an overall operative visceral vessel perfusion rate of 94% (82/87). Cumulative visceral branch patency was 92% at 46 months. Stent occlusions, when they did occur, all happened within the first postoperative year. All postoperative occlusions occurred in unstented fenestrations or scallops. No occlusions occurred in stented vessels. The difference in serum creatinine preoperatively and postoperatively at 6 months, 1, 2, and 3 years was not significant ($P = $ NS). No patient required dialysis. The aneurysm sac size decreased significantly during the first year and then remained stable ($P < .05$). Limb perfusion as assessed by the ankle/brachial index was not affected by the presence of a fenestrated or branched endograft.

Conclusions.—The intermediate-term results of fenestrated and branched endografts support their continued use in patients with anatomic contraindications for standard EVAR. Close surveillance is mandatory for early identification of visceral or branched vessel stenosis and preocclusion. All cases of failure appear to occur during the first year and then level off in subsequent longer-term follow-up. This includes death, secondary interventions, branch vessel patency, and complications. As the procedure matures, long-term results and randomized clinical trials will ultimately be required to determine the safety, efficacy, and stability of this system.

▶ Early results of fenestrated aortic grafts were associated with an increased risk of renal complications. Concern that aneurysmal morphology changes would increase branch vessel complications may be unfounded beyond the first year. In Europe, where devices have CE approval, patient selection is crucial, and when unfavorable neck anatomy is present, fenestrated or branched devices are being employed. Midterm results support the use of these devices preferentially over current nonfenestrated devices when short (<15 mm), angled, or conical necks are present.

G. L. Moneta, MD

Complex thoracoabdominal aortic aneurysms: Endovascular exclusion with visceral revascularization
Black SA, Wolfe JHN, Clark M, et al (St Mary's Hosp, London)
J Vasc Surg 43:1081-1089, 2006

Objective.—We review our ongoing experience with a transabdominal stent repair of complex thoracoabdominal aneurysms (Crawford type I, II, and III) with surgical revascularization of visceral and renal arteries.

Methods.—A retrospective review was conducted of prospectively collected data from 29 consecutive patients who underwent an attempted visceral hybrid procedure between January 2002 and April 2005. Twenty-two patients were elective, four were urgent (symptomatic), and three were emergent (true rupture). The median patient age was 74 years (range, 37 to 81 years). The aneurysms were Crawford type I in 3, type II in 18, type III in 7,

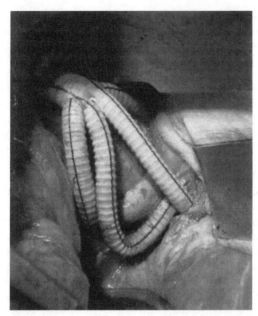

FIGURE 1.—Completed visceral and renal retrograde revascularization grafts show the "lazy C" configuration of the graft to the superior mesenteric artery. (Courtesy of Black SA, Wolfe JHN, Clark M, et al. Complex thoracoabdominal aortic aneurysms: endovascular exclusion with visceral revascularization. *J Vasc Surg.* 2006;43:1081-1089. Copyright 2006 by Elsevier. Reprinted by permission.)

and type IV in 1. Previous aortic surgery had been performed in 13 (45%) of 29 and included aortic valve and root replacement in 3, TAA repair in 1, type I repair in 1), type IV repair in 3, type B dissection in 2, infrarenal aneurysm in 5, and right common iliac aneurysm in 1. Severe preoperative comorbidity was present in 23 (80%) of 29: chronic renal impairment in 5, severe chronic obstructive pulmonary disease in 6, myocardial disease in 11 at New York Heart Association grade II (6) and grade III (5), and Marfan's syndrome in 6. Twenty-six patients (90%) had a completed procedure. In two patients, myocardial instability prevented completion of the procedure despite extensive preoperative cardiac assessment, and in one, poor flow in the true lumen of a chronic type B dissection prevented anastomosis of the revascularization grafts. Exclusion of the full thoracoabdominal aorta was achieved in all 26 completed procedures and extended to include the iliac arteries in four, with revascularization of coeliac in 26, superior mesenteric artery in 26, left renal artery in 21, and right renal artery in 21).

Results.—There was no paraplegia ≤30 days or during inpatient admission, and elective and urgent mortality was 13% (3/23). All of the patients with ruptured thoracoabdominal aneurysms died ≤30 days. Major complications included prolonged respiratory support (>5 days) in 9, inotropic support in 4, renal impairment requiring temporary support in 2 and not requiring support in 2, prolonged ileus in 2, resolved left hemispheric stroke in 1, and resection of an ischemic left colon in 1. Median blood loss was 3.9 liters (range, 1.2 to 13 liters). The median ischemia time was 15 minutes (range, 13 to 27 minutes) for the superior mesenteric and coeliac arteries and 15 minutes for the renal arteries (range, 13 to 21 minutes). The median hospital stay was 27 days (range, 16 to 84 days). Follow-up was a median of 8 months (range, 2 to 31 months), with 92 of 94 grafts patent. Six patients were found to have a type I endoleak. In four, this was a proximal leak, and stent extension in three reduced, but did not cure, the endoleak. One patient with a distal type I endoleak was successfully treated by embolization. Four type II endoleaks resolved without intervention, and one was treated by occlusion coiling of the origin of the left subclavian artery. A single late type III endoleak was found.

Conclusion.—Early results of visceral hybrid stent-grafts for types I, II, and III thoracoabdominal aneurysms are encouraging, with no paraplegia in this particularly high-risk group of patients. These results have encouraged us to perform the new procedure, in preference to open surgery, in Crawford type I, II, and III thoracoabdominal aortic aneurysms (Fig 1).

▶ Except in selected centers, open thoracoabdominal aortic aneurysm repair is associated with a high morbidity and mortality. Hybrid techniques avoid aortic cross-clamping and visceral ischemia, which appear to reduce major complications and paraplegia rates. These are not by any means "cheap shot" operations. These procedures can be long and tedious, but may offer improved results in selected centers. As fenestrated and branched endovascular aneurysm repair continues to improve, these techniques will aid in bridging the gap until the device and technical aspects are improved to allow complete endovascular exclusion to be accomplished.

G. L. Moneta, MD

A Prospective Analysis of Fenestrated Endovascular Grafting: Intermediate-term Outcomes

O'Neill S, Greenberg RK, Haddad F, et al (Cleveland Clinic Found, Ohio)
Eur J Vasc Endovasc Surg 32:115-123, 2006

Purpose.—To assess the intermediate-term outcomes following fenestrated grafting for juxtarenal aneurysms.

Materials and Methods.—A prospective trial was conducted on patients with short proximal necks, who were considered to be high-risk for open repair and unacceptable for conventional endovascular repair. Devices were designed from reconstructed CT data. Follow-up studies included CT, duplex ultrasound, and KUB and occurred at hospital discharge, 1, 6, and 12 months and annually thereafter.

Results.—One hundred and nineteen patients were treated (2001–2005). Mean age and aneurysm size were 75 years and 65 mm, respectively, and 82% were male. A total of 302 visceral vessels were inferior to the fabric seal (a mean of 2.5 vessels per patient), with the most common design incorporating two renal arteries and the SMA (58%). All prostheses were implanted successfully without any acute visceral artery loss. The mean follow-up was 19 months (0–42 months). One patient died within 30 days of device implantation. Kaplan–Meier estimates of survival at 1, 12, 24, and 36 months are 0.99, 0.92, 0.83 and 0.79. There were no ruptures or conversions. Predischarge imaging noted 11 type I and type III endoleaks. The 30-day endoleak rate was 10% (all type II). Aneurysm sac size decreased (>5 mm) in 51, 79 and 77% at 6, 12 and 24 months, respectively. One patient had sac enlargement within the first year, associated with a persistent type II endoleak. In-stent stenoses occurred in 12 renal arteries and one SMA. Six renal arteries and the SMA stenosis were treated and two renal stenoses are awaiting treatment. Ten of 231 stented renal arteries occluded (three prior to discharge), one of which was recanalized. One component separation was treated with an extension at 2 years.

Conclusions.—The placement of endovascular prostheses with graft material incorporating the visceral arteries is safe and appears to be effective at preventing rupture. Continued follow-up to assess the long-term benefit, aneurysm sac behavior and effect of stenting upon the visceral ostia remains critical.

▶ Outside a few selected centers, progress has been slow in the development of fenestrated endovascular grafts. This is likely because the grafts thus far must be individually designed. There is also a high level of technical skill required for successful placement. Acceptance of this technology will require conclusive evidence that the graft body itself does not migrate. As pointed out by the authors, even minimum migration of a fenestrated graft will result in significant renal and mesenteric artery complications.

G. L. Moneta, MD

Hybrid approach to complex thoracic aortic aneurysms in high-risk patients: Surgical challenges and clinical outcomes
Zhou W, Reardon M, Peden EK, et al (Baylor College of Medicine; Methodist Hosp, Houston)
J Vasc Surg 44:688-693, 2006

Background.—Endovascular therapy is a less invasive alternative treatment for high-risk patients with thoracic aortic aneurysms. However, this technology alone is often not applicable to complex aneurysmal morphology. The purpose of this study was to evaluate the utility of hybrid strategies in high-risk patients who are otherwise unsuitable for endovascular therapy alone.

Methods.—During an 18-month period, 31 high-risk patients (mean age, 69 years; range, 52-89 years) underwent combined open and endovascular approaches for complex aneurysms, including 16 patients with ascending and arch aneurysms and 15 patients with aneurysms involving visceral vessels. Among them, 11 patients had histories of aneurysm repairs. To over-

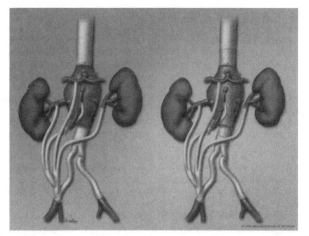

FIGURE 2.—Schematic demonstration of an aortic aneurysm involving visceral branches. Visceral vessel debranching procedures, including iliac to celiac and superior mesenteric artery bypasses and iliac to bilateral renal artery bypasses, were performed to render the endovascular treatment a feasible option. (Courtesy of Zhou W, Reardon M, Peden EK, et al. Hybrid approach to complex thoracic aortic aneurysms in high-risk patients: surgical challenges and clinical outcomes. *J Vasc Surg*. 2006;44:688-693. Copyright 2006 by Elsevier. Reprinted by permission.)

come the anatomic limitations of endovascular repairs, various adjunctive surgical maneuvers were used, including aortic arch reconstruction in 3 patients, supra-aortic trunk debranching in 13 patients (including 8 patients who required aortas as inflow sources), and visceral vessel bypasses in 15 patients (including 10 patients who required bypasses to all 3 visceral branches) (Fig 2). Additionally, carotid artery access was obtained in 1 patient, and iliac artery conduits were created in 12 patients.

Results.—Technical success was achieved in all patients. There was one perioperative death (3.2%) due to postoperative bleeding. Two patients (6.4%) had immediate type II endoleaks, which were resolved by the 1-month follow-up. Other procedure-related complications occurred in three patients (9.6%), including renal bypass thromboses in two patients and retroperitoneal hematoma, which was successfully managed conservatively, in one patient. During a mean follow-up of 16 months, two patients died of unrelated causes, whereas the remainder of patients were asymptomatic, without aneurysm enlargement.

Conclusions.—Our study highlights how hybrid strategies incorporating surgical and endovascular approaches can be used successfully in treating patients with complex thoracic aortic aneurysms. This combined approach potentially expands the field of endovascular stent grafting and is an attractive solution for patients with poor cardiopulmonary reserves.

▶ This is another in a series of articles from one of the major thoracic centers detailing their initial experience with hybrid approaches and touting their benefit in high-risk patients. The only thing lacking is a prospective, randomized trial; however, ethically and practically this would be difficult to accomplish. By the time any such trial could be completed, alternative approaches will hopefully be available. Black et al and O'Neill et al wrote articles closely relating to this one. Black et al wrote about complex thoracoabdominal aortic aneurysms and endovascular exclusion with visceral revascularization,[1] while O'Neill et al wrote about a prospective analysis of fenestrated endovascular grafting and intermediate-term outcomes.[2]

G. L. Moneta, MD

References

1. Black SA, Wolfe JH, Clark M, Hamady M, Cheshire NJ, Jenkins MP. Complex thoracoabdominal aortic aneurysms: endovascular exclusion with visceral revascularization. *J Vasc Surg.* 2006;43:1081-1089.
2. O'Neill S, Greenberg RK, Haddad F, Resch T, Sereika J, Katz E. A prospective analysis of fenestrated endovascular grafting: intermediate-term outcomes. *Eur J Vasc Endovasc Surg.* 2006;32:115-123.

Results of endovascular repair of the thoracic aorta with the Talent Thoracic stent graft: The Talent Thoracic Retrospective Registry
Fattori R, Nienaber CA, Rousseau H, et al (Univ Hosp S Orsola, Bologna, Italy; Univ Hosp Rostock, Germany; Hôpital de Rangueil, Toulouse, France; et al)
J Thorac Cardiovasc Surg 132:332-339, 2006

Background.—Endovascular treatment of thoracic aortic diseases demonstrated low perioperative morbidity and mortality when compared with conventional open repair. Long-term effectiveness of this minimally invasive technique remains to be proven. The Talent Thoracic Retrospective Registry was designed to evaluate the impact of this therapy on patients treated in 7 major European referral centers over an 8-year period.

Methods.—Data from 457 consecutive patients (113 emergency and 344 elective cases) who underwent endovascular thoracic aortic repair with the Medtronic Talent Thoracic stent graft (Medtronic/AVE, Santa Rosa, Calif) were collected. Follow-up analysis (24 ± 19.4 months, range 1-85.1 months) was based on clinical and imaging findings, including all adverse events. To ensure consistency of data interpretation and event reporting, one physician reviewed all adverse events and deaths for the whole cohort of patients. In the case of discrepancies, the treating physicians were queried.

Findings.—Among 422 patients who survived the interventional procedure (in-hospital mortality 5%, 23 patients), mortality during follow-up was 8.5% (36 patients), and in 11 of them the death was related to the aortic disease. Persistent endoleak was reported at imaging follow-up in 64 cases: 44 were primary (9.6%) and 21 occurred during follow-up (4.9%). Seven patients with persistent endoleak had aortic rupture during follow-up, at a variable time from 40 days to 35 months, and all subsequently died. A minor incidence of migration of the stent graft (7 cases), graft fabric alteration (2 cases), and modular disconnection (3 cases) was observed at imaging. Kaplan-Meier overall survival estimate at 1 year was 90.97%, at 3 years was

85.36%, and at 5 years was 77.49%. At the same intervals, freedom from a second procedure (either open conversion or endovascular) was 92.45%, 81.3%, and 70.0%, respectively.

Conclusion.—Endovascular treatment for thoracic aortic disease with the Talent stent graft is associated with low early morbidity and mortality rates also for patients who are at high risk and treated on an emergency basis. Follow-up data indicate a substantial durability of the procedure with a high freedom from related death and secondary interventions.

▶ These are registry data. They are subject to all the limitations of such data. Patients were treated for a variety of acute and chronic conditions. Patients were acquired over 8 years, but more than 3 years of clinical and imaging follow-up was available in only 95 patients. The data suggest that the Talent thoracic aortic stent-graft can be deployed with a reasonable rate of complications for a variety of thoracic pathologies. Further follow-up is obviously required to establish long-term efficacy.

G. L. Moneta, MD

Early outcomes after elective and emergent endovascular repair of the thoracic aorta
Iyer VS, MacKenzie KS, Tse LW, et al (McGill Univ, Montréal)
J Vasc Surg 43:677-683, 2006

Background.—Endovascular treatment of thoracic aortic pathology has emerged as a viable alternative to open surgical repair in both the elective and emergent settings. The aim of this study was to evaluate preoperative work-up, intra-operative strategy, and outcomes of endovascular stent-grafting of the thoracic aorta in patients undergoing elective repair and those undergoing emergent repair.

Methods.—All patient information was obtained by a retrospective review of an established clinical database for all endovascular thoracic stent-graft cases. From October 1999 to August 2005, 70 patients were treated with endovascular stent-grafts for lesions of the thoracic aorta. Thirty-five patients had an elective endovascular procedure, and 35 patients had an emergent procedure.

Results.—Thirty-five patients in the endovascular (EL) group were treated for aneurysm (n = 34) and type B dissection (n = 1). Thirty-five patients in the emergent (EM) group were treated for aneurysm (n = 10), intramural hematoma (n = 10), type B dissection (n = 7), traumatic rupture (n = 7), and aortoesophageal fistula (n = 1). Preoperative angiography was performed in 94.3% (33/35) of EL patients but in only 45.7% (16/35) EM patients ($P < .005$). The EM procedures had significantly shorter operative times, used lower contrast volumes, used fewer stent-graft components (mode 2, range 1 to 5 vs mode 1, range 1 to 3; $P = .02$), and spinal cerebrospinal fluid drains were used significantly less often (82.9% vs 57.1%, $P = .04$). Both groups had similar 30-day morbidity, mortality (0/35 EL vs 1/35

[2.9%] EM, $P = .99$), postoperative endoleak ($9/35$ [25.7%] EL vs $7/35$ [20.0%] EM, $P = .78$), endovascular failure ($3/35$ [8.6%] EL vs $5/35$ [14.3%] EM, $P = .71$), and patient survival.

Conclusion.—There are significant differences in the underlying pathology, preoperative evaluation, and operative course between elective and emergency treatment endovascular procedures for lesions of the thoracic aorta. Endovascular repair of thoracic aortic lesions can be accomplished with low perioperative mortality and morbidity rates, as well as acceptable endoleak and endovascular failure rates for both elective and emergency procedures.

▶ Like most articles that evaluate outcomes for emergent aortic procedures, this report classifies patients treated urgently as having had emergent procedures. This continues to confound the data and makes it difficult to truly analyze results. That having been said, this article, along with several others, is demonstrating the expected improved outcomes for emergent thoracic endovascular aortic repair procedures in most patients, unless multisystem organ failure has occurred before treatment.

G. L. Moneta, MD

Endovascular Thoracic Aortic Repair and Previous or Concomitant Abdominal Aortic Repair: Is the Increased Risk of Spinal Cord Ischemia Real?

Baril DT, Carroccio A, Ellozy SH, et al (Mount Sinai School of Medicine, New York)
Ann Vasc Surg 20:188-194, 2006

Spinal cord ischemia after endovascular thoracic aortic repair remains a significant risk. Previous or concomitant abdominal aortic repair may increase this risk. This investigation reviews the occurrence of spinal cord ischemia after endovascular repair of the descending thoracic aorta in patients with previous or concomitant abdominal aortic repair. Over an 8-year period, 125 patients underwent endovascular exclusion of the thoracic aorta at the Mount Sinai Medical Center. Twenty-eight of these patients had previous or concomitant abdominal aortic repair. The 27 patients who underwent staged repairs all had cerebrospinal fluid (CSF) drainage during and following repair. This population was analyzed for the complication of spinal cord ischemia and factors related to its occurrence. Mean follow-up was 19.3 months (range 1-61). Spinal cord ischemia developed in four of the 28 patients (14.3%) who underwent endovascular thoracic aortic repair with previous or concomitant abdominal aortic repair, while one of 97 patients (1.0%) developed ischemia among the remaining thoracic endograft population. One patient with concomitant abdominal aortic repair developed cord ischemia that manifested 12 hr following the procedure. The remaining three patients with previous abdominal aortic repair developed more delayed-onset paralysis ranging from the third postoperative day to 7 weeks following repair. Irreversible cord ischemia occurred in three patients, with full recovery in one patient. Major complications from CSF drainage occurred in one patient (3.7%). Spinal cord ischemia occurred at a markedly higher rate in patients with previous or concomitant abdominal aortic repair. This risk continued beyond the immediate postoperative period. The benefit of perioperative and salvage CSF drainage remains to be determined.

▶ Many patients undergoing thoracic endovascular aortic repair have undergone prior abdominal aortic aneurysm (AAA) repair or have concomitant AAAs. This article adds additional data, suggesting that these patients have a higher incidence of paraplegia compared with those without prior AAA repairs. Despite close blood pressure monitoring and CSF drainage, this dreaded complication cannot be completely eliminated and may occur even weeks after the procedure. Careful attention should be directed towards evaluating the contribution of blood flow to the spinal cord from the vertebral and hypogastric arteries, as well as the visceral ischemic impact, along with the extent of aorta being treated.

G. L. Moneta, MD

Coverage of the left subclavian artery during thoracic endovascular aortic repair
Riesenman PJ, Farber MA, Mendes RR, et al (Univ of North Carolina, Chapel Hill)
J Vasc Surg 45:90-95, 2007

Background.—Thoracic aortic stent grafts require proximal and distal landing zones of adequate length to effectively exclude thoracic aortic lesions. The origins of the left subclavian artery and other aortic arch branch vessels often impose limitations on the proximal landing zone, thereby disallowing endovascular repair of more proximal thoracic lesions.

Methods.—Between October 2000 and November 2005, 112 patients received stent grafts to treat lesions involving the thoracic aorta. The proximal aspect of the stent graft partially or totally occluded the origin of at least one great vessel in 28 patients (25%). The proximal attachment site was in zone 0 in one patient (3.6%), zone 1 in three patients (10.7%), and zone 2 in 24 patients (85.7%). Patients with proximal implantation in zones 0 or 1 underwent debranching procedures of the supra-aortic vessels before stent graft repair. In one patient who underwent zone 1 deployment, the left subclavian artery was revascularized before stent graft deployment. Among patients who underwent zone 2 deployment with partial or complete occlusion of the left subclavian artery, none underwent prior revascularization. Patients were assessed postoperatively and at follow-up for development of neurologic symptoms as well as symptoms of left upper extremity claudication or ischemia.

Results.—Mean follow-up was 7.3 months. Among the 24 patients with zone 2 implantation, 10 (42%) had partial left subclavian artery coverage at the time of their primary procedure. A total of 19 patients experienced complete cessation of antegrade flow through the origin of the left subclavian artery without revascularization at the time of the initial endograft repair as a result of a secondary procedure or as a consequence of left subclavian artery thrombosis. Left upper extremity symptoms developed in three (15.8%) patients that did not warrant intervention, and rest pain developed in one (5.3%), which was treated with the deployment of a left subclavian artery stent. Two primary (type IA and type III) endoleaks (7.1%) and one secondary endoleak (type IA) (3.6%) were observed in patients who underwent zone 2 deployment. Three cerebrovascular accidents were observed. Thoracic aortic lesions were successfully excluded in all patients who underwent supra-aortic debranching procedures.

Conclusion.—Intentional coverage of the origin of the left subclavian artery to obtain an adequate proximal landing zone during endovascular repair of thoracic aortic lesions is well tolerated and may be managed expectantly, with some exceptions.

▶ The debate concerning left subclavian artery revascularization continues. From an ischemic upper extremity standpoint, coverage is tolerated extremely well, and routine revascularization is not warranted except in certain instances. However, 2 other complications can occur and must be factored into the patient's treatment. First, there is a higher incidence of stroke when device implantation occurs in more proximal zones. There are, however, no data suggesting that left subclavian artery revascularization decreases this risk. Second, the vertebral artery can contribute to spinal cord perfusion, and some recent data suggest that there may be reduced spinal cord ischemia by maintaining antegrade left subclavian artery flow.

G. L. Moneta, MD

Utility of left subclavian artery revascularization in association with endoluminal repair of acute and chronic thoracic aortic pathology

Peterson BG, Eskandari MK, Gleason TG, et al (Northwestern Univ, Chicago)
J Vasc Surg 43:433-439, 2006

Background.—A rapidly increasing number of thoracic aortic lesions are now treated by endoluminal exclusion by using stent grafts. Many of these lesions abut the great vessels and limit the length of the proximal landing zone. Various methods have been used to address this issue. We report our experience with subclavian artery revascularization in association with endoluminal repair of acute and chronic thoracic aortic pathology.

Methods.—Thirty (43%) of 70 patients undergoing thoracic endovascular stent-graft placement from January 2001 to August 2005 had lesions adjacent to or involving the origin of the subclavian artery. The mean age was 62 years (range, 22-85 years; 63% were men, and 37% were women). This subgroup of 30 patients had indications for repair that included thoracic aortic aneurysm (n = 15), traumatic transection (n = 6), chronic dissection with pseudoaneurysm (n = 5), and acute dissection with intramural hematoma (n = 4). All 30 patients had the subclavian origin covered by the stent graft. In eight cases (27%), no effort was made to revascularize the subclavian artery before or during the endograft placement procedure. Twenty-three (77%) of 30 patients underwent subclavian to carotid artery transposition (n = 21) or bypass (n = 2) before (n = 12; average of 14 days before stent-graft placement), concomitant with (n = 10), or after (n = 1) the endovascular procedure. Physical examination and computed tomography scans were performed after surgery at 1, 6, and 12 months and annually thereafter. The mean follow-up was 18 months (range, 1-51 months).

Results.—Five acute complications occurred in the eight patients (63%) who had the subclavian artery covered without pre-endograft revascularization and included four patients who experienced stroke (accounting for the only death) and one patient who developed symptomatic subclavian-vertebral steal that necessitated transposition 7 months later. Two (9%) of the 23 patients who had subclavian revascularization experienced left-sided vocal cord palsies, and 1 patient (4%) developed lower extremity paraparesis secondary to spinal cord ischemia. No late endoleaks related to retrograde sac perfusion from the most distal great vessel have been identified in any patient.

Conclusions.—Subclavian revascularization procedures can be performed with relatively low risk. Complications are rare, and patient recovery is rapid. Although this is not necessary in all cases, we advocate subclavian to carotid transposition when the aortic lesion is within 15 mm of the left subclavian orifice to prevent type II endoleak or perfusion of a dissected false lumen when the ipsilateral vertebral artery is patent and dominant or when coronary revascularization using an ipsilateral internal mammary artery is anticipated and in cases that necessitate extensive coverage of intercostals that contribute to spinal cord perfusion. Carotid to subclavian artery bypass should be reserved for patients with a patent internal mammary artery conduit perfusing a coronary vessel and should be combined with proximal subclavian ligation.

▶ This is another article discussing the benefits and risks of left subclavian artery revascularization associated with thoracic endovascular aortic repair. One thing is certain; if the left vertebral artery is the dominant artery to the posterior circulation, then coverage without prior revascularization can lead to devastating stroke. While these authors advocate transposition over bypass because of its superior patency, this is not necessarily true. Patency is also impacted by disease process, and these patients are having the procedure performed for proximal landing zone lengthening, not for occlusive disease.

G. L. Moneta, MD

Endoleaks after endovascular repair of thoracic aortic aneurysms

Parmer SS, Carpenter JP, Stavropoulos SW, et al (Univ of Pennsylvania, Philadelphia)
J Vasc Surg 44:447-452, 2006

Objective.—Endoleaks are one of the unique complications seen after endovascular repair of thoracic aortic aneurysms (TEVAR). This investigation was performed to evaluate the incidence and determinants of endoleaks, as well as the outcomes of secondary interventions in patients with endoleaks, after TEVAR.

Methods.—Over a 6-year period, 105 patients underwent TEVAR in the context of pivotal Food and Drug Administration trials with the Medtronic Talent (n = 64) and Gore TAG (n = 41) devices. The medical and radiology records of these patients were reviewed for this retrospective study. Of these, 69 patients (30 women and 39 men) had follow-up longer than 1 month and were used for this analysis. The patients were evaluated for the presence of an endoleak, endoleak type, aneurysm expansion, and endoleak intervention.

Results.—The mean follow-up in this patient cohort was 17.3 ± 14.7 months (range, 3-71 months). Endoleaks were detected in 29% (20/69) of patients, of which 40% (8/20) were type I, 35% (7/20) were type II, 20% (4/20) were type III, and 5% (1/20) had more than one type of endoleak (Fig 1). Patients without endoleaks experienced greater aneurysm sac regression than those with endoleaks (-2.89 ± 9.1 mm vs -0.13 ± 7.2 mm), although this difference was not statistically significant ($P = .232$). All but 2 endoleaks (90%; 18/20) were detected on the initial postoperative computed tomographic scan at 30 days. Two endoleaks (10%; 2/20) developed late. The endoleak group had more extensive aneurysms with significantly larger aneurysms at the time of intervention (69.4 ± 10.5 mm vs 60.6 ± 11.0 mm; $P = .003$). Factors predictive of endoleak included male sex ($P = .016$), larger aneurysm size ($P = .003$), the length of aorta treated by stent grafts ($P = .0004$), and an increasing number of stents used ($P < .0001$). No open conversions were performed for treatment of endoleaks. Four (50%) of the eight type I endoleaks were successfully repaired by using endovascular techniques. None of the type II endoleaks was treated by secondary intervention. During follow-up, the maximum aneurysm diameter in the type II endoleak patients increased a mean of 2.94 ± 7.2 mm (range, -4.4 to 17 mm). Spontaneous thrombosis has occurred in 29% (2/7) of the type II endoleaks. Patients with type III endoleaks experienced a decrease in mean maximal aneurysm diameter of 0.78 ± 3.1 mm during follow-up.

Conclusions.—Endoleaks are not uncommon after TEVAR. Many type I endoleaks may be treated successfully by endovascular means. Short-term follow-up suggests that observational management of type II endoleaks is associated with continued sac expansion, and these patients should be monitored closely.

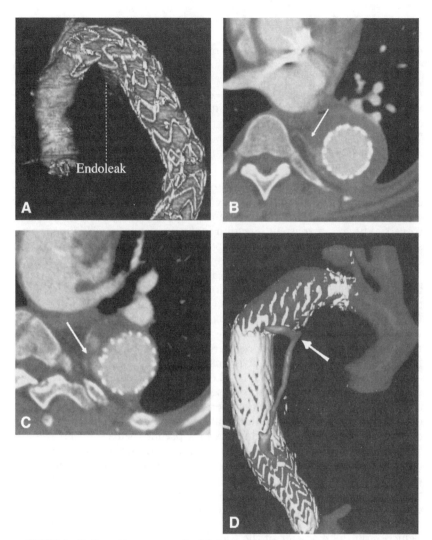

FIGURE 1.—Radiographic appearance of endoleaks. A, Three-dimensional reconstruction demonstrating a proximal type I endoleak. B, A type II endoleak is demonstrated on computed tomographic angiography with contrast filling the aneurysm sac and in communication with an intercostal artery (*arrow*). C, A type III endoleak between endograft components (*arrow*) is demonstrated on computed tomographic angiography. D, Three-dimensional reconstruction of the type III endoleak depicted in C. The aneurysm sac and contained thrombus are not included in the reconstructed image. (Courtesy of Parmer SS, Carpenter JP, Stavropoulos SW, et al. Endoleaks after endovascular repair of thoracic aortic aneurysms. *J Vasc Surg.* 2006;44:447-452. Copyright 2006 by Elsevier. Reprinted by permission.)

▶ The distribution and behavior of endoleaks is, not surprisingly, similar for thoracic aortic aneurysms as compared with abdominal aortic aneurysms. While this series demonstrates that larger aneurysms, as well as those requiring extensive coverage and multiple stents, are at increased risk for endoleak, it would have been an added benefit to the reader to evaluate whether neck diameter or attachment neck length impacted the incidence of endoleaks. Similar to endovascular repair of abdominal aortic aneurysms the significance and management of type II endoleaks remain controversial.

G. L. Moneta, MD

Endovascular stent graft repair for infected thoracic aortic pseudoaneurysms—a durable option?
Ting ACW, Cheng SWK, Ho P, et al (Univ of Hong Kong, China)
J Vasc Surg 44:701-705, 2006

Objective.—Open surgical repair for infected thoracic aortic pseudoaneurysms carries significant mortality and morbidity. Endovascular stent graft repair has been our preferred approach, although its role remains controversial because persistent infection is always a concern. We aimed to assess the efficacy and durability of endovascular stent graft repair in these patients.

Methods.—Between August 2000 and November 2005, seven consecutive patients with eight infected pseudoaneurysms of the thoracic aorta were treated with endovascular stent graft repair. Patients were diagnosed based on a typical appearance of an infected pseudoaneurysm on imaging together with a positive bacteriology culture or clinical evidence of sepsis. The follow-up protocol included regular clinical examination, hematologic tests, and computed tomography scans.

Results.—There were six men and one woman with a median age of 68 years at operation. Three patients presented with an aortoenteric fistula. The operations were performed in the operating room with the image guidance of a mobile C-arm. Endovascular stent grafts were deployed successfully in all patients, with complete exclusion of the pseudoaneurysms. Intravenous antibiotics were continued for 1 to 6 weeks and followed by lifelong maintenance oral antibiotics. The median hospital stay was 27 days, with no hospital deaths. No paraplegia or other major complications occurred. Two patients with aortoesophageal fistula where the fistula tracts were persistent died during follow-up. The other five patients remained well, with no evidence of graft infection at a median follow-up of 34 months. A significant reduction in the diameter of the pseudoaneurysm (>5 mm) was noted on computed tomography scans after 12 months.

Conclusion.—Endovascular stent graft repair is effective and may be a durable option for infected pseudoaneurysms of the thoracic aorta.

▶ Endovascular repair of infected thoracic aortic is definitely possible and may reduce the major complications associated with open repair either by extra-anatomic or in situ reconstruction and surgical debridement. However, if debridement of grossly infected tissue or cessation of continued contamination does not occur, sepsis will usually ensue at a later date, as seen in this article in 2 individuals. If surgical debridement is not possible, then percutaneous drainage can be performed to control sepsis, and fistulas can be closed by various minimally invasive techniques to reduce the risk of ongoing contamination. It should not be necessary to reemphasize that these patients should remain on lifelong antibiotics, and long-term complications will not be entirely a surprise.

G. L. Moneta, MD

Timing of endovascular repair of blunt traumatic thoracic aortic transections
Reed AB, Thompson JK, Crafton CJ, et al (Univ of Cincinnati, Ohio)
J Vasc Surg 43:684-688, 2006

Background.—Patients with blunt traumatic thoracic aortic transection (BTTAT) just distal to the takeoff of the left subclavian artery typically have concomitant injuries that make open emergent surgical repair highly risky. Over the past decade, endovascular repair of the injured thoracic aorta with commercially available and custom-made covered stents has developed as a viable option, with reported decreases in short-term morbidity and mortality. If active extravasation of contrast from the injured thoracic aorta is not appreciated on chest computed tomography scan, other concurrent injuries of the head, abdomen, and extremities can often be repaired with careful control of blood pressure. The timing of endovascular repair of the traumatic thoracic aortic transection, however, often comes into question, particularly with the presence of fever, pneumonia, or bacteremia. We sought to identify a time frame during which endovascular repair of BTTAT could safely be performed.

Methods.—Age, concomitant injuries, time from trauma to repair, type of device, and major outcomes were recorded.

Results.—Over a 5-year period (January 2000 to March 2005), 51 patients presented with BTTAT. Twenty-seven (52.9%) patients with BTTAT died shortly after arrival. Of the remaining 24, 9 underwent emergent open repair, with 1 intraoperative death. Two delayed open repairs were performed. Thirteen patients with BTTAT underwent delayed endovascular repair. Successful endovascular repair of BTTAT was performed in all 13 patients, with no intraoperative deaths. Seven patients were treated with commercial devices and six with custom-made covered stents. None of the repairs was performed emergently. The timing of repair ranged from 1 day to 7 months (median, 6 days), and all patients were treated aggressively with β-blockade before surgery. One patient was discharged from the hospital and underwent elective repair at a later date. Three patients died in the postoperative period (30 days): two from multisystem organ failure and one from iliac artery complications encountered at the time of device deployment. The remaining 10 patients were successfully discharged to a rehabilitation facility.

Conclusions.—The opportunity to successfully perform endovascular repair of BTTAT may be possible many days after the initial injury in the hemodynamically stable trauma patient.

▶ The authors suggest that delayed repair of blunt aortic injuries in selected patients may be safe if blood pressure and heart rate can be controlled, which is not always guaranteed. This approach was adopted by many centers for minor intimal injuries of the aorta because of the significant morbidity and mortality of emergent open repair. One must realize, however, that thoracic endovascular aortic repair (TEVAR) for blunt aortic trauma with appropriate-sized devices has a lower complication rate than watchful waiting (2%) in these circumstances. In light of this, the only reason to delay repair would be to treat other more life-threatening conditions, or if the vascular specialist believes that the long-term result of TEVAR for blunt aortic trauma does not warrant performance of the procedure.

G. L. Moneta, MD

The Elephant Trunk Technique for Stage Repair of Complex Aneurysms of the Entire Thoracic Aorta
LeMaire SA, Carter SA, Coselli JS (Texas Heart Inst, Houston; Baylor College of Medicine)
Ann Thorac Surg 81:1561-1569, 2006

Background.—Extensive thoracic aortic aneurysms that involve the ascending, arch, and descending segments require challenging repairs associated with substantial morbidity and mortality. The purpose of this report is to evaluate contemporary outcomes after surgical repair of extensive thoracic aortic aneurysms using a two-stage approach with the elephant trunk technique.

Methods.—During a 15½ -year period, 148 consecutive patients underwent total aortic arch replacement using the elephant trunk technique. Seventy-six of these patients (51%, 76/148) returned for second-stage repair of the descending thoracic or thoracoabdominal aorta 4.9 ± 7.5 months after the first stage.

Results.—Operative mortality after the proximal aortic stage was 12% (18/148). Seven patients (5%) had strokes. Among the patients who subsequently underwent distal aortic repair, operative mortality was 4% (3/76). Two patients (3%) developed paraplegia. Long-term survival after completing the second stage of repair was 70 ± 6% at 5 years and 59 ± 7% at 8 years.

Conclusions.—Contemporary management of extensive thoracic aortic aneurysms using the two-stage elephant trunk technique yields acceptable short-term and long-term outcomes. This technique remains an important component of the surgical armamentarium.

▶ This article represents an extensive experience with thoracoabdominal aortic aneurysms. These detailed outcome results serve as a basis for which future endovascular therapies will be compared and include stroke, paraplegia, and mortality associated with the elephant trunk repair. As endovascular therapies develop, it will be important to see whether modifications in surgical techniques develop to help accommodate and plan future procedures that may involve endovascular methods.

G. L. Moneta, MD

Midterm results of extensive primary repair of the thoracic aorta by means of total arch replacement with open stent graft placement for an acute type A aortic dissection
Uchida N, Ishihara H, Shibamura H, et al (Hiroshima-city Asa Gen Hosp, Japan)
J Thorac Cardiovasc Surg 131:862-867, 2006

Objectives.—We sought to describe the midterm results of extensive primary repair of the thoracic aorta by means of the modified elephant trunk technique with a stent graft for acute type A aortic dissection, particularly the changes of the false lumen shown by enhanced computed tomographic scanning.

Methods.—The subjects were 35 consecutive patients who received arch replacement with open stent grafting for type A acute aortic dissection between December 1997 and April 2002. The mean follow-up period was 55 months (range, 30-83 months). Computed tomographic scanning was performed at 1, 3, 12, and 36 months postoperatively to detect thrombosis and obliteration of the false lumen after its exclusion by the stent graft (Fig 1). The diameter of the aorta was measured at 3 levels: the distal edge of the stent graft, the diaphragm, and the origin of the superior mesenteric artery.

Results.—Two patients died in the initial operation, but no patients required additional surgical treatment of the thoracic aorta. The mean diameter of the stent grafts was 26.2 mm, and the mean length was 8.9 cm. Thrombus formation in the false lumen was recognized at the distal edge of the graft in all patients, at the diaphragmatic level in 26 patients, and at the superior mesenteric artery level in 15 patients. Obliteration of the false lumen was recognized at the distal edge of the graft in all patients, at the diaphragmatic level in 20 patients, and at the superior mesenteric artery level in 15 patients. The aorta distal to the stent graft showed minimal changes.

Conclusions.—In patients with acute type A aortic dissections, it is possible to perform extensive primary repair of the thoracic aorta with relative safety by using a synthetic graft with a self-expanding stent, and this method might reduce the necessity of further operations not only for the distal descending aorta but also for the thoracoabdominal aorta.

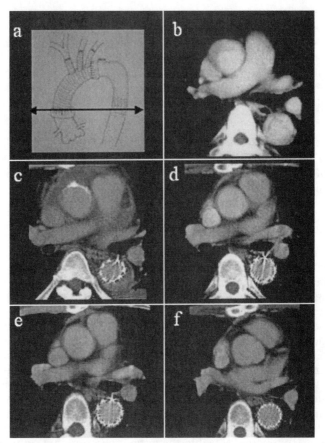

FIGURE 1.—Postoperative CT follow-up study. A, Level examined: edge of the stent graft. B, Preoperative findings. C, One month postoperatively. D, Three months postoperatively. E, One year postoperatively. F, Three years postoperatively. (Courtesy of Uchida N, Ishihara H, Shibamura H, Yoshiki K, Ozawa M. Midterm results of extensive primary repair of the thoracic aorta by means of total arch replacement with open stent graft placement for an acute type A aortic dissection. *J Thorac Cardiovasc Surg.* 2006;131:862-867. Copyright 2006 with permission from The American Association for Thoracic Surgery.)

▶ This is a clever use of the combination of endovascular and open surgery. It is essentially a 1-step elephant trunk procedure. The technique appears to represent a significant advance over a 2-stage open repair of type A aortic dissection. Hopefully, this approach can significantly reduce the number of patients requiring late descending thoracic aortic repair after the repair of type A dissection.

G. L. Moneta, MD

Combined surgical and endovascular treatment of aortic arch aneurysms
Saleh HM, Inglese L (Ain Shams Univ, Cairo; S Donato Hosp, Milan, Italy)
J Vasc Surg 44:460-466, 2006

Background.—Traditional repair of aortic arch aneurysms requires cardiopulmonary bypass, hypothermia, and circulatory arrest and is associated with considerable morbidity and mortality. Endovascular stent-graft placement has developed as a safe and effective treatment for various diseases of the descending aorta and, recently, even in delicate anatomic regions such as the aortic arch. The aim of this study is to review our clinical experience with endovascular treatment of aortic arch aneurysms after surgical transposition of supra-aortic vessels (Fig 1).

Methods.—Fifteen patients received thoracic stent-graft implants after aortic debranching for repair of aortic arch aneurysms during the 3-year period ending December 31, 2005. All patients were not candidates for stan-

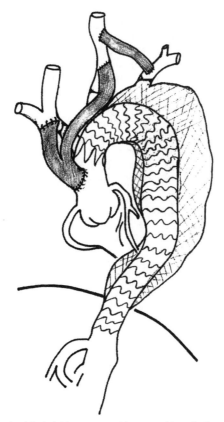

FIGURE 1.—Schematic of the hybrid treatment with transposition of epiaortic vessels, banding of ascending aorta and deployment of an endograft. (Courtesy of Saleh HM, Inglese L. Combined surgical and endovascular treatment of aortic arch aneurysms. *J Vasc Surg.* 2006;44:460-466. Copyright 2006 by Elsevier. Reprinted by permission.)

dard endovascular repair due to inadequate proximal landing zones on the aortic arch. Device design and implant strategy were determined by an evaluation of aortic morphology with angiography and computed tomography (CT) scanning. Stent-grafts were used to repair the arch after supra-aortic vessel transposition was performed. The endografts were implanted transfemorally or via an iliac Dacron conduit graft using standardized endovascular techniques. Follow-up was 100% complete (mean, 18 ± 2.5 months; range, 12 to 36 months). Outcome variables included death and treatment failure (endoleak, aortic rupture, reintervention, or aortic-related or sudden death). Follow-up included clinical examination, chest radiograph, and CT at discharge, 6 months after stent-graft placement, and yearly thereafter.

Results.—Stent-graft deployment success was 100% after staged supra-aortic vessel transposition. Patency of all endografts and conventional bypasses was 100%. No endoleak or graft migration was observed. There were no neurologic complications. One patient died 2 months after the procedure from pulmonary complications.

Conclusion.—Repair of aortic arch aneurysms by sequential transposition of the supra-aortic branches and endovascular stent-graft placement is feasible. Extended application of this technique will enable safe and effective treatment of a highly selected subgroup of patients with aortic aneurysms by avoiding conventional arch aneurysm repair in deep hypothermia and circulatory arrest.

▶ This represents one of the larger series of great vessel relocation to facilitate thoracic endovascular aortic aneurysm repair. It is surprising that no neurologic complications were identified given the increased risk with more proximal implantation. The optimal method for conducting these procedures—simultaneous, sequential, antegrade, retrograde, with or without cerebral bypass—remains to be determined. However, one thing appears to be certain; compared with hypothermic arrest and repair, the morbidity and mortality are reduced.

G. L. Moneta, MD

11 Leg Ischemia

High prevalence of proximal claudication among patients with patent aortobifemoral bypasses
Jacquinandi V, Picquet J, Bouyé P, et al (Univ Hosp of Angers, France)
J Vasc Surg 45:312-318, 2007

Background.—Proximal (ie, buttock, hip) claudication can result from impaired perfusion in the hypogastric area after aortobifemoral bypass (ABF) despite normal femorodistal blood flow provided by the patent bypass. The proportion of patients that experience proximal claudication after ABF is unknown, and arguments for the vascular origin of symptoms specifically at the proximal level have never been reported.

Methods.—This was a prospective study set in an institutional practice of ambulatory patients referred for a systematic survey of their previous ABF bypass. Among the 131 eligible patients, 10 refused to participate and 16 were unable to walk on a treadmill. The 105 studied patients (94 men, 11 women) were a mean age of 63 ± 10 years, and the median delay from surgery was 2 years (range, 4 months to 26 years). We used a modified version of the San Diego Claudication Questionnaire administered both at rest before the treadmill study and again after the treadmill test. Transcutaneous oxygen pressure ($TcPO_2$) at the buttock level was used to evaluate blood flow impairment during exercise at the proximal level, with blood flow impairment defined as buttock minus chest $TcPO_2$ decrease in excess of −15 mm Hg.

Results.—Thirty patients reported proximal exercise-related pain consistent with vascular criteria by history before exercise. However, 59 patients (56%) reported symptoms compatible with proximal claudication, and $TcPO_2$ values were abnormal on one or both sides in 52. The persistence of at least one (prograde or retrograde) pathway to the hypogastric circulation, determined by review of operative details from the aortobifemoral bypass and angiography, did not significantly decrease the proportion of patients reporting proximal claudication by history (26%) or on treadmill (55%) compared with those with bilateral hypogastric occlusion (33% by history, $P = .51$ compared with at least one prograde hypogastric pathway and 61% based on treadmill test, $P = .65$ compared with at least one prograde hypogastric pathway).

Conclusion.—The present study shows that (1) the proportion of ABF patients with a median bypass age of 2 years that report proximal claudication is high (28%), (2) this proportion is significantly higher when claudication is detected by treadmill exercise tests, (3) a vascular origin (or at least contribution) is likely 88% of the proximal symptoms observed on treadmill, (4) the presence of proximal claudication with associated abnormal $TcPO_2$ results increases the risk of walking impairment in affected patients, and (5) preservation of at least one internal iliac artery to allow prograde or retrograde flow to the hypogastric vascular bed does not decrease the risk of proximal claudication after ABF surgery. A vascular origin of (or at least contribution to) most of the proximal exercise-related symptoms should always be discussed in patients with patent ABF bypass.

▶ This article certainly calls into question a number of our basic tenets regarding ABF grafting for occlusive disease. Tenet 1: ABF grafting cures claudication; actually, no. One quarter of the patients here have buttock and hip exercise-induced symptoms and more than 50% have treadmill and transcutaneous PO_2 abnormalities. Tenet 2: Residual symptoms in patients with patent ABF grafts are not due to vascular disease; actually not. Nearly all are secondary to vascular disease. Tenet 3: Preservation of a hypogastric artery is important in preventing hip and buttock symptoms after ABF bypass grafting; actually, not really. It did not seem to matter in this article. It is sort of amazing what you see when you look. Yogi was correct!

G. L. Moneta, MD

Percutaneous angioplasty of the superior gluteal artery for buttock claudication: A report of seven cases and literature review
Batt M, Baque J, Bouillanne P-J, et al (Hôpital Saint-Roch, Nice, France)
J Vasc Surg 43:987-991, 2006

Background.—Buttock claudication due to stenosis or occlusion of the superior gluteal artery is infrequent. The recent development of noninvasive gluteal duplex scanning, combined with aortoiliac angiography using oblique projections and the availability of low-profile devices for percutaneous transluminal angioplasty (PTA), led us to review our recent experience concerning the diagnosis and mid-term results of PTA for superior gluteal artery stenosis or occlusion.

Methods.—The files of all patients who had been treated in our department by PTA for superior gluteal artery stenosis or occlusion with buttock claudication were analyzed retrospectively, and any associated arterial lesions, morbidity, restenosis, or recurrent buttock claudication were noted. Outcomes were compared with published reports.

Results.—Retrospective review identified six patients (5 men, 1 woman; mean age, 64 years) with seven cases of buttock claudication (1 bilateral localization) who had undergone PTA within the past 2 years. There was no case of isolated buttock claudication. Buttock claudication was associated with impotence, thigh claudication, or calf claudication in seven cases. Gluteal duplex scans were performed for three of the patients diagnosed with

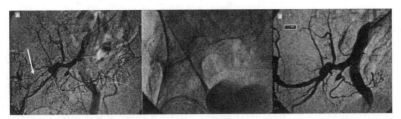

FIGURE 2.—Recanalization with percutaneous angioplasty for superior gluteal artery occlusion (*arrow*). (Reprinted by permission of the publisher from Batt M, Baque J, Bouillanne P-J, et al. Percutaneous angioplasty of the superior gluteal artery for buttock claudication: a report of seven cases and literature review. *J Vasc Surg.* 2006;43:987-991.)

two stenoses and one occlusion. Aortoiliac angiography revealed five superior gluteal artery stenoses and two occlusions (Fig 2). PTA without stenting was successful in all cases, without morbidity or mortality. During a mean follow-up of 13 months, restenosis occurred in one patient. A repeat PTA without stenting was successful, with resolution of the buttock claudication.

Conclusions.—Buttock claudication due to superior gluteal artery stenosis is probably underestimated when gluteal duplex scanning and aortoiliac angiography with oblique projections are not performed. PTA gives good results, and the procedure can be repeated should restenosis occur.

▶ Although not common, there are certainly some patients with buttock claudication on the basis of internal iliac artery occlusion or stenosis. However, I must admit I had not before considered superior gluteal artery disease alone as a source of buttock claudication. Perhaps this is an unrecognized problem: it is 29% of the patients with buttock claudication in these authors' experience. Another alternative is that this is a "regional disease" endemic to the authors' institution. The authors postulate essentially mechanical damage of the superior gluteal artery in the gluteal canal. It is interesting to speculate that perhaps this is the cause of continued claudication of some of the patients described in the previous abstract.

G. L. Moneta, MD

Variability in Responsiveness to Clopidogrel in Patients with Intermittent Claudication

Cassar K, Bachoo P, Ford I, et al (Univ of Aberdeen, Scotland, England)
Eur J Vasc Endovasc Surg 32:71-75, 2006

Objective.—The concept of clopidogrel resistance is frequently evoked in the cardiac literature. The variability of antiplatelet response in patients with intermittent claudication has not been investigated. The aim of this study was to describe the effect of the addition of clopidogrel to aspirin using *ex vivo* measures of platelet activation in patients with life-style limiting intermittent claudication.

Design of Study.—Data from randomised controlled trial.

Materials.—Data from 67 patients with intermittent claudication taking part in a randomised controlled trial and who received clopidogrel in addition to aspirin was analysed.

Methods.—Platelet activation was measured using whole-blood flow cytometric measurement of ADP-stimulated fibrinogen binding at baseline and 12h after administration of a loading dose of 300 mg clopidogrel. Patients continued to receive 75 mg clopidogrel daily for 30 days and platelet activation was again measured at day 30. Compliance with treatment was assessed by counting returned tablets.

Results.—Six patients were excluded from analysis because of incomplete compliance with treatment. Six of the sixty-one patients (9.8%) showed no reduction in platelet activation 12 h after administration of the loading dose of clopidogrel. At 30 days these six patients still showed no response to clopidogrel. Amongst the remaining 55 patients, the mean reduction in fibrinogen binding after clopidogrel administration was 51.5% (95% CI: 43.8–59.2). Amongst responders there was a wide variability in reduction of fibrinogen binding in response to clopidogrel (range 8.11–97.7%). Four of these patients (6.6%) showed a reduction of more than 95% in fibrinogen binding.

Conclusions.—Patients with intermittent claudication show a wide variability in their response to clopidogrel. While a small proportion of these patients shows no response at all, another small group appears to respond excessively to clopidogrel. Clinical studies are required to identify whether hyper-responders are at increased risk of bleeding complications and whether hyporesponders are at a higher risk of thrombotic events.

▶ The results of this study are not all that surprising. All subgroups of patients studied previously have shown variable response to both aspirin and clopidogrel administration. The implication of data such as this is that patients who have cardiovascular events on aspirin or clopidogrel therapy should perhaps be tested as to whether the drug itself is actually inducive of antiplatelet affects in that particular patient.

G. L. Moneta, MD

The Novel Phosphodiesterase Inhibitor NM-702 Improves Claudication-Limited Exercise Performance in Patients With Peripheral Arterial Disease
Brass EP, Anthony R, Cobb FR, et al (Harbor-UCLA Med Ctr, Torrance, Calif; Catalyst Pharmaceutical Research, Inc, Pasadena, Calif; Nissan Chemical America, Pasadena, Calif; et al)
J Am Coll Cardiol 48:2539-2545, 2006

Objectives.—The current study tested the hypothesis that NM-702 improves treadmill exercise performance in peripheral arterial disease patients with claudication-limited exercise performance.

Background.—Patients with claudication experience significant disability, owing to their exercise limitation. Therapeutic options to improve exercise performance in these patients are limited. NM-702 is a novel drug that inhibits phosphodiesterase as well as thromboxane A_2 synthase.

Methods.—This study was a randomized, multi-center, placebo-controlled, double-blind trial. Patients were randomized to receive 24 weeks of twice-daily treatment with either placebo (intent to treat population, n = 130), 4 mg NM-702 (n = 126), or 8 mg NM-702 (n = 130).

Results.—After 24 weeks of treatment, 8 mg NM-702 was associated with a statistically significant increased peak walking time on a graded treadmill as compared with placebo (p = 0.004). Peak walking time after 24 weeks was increased by 17.1 ± 49.0% in the placebo arm, 22.1 ± 60.1% in the 4-mg NM-702 arm, and 28.1 ± 50.5% in the 8-mg NM-702 arm. NM-702 at the 8-mg dose for 24 weeks was associated with statistically significant improvements in the treadmill claudication onset time as compared with placebo. In addition, as compared with placebo, NM-702 improved the physical component and physical functioning scores of the Medical Outcomes Study 36-Item Short Form and the walking distance and stair climbing domains of the Walking Impairment Questionnaire. NM-702 was generally well tolerated, but adverse events typical of vasodilators were common.

Conclusions.—NM-702 used for 24 weeks by patients with claudication was associated with improvements in laboratory- and ambulatory-based exercise performance.

▶ The 8 mg NM-702 dosage was associated with a magnitude of improvement in both treadmill performance and questionnaire assessments similar to that of cilostazol. This suggests NM-702 produces potentially clinically meaningful changes. Like cilostazol, NM-702 is a phosphodiesterase inhibitor. Inhibition of phosphodiesterase may, therefore, be a reasonable target mechanism for drug therapy for intermittent claudication.

G. L. Moneta, MD

Natural history of limbs with arterial insufficiency and chronic ulceration treated without revascularization

Marston WA, Davies SW, Armstrong B, et al (Univ of North Carolina at Chapel Hill)

J Vasc Surg 44:108-114, 2006

Objectives.—The natural history of limbs affected by ischemic ulceration is poorly understood. In this report, we describe the outcome of limbs with stable chronic leg ulcers and arterial insufficiency that were treated with wound-healing techniques in patients who were not candidates for revascularization.

Methods.—A prospectively maintained database of limb ulcers treated at a comprehensive wound center was used to identify patients with arterial insufficiency, defined as an ankle-brachial index (ABI) <0.7 or a toe pressure <50 mm Hg. Patients were treated without revascularization when medical comorbidity or anatomic considerations did not allow revascularization with acceptable risk. Ulcers were treated with a protocol emphasizing pressure relief, debridement, infection control, and moist wound healing. Risk factors analyzed for their affect on healing and amputation risk included age, gender, diabetes mellitus, chronic renal insufficiency (serum creatinine > 2.5 mg/dL), severity of ischemia measured by ABI or toe pressure, wound grade, wound size, and wound location.

Results.—Between January 1999 and March 2005, 142 patients with 169 limbs having arterial insufficiency and full-thickness ulceration were treated without revascularization. Mean patient age was 70.8 ± 4.5. Diabetes mellitus was present in 70.4% of limbs and chronic renal insufficiency in 27.8%. Toe amputations or other foot-sparing procedures were performed in 28% of limbs. Overall, limb loss occurred in 37 patients. By life-table analysis, 19% of limbs required amputation ≤6 months of initial treatment and 23% at 12 months. Complete wound closure was achieved in 25% by 6 months and in 52% by 12 months. Statistical analysis showed a correlation between ABI and the risk of limb loss. In patients with an ABI <0.5, 28% and 34% of limbs experienced limb loss at 6 and 12 months, respectively, compared with 10% and 15% of limbs in patients with an ABI >0.5 ($P = .01$). The only risk factor associated with wound closure was initial wound size ($P < .005$).

Conclusions.—Limb salvage can be achieved in most patients with arterial insufficiency and uncomplicated chronic nonhealing limb ulcers using a program of wound management without revascularization. Healing proceeds slowly, however, requiring more than a year in many cases. Patients with an ABI <0.5 are more likely to require amputation. Interventions designed to improve outcomes in critical limb ischemia should stratify outcomes based on hemodynamic data and should include a comparative control group given the natural history of ischemic ulcers treated in a dedicated wound program.

▶ Patients with lower extremity wounds, who were not candidates for revascularization were monitored for an average of 18 months. This study was performed to help better define the natural history of lower extremity arterial occlusive disease. Risk of major amputation is negatively related to ABI, but wound healing was achievable for a large number of patients.

G. L. Moneta, MD

Spinal Cord Stimulation is not Cost-effective for Non-surgical Management of Critical Limb Ischaemia

Klomp HM, for the ESES Study Group (Erasmus Univ, Rotterdam, The Netherlands; Netherlands Cancer Inst Antoni van Leeuwenhoek Hosp, Amsterdam)
Eur J Vasc Endovasc Surg 31:500-508, 2006

Objective.—To quantify the costs of treatment in critical limb ischaemia (CLI) and to compare costs and effectiveness of two treatment strategies: spinal cord stimulation (SCS) and best medical treatment.

Methods.—One hundred and twenty patients with CLI not suitable for vascular reconstruction were randomised to either SCS in addition to best medical treatment or best medical treatment alone. Primary outcomes were mortality, amputation and cost. Cost analysis was based on resources used by patients for 2 years after randomisation. Both medical and non-medical costs were included.

Results.—Patient and limb survival were similar in the two treatment groups (Fig 1). Costs of in-hospital-stay and institutional rehabilitation constituted the predominant part (±70%) of the total costs of medical care in CLI. Cost of SCS-implantation and complications (€7950 per patient) exceeded by far cost due to amputation procedures (€410 per patient). The total costs of treatment were €36,600 per patient over 2 years for the SCS-group vs. €28,700 for best medical treatment alone (28% higher for SCS-group, p = 0.009).

Conclusions.—Total costs of treatment in CLI are high. Major components are hospital and rehabilitation costs. In contrast to recent reviews, there were no long-term benefits of SCS-treatment. Therefore, cost-

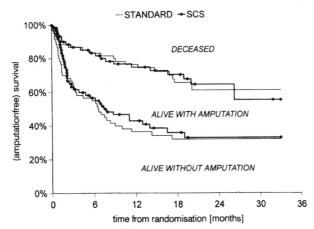

FIGURE 1.—Mortality and amputation in CLI. The upper curves indicate patient survival for both treatment groups ("SCS" and 'standard treatment'). The area between the upper and lower curves represents the proportion of patients alive with major amputation. Patients at risk: at 12 months 47/44, at 24 months 21/19. (Courtesy of Klomp HM, for the ESES Study Group. Spinal cord stimulation is not cost-effective for non-surgical management of critical limb ischaemia. *Eur J Vasc Endovasc Surg.* 2006;31:500-508. Reprinted by permission of the publisher W B Saunders Company Limited London.)

effectiveness is reduced to cost-minimisation and SCS-treatment is considerably more expensive than best medical treatment.

▶ If you do the math pertaining to the results of this randomized trial, SCS as treatment for unreconstructable lower limb ischemia is not effective. No more limbs are saved than with medical management and the number needed to treat to potentially save 1 limb is 13 at a projected cost over $200,000 per limb saved. This does not pencil out in anyone's calculations of cost effectiveness.

G. L. Moneta, MD

One-year prospective quality-of-life outcomes in patients treated with angioplasty for symptomatic peripheral arterial disease
Kalbaugh CA, Taylor SM, Blackhurst DW, et al (Greenville Hosp System, SC)
J Vasc Surg 44:296-303, 2006

Background.—Despite lower reported patency rates than open bypass, percutaneous transluminal angioplasty (PTA) may result in symptom relief, limb salvage, maintenance of ambulation and independent living, and overall improved quality of life. The goal of this study was to prospectively assess quality of life and functional outcomes after angioplasty and stenting in patients with chronic leg ischemia.

Methods.—From August to December 2002, 84 patients with 118 chronically ischemic limbs underwent PTA with or without stenting as part of an ongoing prospective project performed to examine management of symptomatic peripheral arterial disease. All patients completed a preprocedure health questionnaire (Short Form 36) to provide adequate baseline data. Each patient was followed up every 3 months after treatment for 1 year to determine traditional outcomes of arterial patency, limb salvage, survival and amputation-free survival, and functional outcomes assessed according to improvement in quality of life, maintenance of ambulatory status, and maintenance of independent living status. The entire cohort was analyzed, as were subgroups of patients with lifestyle-limiting claudication and those with critical limb ischemia. Outcomes were analyzed by using Kaplan-Meier life-table analysis, the log-rank test for survival curves, and the one-sample *t* test. A Cox proportional hazard model was used to determine whether presentation and level of disease were independent predictors of outcome.

Results.—Of the 84 patients, 54 (64.3%) were treated for claudication (34 aortoiliac occlusive disease and 20 infrainguinal disease), and 30 (35.7%) were treated for critical limb ischemia (11 aortoiliac occlusive disease and 19 infrainguinal disease). One-year results for the 54 patients with claudication were as follows: primary patency, 78.5%; limb salvage, 100%; amputation-free survival, 96.3%; survival, 96.3%; maintenance of ambulation status, 100%; and maintenance of independence, 100%. There was statistical improvement in all physical function categories, including physical function (29.4 ± 8.9 vs 37.1 ± 11.3; $P < .0001$), role-physical (32.5 ± 11.3 vs 39.5 ± 13.0; $P = .0001$), bodily pain (35.8 ± 8.5 vs 42.9 ± 10.9; $P < .0001$), and aggregate physical scoring (31.1 ± 9.7 vs 38.1 ± 11.5; $P < .0001$). One-year results for the 30 patients with critical limb ischemia were as follows: primary patency, 35.2%; limb salvage, 77.2%; amputation-free survival, 50.0%; survival, 60.0%; maintenance of ambulation status, 75.8%; and maintenance of independence, 92.8%. There was statistical improvement in bodily pain resolution (35.3 ± 12.0 vs 46.6 ± 12.0; $P = .0009$). Cox models with hazard ratios (HRs) revealed that presentation was a significant predictor for outcomes of primary patency (HR, 4.2; $P= .0002$), secondary patency (HR, 6.0; $P < .0001$), limb salvage (HR, 20.2; $P = .0047$), survival (HR, 10.9; $P = .0002$), and amputation-free survival (HR, 11.2; $P < .0001$). Conversely, the level of disease was predictive of outcome only for primary patency (HR, 1.8; $P = .00289$).

Conclusions.—Despite inferior reconstruction patency rates when compared with the historical results of open bypass, PTA provides excellent functional outcomes with good patient satisfaction, especially for treating claudication. These findings support a more liberal use of PTA intervention for patients with vasculogenic claudication.

▶ The only good thing about this article is that the authors' tried to provide some data reflecting the patient's perception of outcome. There are better quality-of-life and more disease-specific instruments for vascular patients than the SF36. And the follow-up is way too short to assess benefit for claudication. Also, there was no control group and no cost analysis. Overall, the results were as expected. Patients with claudication and treatment of aortoiliac segments did the best in terms of procedure durability and improved quality of life. Patients with critical limb ischemia and infrainguinal reconstructions did poorly with 1-year primary patency rates of 23%.

G. L. Moneta, MD

Analysis of Outcomes Following Failed Endovascular Treatment of Chronic Limb Ischemia
Ryer EJ, Trocciola SM, DeRubertis B, et al (Cornell Univ, New York; Columbia Univ, New York)
Ann Vasc Surg 20:440-446, 2006

Despite recent studies highlighting the advantages of endoluminal intervention in the management of chronic limb ischemia (CLI), outcomes following failed peripheral angioplasty remain less well described. We present a retrospective analysis of failed transluminal infrainguinal percutaneous arterial angioplasty with or without stenting (PTA/S) in patients with CLI. A database of patients undergoing infrainguinal PTA/S between 2002 and 2005 was maintained. Patients underwent duplex scanning follow-up at 2 weeks, 3 months, and every 6 months after the intervention. Angiograms were reviewed in all cases to assess lesion characteristics. Results were standardized to current Transatlantic Inter-Society Consensus (TASC) criteria. Kaplan-Meier survival analyses were performed to assess time-dependent outcomes. In total, our analysis involved 246 patients who underwent treatment for CLI using PTA/S. Eighteen percent of procedures ($n = 46$) were considered an intervention failure secondary to restenosis by duplex ultrasound, returning clinical symptoms, a nonhealing foot lesion, or the absence of a prior palpable pulse. Indications for the original procedure in patients whose PTA/S failed were tissue loss in 44%, claudication in 44%, and rest pain in 12%, while TASC lesion grades were A (0%), B (18%), C (18%), and D (64%). Of patients failing PTA/S, 4% failed in the first 30 days, 78% failed between 1 and 18 months, while 18% failed following 18 months, with a mean time to failure of 8.7 months. Also, 82% of PTA/S failures were candidates for a second endovascular procedure, 11% were suitable for only traditional open bypass, and 4% demonstrated progression of disease necessitating amputation. Of patients undergoing a second endovascular procedure, limb salvage rates were 86% at 12-month follow-up and there was a single periprocedural mortality and complication rate of 6.6%. Of patients requiring open surgical bypass after failed PTA/S, 20% ($n = 1$) required a major amputation and there were no mortalities. Failure of endoluminal therapy for treatment of lower extremity arterial occlusive disease is amenable to subsequent endovascular intervention for limb salvage with limited morbidity and mortality.

▶ Failure of endovascular therapy for the treatment of lower extremity occlusive disease does not predict limb loss in 12 months of follow-up. Failure of initial endovascular therapy typically occurs between 1 and 18 months after the procedure, and secondary endovascular therapy or surgical bypass graft may be used to maintain limb salvage.

G. L. Moneta, MD

Balloon Angioplasty versus Implantation of Nitinol Stents in the Superficial Femoral Artery

Schillinger M, Sabeti S, Loewe C, et al (Med Univ of Vienna)
N Engl J Med 354:1879-1888, 2006

Background.—Because stent implantation for disease of the superficial femoral artery has been associated with high rates of late clinical failure, percutaneous transluminal angioplasty is preferred for endovascular treatment, and stenting is recommended only in the event of suboptimal technical results. We evaluated whether primary implantation of a self-expanding nitinol (nickel–titanium) stent yielded anatomical and clinical benefits superior to those afforded by percutaneous transluminal angioplasty with optional secondary stenting.

Methods.—We randomly assigned 104 patients who had severe claudication or chronic limb ischemia due to stenosis or occlusion of the superficial femoral artery to undergo primary stent implantation (51 patients) or angioplasty (53 patients). Restenosis and clinical outcomes were assessed at 6 and 12 months.

Results.—The mean (±SD) length of the treated segment was 132±71 mm in the stent group and 127±55 mm in the angioplasty group. Secondary stenting was performed in 17 of 53 patients (32 percent) in the angioplasty group, in most cases because of a suboptimal result after angioplasty. At 6 months, the rate of restenosis on angiography was 24 percent in the stent group and 43 percent in the angioplasty group (P=0.05) (Fig 1); at 12 months the rates on duplex ultrasonography were 37 percent and 63 per-

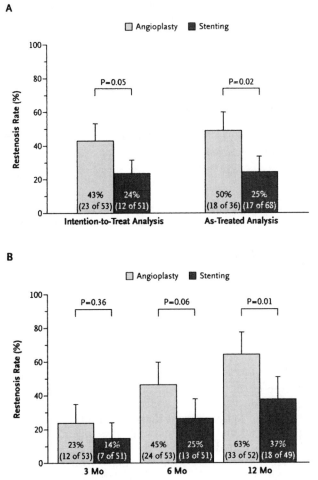

FIGURE 1.—Rates of Restenosis on Angiography (Panel A) and Duplex Ultrasonography (Panel B). Restenosis was defined as stenosis of more than 50 percent. Panel A shows the rates as determined by angiography at six months, analyzed according to the intention-to-treat principle and according to the treatment actually received. Panel B shows the rates of restenosis in the same patients as determined by duplex ultrasonography at 3, 6, and 12 months, analyzed according to the intention-to-treat principle. I bars indicate 95 percent confidence intervals. (Reprinted by permission of the New England Journal of Medicine. From Schillinger M, Sabeti S, Loewe C, et al. Balloon angioplasty versus implantation of nitinol stents in the superficial femoral artery. *N Engl J Med.* 2006;354:1879-1888. Copyright 2006, Massachusetts Medical Society. All rights reserved.)

cent, respectively (P=0.01). Patients in the stent group were able to walk significantly farther on a treadmill at 6 and 12 months than those in the angioplasty group.

Conclusions.—In the intermediate term, treatment of superficial-femoral-artery disease by primary implantation of a self-expanding nitinol stent yielded results that were superior to those with the currently recommended approach of balloon angioplasty with optional secondary stenting.

▶ This study suggests that the primary use of nitinol stents may improve what is a relatively poor result of angioplasty and secondary stenting of the superficial femoral artery. Given that there have been previous studies suggesting that an exercise program is as effective or more effective than angioplasty of the superficial femoral artery, it is a shame that the authors did not include a control group in their trial. It would also have been nice to know whether the increased walking distance measured on the treadmill translated to increased quality of life for the patients in this study. Nevertheless, it can be said that given the endpoints of this trial, the use of primary stenting with nitinol stents for angioplasty of the superficial femoral artery was superior to selective stenting after angioplasty of the superficial femoral artery.

G. L. Moneta, MD

Low-molecular-weight heparin for prevention of restenosis after femoropopliteal percutaneous transluminal angioplasty: A randomized controlled trial
Koppensteiner R, Spring S, Amann-Vesti BR, et al (Univ Hosp Zurich, Switzerland; Univ of Zurich, Switzerland)
J Vasc Surg 44:1247-1253, 2006

Background.—Restenosis after angioplasty is essentially due to intimal hyperplasia. Low-molecular-weight heparins (LMWHs) have experimentally been shown to have antiproliferative effects in addition to their antithrombotic properties. Their potential in reducing restenosis remains to be established. Therefore, we wanted to test the hypothesis that LMWH plus aspirin is more effective than aspirin alone in reducing the incidence of restenosis/reocclusion in patients undergoing percutaneous transluminal angioplasty (PTA) of femoropopliteal arteries. Further, different effects of LMWH in patients treated for critical limb ischemia (CLI) or claudication only should be investigated.

Methods.—After successful PTA, 275 patients with symptomatic peripheral arterial disease (claudication or critical limb ischemia) and femoropopliteal obstructions were randomized to receive either 2500 IU of dalteparin subcutaneously for 3 months plus 100 mg of aspirin daily (n = 137), or 100 mg aspirin daily alone (n = 138). The primary end point was restenosis or reocclusion documented by duplex ultrasonography imaging at 12 months.

Results.—Restenosis/reocclusion occurred in 58 patients (44%) in the dalteparin group and in 62 patients (50%) in the control group (P = .30). In a subgroup analysis according to the severity of peripheral arterial disease, we found that in patients treated for claudication, restenosis/reocclusion developed in 43 (43%) in the dalteparin group, and in 35 (41%) in the control group ($P = .70$); in patients treated for CLI, restenosis/reocclusion was significantly lower in the dalteparin group (15, 45%) than in the control group (27, 72%; $P = .01$). No major bleeding events occurred in either group.

Conclusions.—Treatment with 2500 IU dalteparin subcutaneously given for 3 months after femoropopliteal PTA failed to reduce restenosis/reocclusion at 12 months. However, dalteparin may be beneficial in the subgroup of patients with CLI at 12 months follow-up.

▶ Despite favorable animal data, LMWHs have previously not been found to decrease intimal hyperplasia after femoropopliteal bypass as well. The numbers here are too small to conclude favorable effect for LMWH in reducing recurrent stenosis in patients with CLI after angioplasty. More than 50% have a restenosis or occlusion develop by 1 year. The whole field of femoropopliteal angioplasty is a bit of the "cart before the horse," (ie, everyone keeps thinking new devices are the answer to greater durability of infrainguinal percutaneous reconstructions). However, these same people continue to ignore the great elephant of intimal hyperplasia that is also in the room.

G. L. Moneta, MD

Long-Term Results After Directional Atherectomy of Femoro-Popliteal Lesions

Zeller T, Rastan A, Sixt S, et al (Herz-Zentrum Bad Krozingen, Germany; Univ Hosp Basel, Switzerland; Univ Hosp Tübingen, Germany)
J Am Coll Cardiol 48:1573-1578, 2006

Objectives.—Our objective in this research was the evaluation of the long-term results after directional atherectomy using the Silverhawk device (FoxHollow Technologies, Redwood City, California) of femoro-popliteal lesions.

Background.—Considering reports on stent fractures in femoro-popliteal arteries, atherectomy may be a valuable alternative to stenting.

Methods.—Eighty-four patients with 100 legs and 131 lesions with peripheral occlusive disease Rutherford categories 2 to 5 were included in a prospective registry. Forty-five lesions were de novo lesions (group 1; 34%), 43 lesions native vessel restenoses (group 2; 33%), and 43 lesions in-stent restenoses (group 3; 33%). Additional low pressure balloon angioplasty was used in 78 of 131 lesions (59%) and stenting in 8 lesions (6%).

Results.—Technical success rate was 86% for atherectomy only and 100% after additional therapy. Mean lesion length was 43 ± 54 mm, 105 ± 122 mm, and 131 ± 111 mm for group 1, group 2, and group 3, respectively ($p < 0.001$). Primary patency, defined as freedom of a >50% restenosis detected by duplex, was 84%, 54%, and 54% at 12 months ($p = 0.002$) and 73%, 42%, and 49%, at 18 months ($p = 0.008$); secondary patency rates

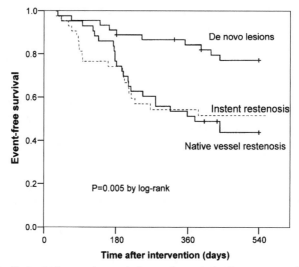

FIGURE 2.—Kaplan-Meier event-free survival curves for survival without target vessel revascularization. (Reprinted with permission from the American College of Cardiology from Zeller T, Rastan A, Sixt S, et al. Long-term results after directional atherectomy of femoro-popliteal lesions. *J Am Coll Cardiol.* 2006;48:1573-1578.)

were 100%, 93%, and 91% at 12 months (p = NS) and 89%, 67%, and 79% at 18 months (p = 0.001), respectively; and target lesion revascularization rate was 16%, 44%, and 47% at 12 months and 22%, 56%, and 49% at 18 months (p = 0.003 each) for group 1, group 2, and group 3, respectively (Fig 2). The only independent predictor for restenosis was treatment of restenotic lesions. Ankle-brachial index was significantly improved after 12 months and 18 months in all groups.

Conclusions.—Long-term technical and clinical results after directional atherectomy of femoro-popliteal lesions are in favor of de novo lesions compared with restenotic lesions.

▶ The results presented here for use of the Silverhawk catheter (FoxHollow Technologies, Redwood City, CA) for treatment of de novo femoral-popliteal lesions are similar to results obtained treating femoropopliteal lesions with bare and drug-coated stents.[1] The number of devices and techniques available for catheter-based treatment of femoropopliteal arteries is expanding expeditiously. Without direct head-to-head randomized trials, we have no way of knowing which device or technique will provide the best results. However, with the proprietary interest of industry, the financial interest of stockholders, and the current enthusiasm for catheter-based treatments, such trials are unlikely to be conducted.

G. L. Moneta, MD

Reference

1. Oliva VL, Soulez G. Sirolimus-eluting stents versus the superficial femoral artery: second round. *J Vasc Interv Radiol.* 2005;16:331-338.

Remote Superficial Femoral Endarterectomy: Long-term Results
Devalia K, Magee TR, Galland RB (Royal Berkshire Hosp, Reading, England)
Eur J Vasc Endovasc Surg 31:262-265, 2006

Purpose.—The aim of this study was to determine long-term results following successful remote superficial femoral endarterectomy (RSFE).

Methods.—RSFE is a minimally invasive technique of revascularising the superficial femoral artery. A single incision was made over the origin of the superficial femoral artery. The endarterectomy was carried out in a closed fashion from above. The cut end of distal atheroma was secured with a stent. Following RSFE patients were followed up with intravenous digital subtraction angiography (IVDSA) and 3-monthly duplex scans. IVDSA was repeated if any abnormality was found.

Results.—RSFE was attempted on 30 patients with 33 symptomatic legs to treat tissue loss ($n = 3$), rest pain ($n = 3$) or intermittent claudication ($n = 27$). In 26 limbs it was possible to complete the RSFE satisfactorily (technical success 79%), but during follow-up 18 later developed stenoses. Of 31 stenoses detected, 27 were treated by angioplasty. Primary patency at 1, 2 and 5 years was 38, 31 and 16%, respectively (Fig 3). Primary-assisted patency at 1, 2 and 5 years was 77, 65 and 60%.

Conclusions.—Primary-assisted patency following RSFE is reasonable, however, it is only achieved with life-long surveillance and intervention. Un-

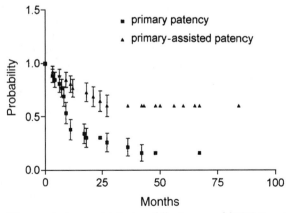

FIGURE 3.—Primary and primary-assisted patency following successful RSFE. Bars represent standard errors of the mean. (Courtesy of Devalia K, Magee TR, Galland RB. Remote superficial femoral endarterectomy: long-term results. *Eur J Vasc Endovasc Surg.* 2006;31:262-265. Copyright 2006 by permission of the publisher W B Saunders Company Limited London.)

til results can be improved the widespread use of RSFE cannot be recommended.

▶ Another nail for the coffin enveloping this procedure is provided. Remote superficial femoral endarterectomy is losing the battle with other less-invasive procedures that do not require arterial cutdown, provide improved initial technical success, higher patency rates, and allow treatment of more than 1 arterial segment during the index procedure.

G. L. Moneta, MD

Subintimal Angioplasty of Supra- and Infrageniculate Arteries
Aarts F, Blankensteijn JD, van der Vliet JA, et al (Radboud Univ, Nijmegen, The Netherlands)
Ann Vasc Surg 20:620-624, 2006

We retrospectively reviewed our experience with subintimal angioplasty for chronic limb ischemia. Hospital records and films of all subintimal angioplasty procedures performed between October 2002 and December 2004 were reviewed and analyzed for demographic data, clinical data, and comorbid condition status. Thirty-nine subintimal angioplasties were performed in 37 patients (65% male, 35% female), with a median age of 73 years. Median follow-up was 9 months. The 30-day mortality rate was 8%. All-cause mortality was 33% after 24 months. In 23 cases (59%), a subintimal angioplasty of the superficial femoral artery (SFA) alone was performed. Both the SFA and popliteal/crural vessels were used in nine limbs (23%), the popliteal artery alone in three limbs (8%), and the crural arteries alone in four limbs (10%). Initial technical and clinical success rates were 67% and 49%, respectively. The complication rate was 28%. Twenty-four additional surgical interventions were performed after the initial angioplasty procedure, of which 12 were major amputations. Amputation-free survival (limb-salvage rate) was 69% at 12 months [95% confidence interval (CI) 52-85%], and overall survival was 69% (95% CI 52-85%) at 12 months. In patients with critical limb ischemia, subintimal angioplasty is feasible and in most cases technically successful. In these high-risk patients, often with combined cardiac, pulmonary, and diabetic risk and considered unfit for bypass surgery, subintimal angioplasty offers a safe and effective alternative.

▶ This obviously is a difficult group of patients with a high amputation rate and a poor survival rate. Success rates reported in this study for subintimal angioplasty are somewhat lower than those reported elsewhere. Subintimal angioplasty is a technically demanding procedure. It may be the authors were still on the learning curve. However, I suspect the results reported here are what most would achieve and apply in this procedure to a similarly difficult cohort of patients.

G. L. Moneta, MD

True lumen re-entry devices facilitate subintimal angioplasty and stenting of total chronic occlusions: Initial report

Jacobs DL, Motaganahalli RL, Cox DE, et al (Saint Louis Univ)

J Vasc Surg 43:1291-1296, 2006

Objective.—The acute technical failure of endovascular treatment of chronic total occlusions (CTOs) is most often due to the inability to re-enter the true lumen after occlusion is crossed in a subintimal plane. This study reports our initial experience with true lumen re-entry devices in the treatment of CTOs.

Methods.—Patients with treatment of CTOs were identified from our vascular registry. All patients in whom the Pioneer catheter or the Outback catheter were used were also identified from a prospectively maintained separate database of cases in which true lumen re-entry devices were used. We used procedural data from the prospective database and reviewed the medical records. Lesion character and location, access type, location of true lumen re-entry, stent usage, procedural times, and complications, were tabulated.

Results.—From August 2003 to December 2004, endovascular techniques were used to treat 87 CTOs in 58 iliac and 29 superficial femoral arteries. In 24 (26%), the true lumen could not be re-entered by using standard catheter and wire techniques. The true lumen was not initially re-entered in 20 (34%) of 58 of treated iliac CTOs and four (13%) of 29 of treated super-

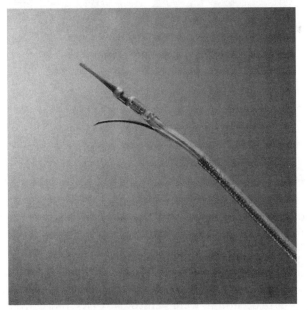

FIGURE 1.—Pioneer intravascular ultrasound true lumen re-entry catheter with needle deployed. (Courtesy of Jacobs DL, Motaganahalli RL, Cox DE, et al. True lumen re-entry devices facilitate subintimal angioplasty and stenting of total chronic occlusions: initial report. *J Vasc Surg.* 2006;43:1291-1296.)

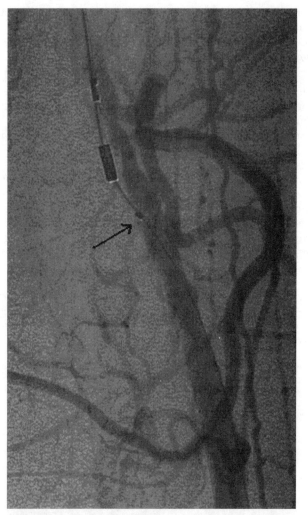

FIGURE 4.—Outback catheter with needle (*arrow*) and wire deployed into true lumen of femoral artery distal to occlusion. (Courtesy of Jacobs DL, Motaganahalli RL, Cox DE, et al. True lumen re-entry devices facilitate subintimal angioplasty and stenting of total chronic occlusions: initial report. *J Vasc Surg.* 2006;43:1291-1296.)

ficial femoral artery CTOs (73% TASC C and D lesions). Intravascular ultrasound-guided true lumen re-entry using the Pioneer catheter (Fig 1) (21 CTOs), or fluoroscopic-guided true lumen re-entry using the Outback catheter (Fig 4) (3 CTOs) was successful in achieving true lumen re-entry in all cases at the location desired. Total time of re-entry catheter manipulation required to achieve re-entry was <10 minutes and was routinely accomplished in <3 minutes. All occlusions were stented. No cases were converted to open repair. Bleeding from the recanalization and angioplasty site occurred in four patients (15%). It was controlled with use of covered stents in two cases, and resolved after placement of uncovered stents in the other two. No significant bleeding occurred at the sites of true lumen re-entry needle deployment. All occlusions treated with true lumen re-entry devices remain clinically patent at a mean follow-up of 5.8 months.

Conclusions.—Endovascular treatment of chronic total occlusions is often limited by the inability to re-enter the true lumen after subintimal crossing of the occluded segment. This occurs more commonly with treatment of iliac occlusions than in superficial femoral artery occlusions. True lumen reentry catheters are very effective at gaining wire passage back to the true lumen and facilitating successful endovascular treatment of chronic total occlusions that would otherwise require open bypass.

▶ Immediate results with 2 percutaneous devices that allow true lumen reentry are reported. No reasons for concern are identified and the authors used these devices efficiently.

G. L. Moneta, MD

Preliminary results of subintimal angioplasty for limbs salvage in lower extremities with severe chronic ischemia and limb-threatening ischemia
Myers SI, Myers DJ, Ahmend A (McGuire Research Inst, Richmond, Va; Virginia Commonwealth Univ, Richmond)
J Vasc Surg 44:1239-1246, 2006

Objective.—This study examined the hypothesis that superficial femoral artery (SFA) subintimal angioplasty (SI-PTA) can maintain limb salvage with minimal complications in patients with symptomatic occlusive arterial disease.

Methods.—From March 1, 2004, until April 28, 2006, 78 patients with rest pain (62.2%), gangrene (25.6%), or severe progressive claudication (12.2%) were treated consecutively with 82 SFA SI-PTAs (4 bilateral). The mean age was 59 ± 1.2 years, and 21 (27%) of the patients were female. All patients were treated in the operating room under local anesthesia by using fluoroscopic guidance, and the percentage SFA that was occluded was measured during the diagnostic portion of the procedure. Selective stent placement was performed after successful recanalization of the occluded arterial segments. Patients were treated with chronic aspirin and clopidogrel bisulfate for 3 months and followed up at 30 days and then every 3 months with physical examination and arterial duplex scan.

Results.—Of the 82 SFA SI-PTA attempts, 76 (92%) were initially successful, with an increase in the ankle-brachial index from 0.46 ± 0.02 to 0.88 ± 0.01 ($P < .001$). Five of the six patients with a failed SFA SI-PTA were female, two of the six had had previous bypass attempts, and one of the six had had a previous SFA SI-PTA attempt by another physician. Forty-nine (64%) of the 76 initially successful SFA SI-PTAs required placement of a stent, and 43 (56.5%) of the successful 76 SFA SI-PTAs required additional PTA of 1 or more arterial segments. The group treated with a successful SFA SI-PTA had

42.5% ± 3.5% SFA occlusion, compared with 82% ± 10% ($P < .05$) in the group with a failed attempt at SFA SI-PTA. Two of the six patients with initial SI-PTA failure underwent leg amputation within 30 days, three were treated with successful leg bypass surgery, and one was lost to follow-up. Of the 76 successful SFA SI-PTAs, 5 (6.5%) failed within 90 days, and the patients were treated successfully with leg bypass surgery. Of the 71 limbs with patent SI-PTAs at 90 days, 68 have remained patent with a mean follow-up 10.4 ± 0.7 months (range, 2-24 months). Three of the 71 SFA SI-PTAs failed between 4 and 7 months (mean, 5 ± 0.7 months): 1 patient was treated with successful bypass surgery, 1 patient is currently considering further intervention, and 1 patient was treated with amputation. Ten (14%) of the 71 successful SFA SI-PTAs required limited PTA for asymptomatic restenosis, as identified by the arterial duplex scan (7.4 ± 1.4 months; range, 2-16 months). There were no perioperative deaths, and three patients have died during follow-up with patent SFA SI-PTAs (9.3 ± 1.4 months).

Conclusions.—These data suggest that SFA SI-PTA can be successfully used for limb salvage with minimal morbidity and mortality in a group of patients with severe lower extremity occlusive vascular disease.

▶ This report demonstrates good outcomes with SI-PTA of the SFA, shortly after the treatment team completed endovascular training. Length of occlusion in the SFA was related to lower initial success and increased frequency of failure less than 90 days after treatment. The need for reintervention was related to length of stenotic SFA.

G. L. Moneta, MD

Postoperative outcomes for patients undergoing elective revascularization for critical limb ischemia and intermittent claudication: A subanalysis of the Coronary Artery Revascularization Prophylaxis (CARP) trial
Raghunathan A, for the CARP Investigators (Univ of California, San Francisco; et al)
J Vasc Surg 43:1175-1182, 2006

Objective.—To determine the perioperative mortality, myocardial infarction rate, and long-term survival of patients with critical limb ischemia (CLI) compared with those with intermittent claudication (IC) within a cohort selected for significant coronary artery disease, a secondary analysis was conducted of a prospective, randomized, multicenter trial of Coronary Artery Revascularization Prophylaxis (CARP) before peripheral vascular surgery. This multicenter trial was sponsored by the Cooperative Studies Program of the Department of Veterans Affairs.

Methods.—Of the 510 patients enrolled in the CARP trial and randomized to coronary revascularization or no revascularization before elective vascular surgery, 143 had CLI and 164 had IC as an indication for lower limb revascularization; >95% of each group were men. The presence of coronary artery disease was determined by cardiac catheterization. Eligible pa-

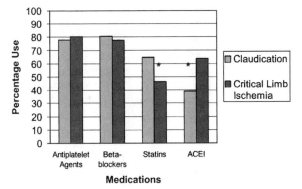

Medications

FIGURE 2.—The medication usage patients reported ≤24 hours before surgery. Comparing the patients with critical limb ischemia and claudication, *p* values were: antiplatelet use = .595; β-blocker use = .534; statins use < .001; and angiotensin-converting enzyme inhibitors (*ACEI*) USE *p* < .001*. (Reprinted by permission of the publisher from Raghunathan A, for the CARP Investigators. Postoperative outcomes for patients undergoing elective revascularization for critical limb ischemia and intermittent claudication: a subanalysis of the Coronary Artery Revascularization Prophylaxis (CARP) trial. *J Vasc Surg.* 2006;43: 1175-1182.)

tients had at least one treatable coronary lesion of ≥70%. Those with significant left main disease, ejection fraction of <20%, and aortic stenosis were excluded. Patients were randomized to coronary artery disease revascularization or no revascularization before vascular surgery and followed for mortality and morbidity perioperatively and for a median of 2.7 years postoperatively. Medical treatment of coronary artery disease was pursued aggressively.

Results.—Patients with IC had a longer time from randomization to vascular surgery (*p* = .001) and more abdominal operations (*p* < .001). Patients with CLI had more urgent operations (*p* = .006), reoperations (*p* < .001), and limb loss (*p* = .008) as well as longer hospital stays (*p* < .001). The IC group had more perioperative myocardial infarctions (CLI, 8.4%; IC, 17.1%; *p* = .024), although perioperative mortality was similar (CLI, 3.5%; IC, 1.8%; *p* = .360). In follow-up, the IC group also had numerically more myocardial infarctions (CLI, 16.8%; IC, 25%; *p* = .079), but mortality was not different (CLI, 21%; IC, 22%; *p* = .825) (Fig 2). Coronary artery revascularization did not lower perioperative or long-term mortality in either group.

Conclusions.—Our data indicate that patients with significant coronary artery disease and either CLI or IC can undergo vascular surgery with low mortality and morbidity, and these results are not improved by coronary artery revascularization before vascular surgery. Furthermore, when selected for the presence of symptomatically stable, severe coronary artery disease, there is no difference in long-term survival between patients with CLI and IC. Finally, the better-than-predicted outcomes for these patients with advanced systemic atherosclerosis may be due to aggressive medical management with beta-blockers, statins, and acetylsalicylic acid.

▶ Initially, the outcome of this study seems unexpected. We normally expect patients with CLI to have higher mortality than patients with IC. In this case, however, long-term mortality was the same for these 2 groups. To me, the results of this study actually make sense; it is coronary disease, by and large, that kills patients with peripheral vascular disease—not leg artery disease. The CLI patients and patients with IC in this study had about the same degree of coronary artery disease. Recent reports in the lay press indicate significant declines in death from cardiac disease. I wonder if this applies to vascular patients as well. If this does not apply to vascular patients, then why not?

G. L. Moneta, MD

Results of percutaneous subintimal angioplasty using routine stenting
Treiman GS, Treiman R, Whiting J (Univ of Utah, Salt Lake City; VA Salt Lake City Health Care System)
J Vasc Surg 43:513-519, 2006

Objective.—To assess the long-term patency and clinical success of subintimal angioplasty in patients with limb-threatening ischemia.

Methods.—From 1999 through 2004, 29 patients with superficial femoral artery (SFA) or popliteal artery occlusion and rest pain or tissue loss underwent subintimal angioplasty. Patients had subintimal wire placement followed by percutaneous transluminal angioplasty and stent placement. From 1 to 10 stents were placed. Technical success required stenosis less than 30% by arteriography, a velocity ratio less than 1.5 by duplex scan, and improvement of the ankle-brachial index greater than 0.15. Follow-up duplex scanning was performed every 3 months for 2 years and then every 6 months thereafter.

Results.—Initial success was obtained in 26 (90%) of the 29 patients, with an improvement in the mean ankle-brachial index of 0.25. Mean follow-up was 38 months (range, 28-54 months). During follow-up, 16 arteries reoccluded. Six of the 16 patients had recurrent symptoms, four required below-knee amputation, two required above-knee amputation, and four died with an intact limb. After treatment failure, two patients had attempted tissue plasminogen activator (TPA), and four had prosthetic tibial bypass. Overall, 15 patients died, and only 2 of the 14 who lived had a patent artery. One of the two required percutaneous transluminal angioplasty of the recanalized artery. By life-table analysis, success was 85%, 64%, 18%, and 9% at 1, 2, 3, and 4 years, respectively. Periprocedural complications occurred in four patients. Of the 13 patients with wounds, six died (four healed), two were alive with healed wounds, and five had limb loss. Of 16 patients with rest pain, 14 developed recurrent symptoms after reocclusion, 1 was alive without pain, and 1 underwent amputation.

Conclusions.—Subintimal angioplasty is technically successful in most patients, with few complications. Most procedures provide short-term clinical success and have allowed for successful wound healing and temporary relief of rest pain. However, late arterial patency is poor, with a high rate of symptom recurrence. Many patients will have recurrent pain, and some will require major amputation. Nevertheless, limb-salvage rates are significantly better than arterial patency. Intermediate-term patency is higher than that commonly reported for prosthetic bypass, and despite the lack of durable long-term patency, the procedure offers an additional potentially effective therapeutic option in the treatment of patients with limb-threatening ischemia and femoropopliteal occlusion.

▶ This article supports my theory that most people are not lining their entire subintimal dissection tracts with stents. Certainly not 10 stents! This is a sick group of patients and the results are sobering. There are only 2 patent arteries in surviving patients. The results, no matter how you try to spin them, cannot justify routine stenting of subintimal angioplasty tracts. The authors ought to be congratulated for their willingness to report poor results. Good for them.

G. L. Moneta, MD

Results of PREVENT III: A multicenter, randomized trial of edifoligide for the prevention of vein graft failure in lower extremity bypass surgery
Conte MS, for the PREVENT III Investigators (Brigham and Women's Hosp, Boston; et al)
J Vasc Surg 43:742-751, 2006

Objective.—The PREVENT III study was a prospective, randomized, double-blinded, multicenter phase III trial of a novel molecular therapy (edifoligide; E2F decoy) for the prevention of vein graft failure in patients undergoing infrainguinal revascularization for critical limb ischemia (CLI).

Methods.—From November 2001 through October 2003, 1404 patients with CLI were randomized to a single intraoperative ex vivo vein graft treatment with edifoligide or placebo. After surgery, patients underwent graft surveillance by duplex ultrasonography and were followed up for index graft and limb end points to 1 year. A blinded Clinical Events Classification committee reviewed all index graft end points. The primary study end point was the time to nontechnical index graft reintervention or major amputation due to index graft failure. Secondary end points included all-cause graft failure, clinically significant graft stenosis (>70% by angiography or severe stenosis by ultrasonography), amputation/reintervention-free survival, and nontechnical primary graft patency. Event rates were based on Kaplan-Meier estimates. Time-to-event end points were compared by using the log-rank test.

Results.—Demographics, comorbidities, and procedural details reflected a population with CLI and diffuse atherosclerosis. Tissue loss was the presenting symptom in 75% of patients. High-risk conduits were used in 24% of cases, including an alternative vein in 20% (15% spliced vein and 5% non–great saphenous vein) and 6% less than 3 mm in diameter; 14% of the cases were reoperative bypass grafts. Most (65%) grafts were placed to infrapopliteal targets. Perioperative (30-day) mortality occurred in 2.7% of patients. Major morbidity included myocardial infarction in 4.7% and early graft occlusion in 5.2% of patients. Ex vivo treatment with edifoligide was well tolerated. There was no significant difference between the treatment groups in the primary or secondary trial end points, primary graft patency, or limb salvage. A statistically significant improvement was observed in secondary graft patency (estimated Kaplan-Meier rates were 83% edifoligide and 78% placebo; $P = .016$) within 1 year. The reduction in secondary patency events was manifest within 30 days of surgery (the relative risk for a 30-day event for edifoligide was 0.45; 95% confidence interval, 0.27-0.76; $P = .005$). For the overall cohort at 1 year, the estimated Kaplan-Meier rate for survival was 84%, that for primary patency was 61%, that for primary assisted patency was 77%, that for secondary patency was 80%, and that for limb salvage was 88%.

Conclusions.—In this prospective, randomized, placebo-controlled clinical trial, ex vivo treatment of lower extremity vein grafts with edifoligide did not confer protection from reintervention for graft failure.

▶ The PREVENT III trial was uniformly well-designed and executed. No benefit was identified for the vein grafts treated with edifoligide, except for secondary patency at 1 year follow-up. These data do raise the question of potential benefit of this compound in longer-term follow-up, which was not carried out in this trial and is not going to happen.

G. L. Moneta, MD

Resource utilization in the treatment of critical limb ischemia: the effect of tissue loss, comorbidities, and graft-related events
Nguyen LL, Lipsitz SR, Bandyk DF, et al (Harvard Med School; Univ of South Florida; Univesity of Washington; et al)
J Vasc Surg 44:971-976, 2006

Objective.—Resource utilization (RU) in the care of patients with critical limb ischemia (CLI) is not well quantified. We present a cohort study to quantify in-hospital RU and analyze the role of tissue loss (TL), comorbidities, and vascular graft-related events (GREs) in patients undergoing peripheral bypass for CLI.

Methods.—A retrospective analysis of 1404 patients enrolled in a multicenter clinical trial (PREVENT III) of vein bypass grafting for CLI was performed with analysis of RU during the 1-year follow-up period. Univariate and multivariable linear regressions were performed to determine RU predictors and outcomes.

Results.—Compared with patients with rest pain, patients presenting with TL as the indication for bypass surgery had a longer index length of stay (mean, 9.8 vs 6.2 days), more rehospitalizations (mean, 1.6 vs 1.2), and a longer cumulative length of stay (mean, 27.7 vs 17.3 days; $P < .0001$ for all comparisons). Rehospitalizations over the ensuing year were for additional procedures (37.5%), wound infection (14.6%), graft failure (10.7%), and other cardiovascular (10%) and noncardiovascular (26%) reasons. Early GRE (stenosis ≥70%, thrombosis, revision, or major amputation within 30 days) occurred in 162 (11.5%) patients, resulting in a longer index length of stay (mean, 11.8 vs 8.6 days; $P = .0002$) and cumulative length of stay (mean, 25.9 vs 24.6 days; $P = .0043$), but no difference in the number of rehospitalizations (mean, 1.6 vs 1.5 days; $P = .3272$). During the 1-year follow-up, 554 (39.5%) patients had GREs, and this resulted in more rehospitalizations (mean, 2.1 vs 1.1; $P < .0001$) and a longer cumulative length of stay (mean, 28.2 vs 21.9 days; $P < .0001$) compared with patients without GRE. Multivariable analysis demonstrated the highly positive association of TL (hazard ratio [HR], 1.75) and early GRE (HR, 1.77) with the index length of stay, whereas comorbidities—namely, dialysis dependency (HR, 1.31), nonsmoking status (HR, 1.29), hypertension (HR, 1.26), and increasing age (HR, 1.01)—also had strong effects. The effect of TL and GRE on later RU (number of rehospitalizations and cumulative length of stay) was present but less pronounced than patient comorbidities (namely, dialysis).

Conclusions.—The stage of disease at presentation (TL vs rest pain) and the patency of the bypass graft (freedom from GRE) are critical determinants of RU over the first year after limb-salvage surgery. These effects predominate early (index length of stay) and persist through 1 year. Patient-specific factors, particularly dialysis-dependent renal failure, are also critical comorbidities affecting RU in these patients.

▶ Length of stay and rehospitalizations were measured for subjects recruited from the PREVENT III trial. Initial and cumulative length of stays and number of rehospitalizations were tallied. Presenting symptom of tissue loss, comorbid dialysis dependence, and graft-related events all had significant impact on resource requirements. This is not unexpected but hopefully will influence those who set DRG reimbursements.

G. L. Moneta, MD

Prospective multicenter study of quality of life before and after lower extremity vein bypass in 1404 patients with critical limb ischemia
Nguyen LL, for the PREVENT III Investigators (Brigham and Women's Hosp, Boston; et al)
J Vasc Surg 44:977-984, 2006

Background.—Patients with critical limb ischemia (CLI) have multiple comorbidities and limited life spans. The ability of infrainguinal vein bypass to improve quality of life (QoL) in patients with CLI has therefore been questioned. Prospective preoperative and postoperative QoL data for patients undergoing lower extremity vein bypass for CLI are presented.

Methods.—A validated, disease-specific QoL questionnaire (VascuQoL) with activity, symptom, pain, emotional, and social domains and responses scored 1 (lowest QoL) to 7 (best QoL) was administered before surgery and at 3 and 12 months after lower extremity vein bypass for CLI. Changes in QoL at 3 and 12 months after lower extremity vein bypass and multiple predetermined variables potentially influencing QoL after lower extremity vein bypass were analyzed to determine the effect of lower extremity vein bypass on QoL in CLI patients.

Results.—A total of 1404 patients had lower extremity vein bypass for CLI at 83 centers in the United States and Canada as part of the PREVENT III clinical trial. Surveys were completed in 1296 patients at baseline, 862 patients at 3 months, and 732 patients at 12 months. The global QoL score (mean ± SD) was 2.8 ± 1.1 at baseline and was 4.7 ± 1.4 and 5.1 ± 1.4 at 3 and 12 months, respectively. Mean changes from baseline at 3 and 12 months were statistically significant ($P < .0001$). Improved QoL scores extended across all domains. Diabetes and the development of graft-related events were associated with decreased improvement in QoL scores, though the mean relative change from baseline remained positive.

Conclusions.—Patients with CLI have a low QoL at baseline that is improved at 3 and 12 months after lower extremity vein bypass. QoL improvements are lower in diabetic patients and those who develop graft-related events. Successful revascularization can be expected to improve QoL in patients with CLI, with benefits that are sustained to at least 1 year.

▶ Subjects for this trial were recruited from the PREVENT III trial, and data were collected via questionnaire. Unfortunately, return of the questionnaires tapered off dramatically starting at 3 months of follow-up, and failure-to-return questionnaires was more highly related to patients who had complications related to treatment. Despite this, QoL improves with revascularization and appears to remain if complications are avoided in patients with CLI.

G. L. Moneta, MD

Determinants of functional outcome after revascularization for critical limb ischemia: An analysis of 1000 consecutive vascular interventions
Taylor SM, Kalbaugh CA, Blackhurst DW, et al (Greenville Hosp System, SC)
J Vasc Surg 44:747-756, 2006

Background.—When reporting standards for successful lower extremity revascularization were established, it was assumed that arterial reconstruction, patency, and limb salvage would correlate with the ultimate goal of therapy: improved functional performance. In reality, factors determining improvement of ambulation and maintenance of independent living status after revascularization have been poorly studied. The purpose of this study was to assess the important determinants of functional outcome for patients after intervention for critical limb ischemia.

Methods.—The results of 1000 revascularized limbs from 841 patients were studied. Indications were rest pain, 41.1%; ischemic ulceration, 35.6%; gangrene, 23.3%; infrainguinal, 70.9%; aortoiliac, 24.2%; and both, 4.9%. Treatment was by endovascular intervention, 35.5%; open surgery, 61.7%; and both, 2.8%. Patient were mean age of 68 ± 12 years, and 56.6% were men, 74.7% were white, 54.2% had diabetes mellitus, 67%

were smokers, 13.4% had end-stage renal disease and were on dialysis, and 36% had prior vascular surgery. Patients were treated with conventional therapy by fellowship-trained vascular specialists at a single center and were analyzed according to the type of intervention, the arterial level treated, age, race, gender, presentation, the presence of diabetes, smoking history, end-stage renal disease, coronary disease, hypertension, hyperlipidemia, obesity, chronic obstructive pulmonary disease, previous stroke, dementia, prior vascular surgery, preoperative ambulatory status, limb loss ≤1 year of treatment, and independent living status. The technical outcomes of reconstruction patency and limb salvage as well as the functional outcomes of survival, maintenance of ambulation, and independent living status were measured for each variable using Kaplan-Meier life-table analysis, and differences were assessed using the log-rank test. A Cox proportional hazards model was used to assess independent predictors of outcome and obtain adjusted hazard ratios and 95% confidence intervals.

Results.—At 5 years, 72.4% of the entire cohort had a patent reconstruction and 72.1% had an intact limb. Overall 5-year functional outcomes were 41.9% for survival, 70.6% for maintenance of ambulation, and 81.3% for independent living status. Outcome was not significantly affected by the type of treatment (endovascular or open surgery) or by the level of disease treated (aortoiliac, infrainguinal, or both). The most important independent, statistically significant predictors of particularly poor functional outcome were impaired ambulatory ability at the time of presentation (70% 5-year mortality, hazard ratio, 3.34; 39.5% failure to eventually ambulate, hazard ratio, 2.83; 30% loss of independent living status, hazard ratio, 7.97), and the presence of dementia (73% late mortality, hazard ratio, 1.57; 41.2% failure to eventually ambulate, hazard ratio, 2.20; 46.4% loss of independent living status, hazard ratio, 5.44). These factors were even more predictive than limb amputation alone.

Conclusion.—Functional outcome for patients undergoing intervention for critical limb ischemia is not solely determined by the traditional measures of reconstruction patency and limb salvage, but also by certain intrinsic patient comorbidities at the time of presentation. These findings question the benefit of our current approach to critical limb ischemia in functionally impaired, chronically ill patients—patients who undoubtedly will be more prevalent as our population ages.

▶ This article is a reasonable attempt to assess functional assessment, but represents little progress beyond the type of analysis reported from our institution about 10 years ago. It is, however, about all you can do with a retrospective study design. Standardized instruments and objective methods for assessing quality of life and functional outcome are, however, available and should be used in prospective assessment of any form of treatment for limb ischemia. It is sobering to consider that by the author's analysis vascular intervention had little impact as assessed by functional outcome in one-third of the patients. This suggests additional analysis is required to determine who really should undergo arterial reconstruction for critical limb ischemia. My late partner, Dr John Porter, once said we spent 40 years in vascular surgery learning what we can do and that now we need to focus on what we should do. Smart man, Dr Porter.

G. L. Moneta, MD

Wound healing and functional outcomes after infrainguinal bypass with reversed saphenous vein for critical limb ischemia
Chung J, Bartelson BB, Hiatt WR, et al (Univ of Colorado, Denver; Colorado Prevention Ctr, Denver; Southern Illinois Univ, Springfield)
J Vasc Surg 43:1183-1190, 2006

Objective.—To examine wound healing and the functional natural history of patients undergoing infrainguinal bypass with reversed saphenous vein for critical limb ischemia (CLI).

Methods.—Consecutive patients undergoing infrainguinal bypass for CLI were retrospectively entered into a technical and functional outcomes database. The patients were enrolled from the tertiary referral vascular surgery practices at the University of Colorado Health Sciences Center and Southern Illinois University Medical School. Main outcome variables included wound healing, self-assessed degree of ambulation (outdoors, indoors only, or nonambulatory), and living status (community or structured) after a mean follow up of 30 ± 23 months. These outcome variables were assessed relative to the preoperative clinical characteristics (symptom duration before vascular consultation, lesion severity, and serum albumin level) and graft patency.

Results.—From August 1997 through December 2004, 334 patients (253 men; median age, 68 years) underwent 409 infrainguinal bypasses (157 popliteal, 235 tibial, and 17 pedal) for CLI (159 Fontaine III and 250 Fontaine IV). Perioperative mortality was 1.2%. At 1 and 3 years, respectively, the primary patency was 63% and 50%, assisted primary patency was 80% and 70%, limb salvage was 85% and 79%, and survival was 89% and 74%. Complete wound healing at 6 and 12 months was 42% and 75%, respectively. Thirty-four patients (10%) died before all wounds were healed. Multivariate analysis indicated that extensive pedal necrosis at presentation independently predicted delayed wound healing ($P \leq .01$). At baseline (defined as the level of function within 30 days before the onset of CLI), 91% of patients were ambulatory outdoors, and this decreased to 72% at 6 months ($P \leq .01$). Similarly, 96% of patients lived independently at baseline, and this decreased to 91% at 6 months ($P \leq .01$) Graft patency was associated with better ambulatory status at 6 months. A longer duration of symptoms before vascular consultation was associated with a worse living status at 6 months.

Conclusions.—Despite achieving the anticipated graft patency and limb salvage results, 25% of patients did not realize wound healing at 1 year of follow-up, 19% had lost ambulatory function, and 5% had lost independent living status. Prospective natural history studies are needed to further define the functional outcomes and their predictors after infrainguinal bypass for CLI.

▶ This report is refreshing because it analyses a specific patient population (presenting complaint of CLI) and a single treatment (reversed saphenous vein graft) to determine the effect of preoperative factors on long-term outcomes (wound healing and functional status). Extent of pedal necrosis predicts poor wound healing, and CLI and surgery combine to significantly improve the ambulatory status and independent living for patients.

G. L. Moneta, MD

Outcome After Occlusion of Infrainguinal Bypasses in the Dutch BOA Study: Comparison of Amputation Rate in Venous and Prosthetic Grafts
Smeets L, for the Dutch BOA Study Group (Twenteborg Hosp, Almelo, The Netherlands; et al)
Eur J Vasc Endovasc Surg 30:604-609, 2005

Objective.—To compare the consequences of occlusion of infrainguinal venous and prosthetic grafts.

Methods.—In total, 2690 patients were included in the Dutch BOA study, a multicenter randomised trial that compared the effectiveness of oral anticoagulants with aspirin in the prevention of infrainguinal bypass graft occlusion. Two thousand four hundred and four patients received a femoropopliteal or femorodistal bypass with a venous (64%) or prosthetic (36%) graft. The incidence of occlusion and amputation was calculated according to graft material and the incidence of amputation after occlusion was compared with Cox regression to adjust for differences in prognostic factors.

Results.—The indication for operation was claudication in 51%, rest pain in 20% and tissue loss in 28% of patients. The mean follow up was 21 months.

After venous bypass grafting 171 (15%) femoropopliteal and 96 (24%) femorodistal grafts occluded. After prosthetic bypass grafting 234 (30%) femoropopliteal and 25 (38%) femorodistal grafts occluded. Patients with occlusions in the venous group had more severe ischemia, less runoff vessels and were older than the patients with prosthetic grafts. In the venous occlusion group 54 (20%) amputations were performed compared to 42 (16%) in the prosthetic occlusion group; crude hazard ratio 1.17 (95% CI 0.78–1.75). After adjustment for above mentioned differences in patient characteristics the hazard ratio was 0.86 (95% CI 0.56–1.32).

Conclusion.—The need for amputation after occlusion is not influenced by graft material in infrainguinal bypass surgery.

▶ Data from a trial Dutch BOA (Dutch Bypass Oral anticoagulants or Aspirin) designed to determine whether the administration of aspirin or oral anticoagulants affected bypass graft patency was re-examined to determine whether the type of graft material (saphenous vein or prosthetic) used affects eventual need for amputation. Graft material selection was not randomized originally. Prosthetic grafts occluded more often than venous grafts, leading to a higher overall absolute number of amputations in the prosthetic group. However, the rate of amputation for after prosthetic graft occlusion was the same as the rate of amputation after loss of venous graft patency.

G. L. Moneta, MD

The Outcome of Occluded Above-knee Femoropopliteal Prostheses Implanted for Critical Ischaemia
Pedersen G, Laxdal E, Aune S (Haukeland Univ, Bergen, Norway; Univ of Bergen, Norway)
Eur J Vasc Endovasc Surg 32:680-685, 2006

Objectives.—To investigate the impact of patient characteristics and treatment modality (graft thrombectomy vs thrombolysis) on the results of redo procedures for occluded above-knee prosthetic femoropopliteal grafts implanted for critical ischaemia.

Material and Methods.—Fifty-five procedures (thrombolysis 24 and thrombectomy 31) were performed on 24 prostheses (23 patients, 24 limbs) between January 1990 and December 2001. All cases were prospectively registered. Graft patency, limb salvage and survival rates were studied and subgroups of patients were compared. Risk factors were analysed with the use of log rank test and Cox proportional hazard analysis.

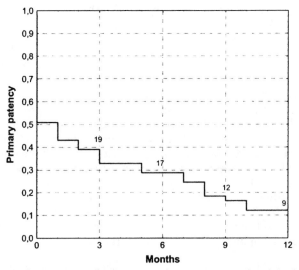

FIGURE 1.—Kaplan-Meier curve: The patency rates of 55 re-opening procedures for occluded prosthetic above-knee femoropopliteal bypass. The numbers above the curve indicate the numbers at risk. (Courtesy of Pederson G, Laxdal E, Aune S. The outcome of occluded above-knee femoropopliteal prostheses implanted for critical ischaemia. *Eur J Vasc Endovasc Surg.* 2006;32:680-685. Copyright 2006 by Elsevier. Reprinted by permission of the publisher.)

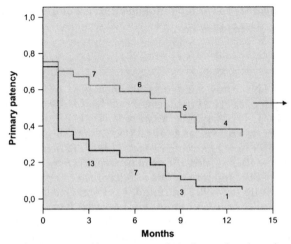

FIGURE 2.—Kaplan-Meier curve: The patency rates of 45 redo procedures for graft occlusions without a graft-related stenosis (lower curve) compared with 10 re-opening procedures in which also an anastomotic revision was done (upper curve). The numbers above and below the curves indicate the numbers at risk. (Courtesy of Pederson G, Laxdal E, Aune S. The outcome of occluded above-knee femoropopliteal prostheses implanted for critical ischaemia. *Eur J Vasc Endovasc Surg.* 2006;32:680-685. Copyright 2006 by Elsevier. Reprinted by permission of the publisher.)

Results.—Half of the 24 initial procedures to restored patency failed within one month. The outcome of second- or third-time redo procedures was similar. The primary patency rates of all 55 redo procedures were 32% at three months, 28% at six months and 12% at 12 months. The results of thrombectomy and thrombolysis were similar. Re-opened grafts additionally treated for an underlying anastomotic stenosis had significantly better patency as compared with re-opened grafts without a pre-existing stenosis on both univariate analysis ($p = 0.024$) and multivariate analysis ($p = 0.027$, hazard ratio 2.813). The one-year limb salvage rate was 76%. The one- and five-year survival rates were 87% and 52%, respectively.

Conclusions.—The results of redo procedures for occluded above-knee prosthetic grafts were disappointing. Grafts in which a graft-related stenosis was treated performed better than grafts in which occlusion could not be attributed to an underlying stenosis. Such cases should most likely be offered conservative treatment, amputation or a new arterial reconstruction (Fig 1, Fig 2).

▶ Re-do procedures directed to the original grafts for occluded above-knee prosthetic grafts (placed for chronic limb ischemia) demonstrate poor (12%) patency rates at one year. The reported limb salvage of 76% at one year is surprising and makes one wonder about how critical the critical limb ischemia actually was. No difference is demonstrated when comparing thrombolysis to thrombectomy. Identification and treatment of a graft stenosis was the only factor that conveyed longer graft patency. Perhaps placement of a new graft is a better way to go.

G. L. Moneta, MD

Does the timing of reoperation influence the risk of graft infection?

Kolakowski S Jr, Dougherty MJ, Calligaro KD (Pennsylvania Hosp, Philadelphia)
J Vasc Surg 45:60-64, 2007

Objective.—This study compared the incidence and characteristics of graft infection in patients who underwent early vs late revisional surgery of lower extremity arterial bypass grafts.

Methods.—Between 1992 and July 2005, 500 revisional procedures were performed on 198 lower extremity bypass grafts. Patients whose revisions were performed <30 days after the primary bypass were in the early revision (ER) group (n = 99), and those done >30 days after bypass were in the late revision (LR) group (n = 99). Infection was defined as cellulitis with graft exposure or purulence in continuity with a graft that required antibiotics and operation for infection control. Mean follow-up was 60 months (range, 2 to 60 months). Groups were compared using Student's *t* test.

Results.—The ER group included 66 autogenous and 33 prosthetic grafts. The LR group consisted of 53 autogenous and 46 prosthetic grafts. Of the 500 revisional procedures performed, 17 graft infections occurred (3.4%). Twelve (70.6%) were prosthetic grafts and five (29.4%) were autogenous grafts (P = .004). Defining the infection rate per graft rather than per revisional procedure, the ER group had a significantly higher graft infection rate at 11% (11/99) compared with 6.1% in the LR group (6/99; P = .012). The risk of infection for prosthetic grafts was significantly higher within the ER group at 27.3% (9/33) compared with autogenous grafts at 3.1% (2/66; P = .0001). Infection developed in three vein grafts and three prosthetic grafts in the LR group (P = NS). For prosthetic graft revisions only, infection risk was 27.3% (9/33) in the ER group and 6.5% (3/46) in the LR group (P = .005). The most common cultured pathogen was methicillin resistant *Staphylococcus aureus* (ER, 6/11 vs LR, 3/6; P = NS). Within the ER group, the prevalence of *Pseudomonas aeruginosa* was significantly higher at 27.3% (3/11) compared with 0% (0/6) in the LR group (P = .04).

Conclusions.—Early revision of lower extremity arterial bypass grafts has a significantly higher risk of graft infection compared with revision >1 month after surgery. Infection will develop in approximately 25% (9/33) of prosthetic grafts that are reoperated on early. If feasible, reoperation should be delayed >1 month for prosthetic grafts needing revision. Endovascular or extra-anatomic interventions should be considered if early revision is mandated in this group.

▶ The main point here is that revising a prosthetic lower extremity bypass <30 days results in an unacceptable rate of graft infection. This likely results from a need to reenter a groin incision where there is often less than perfect healing early on. The best way to avoid such a complication is to avoid the use of a prosthetic graft in the first place. It appears nearly one fourth of this group's infrainguinal bypasses are prosthetic compared to less than 5% in our practice in Oregon. A heightened dedication to autogenous bypass or perhaps more use of endovascular approaches in selected cases may help reduce the infection problem. Also, it is very common in our practice to place muscle flaps over grafts in the groin, whether they be prosthetic or autogenous, when we have to go back through a less than perfectly healed groin incision.

G. L. Moneta, MD

Flow measurement before and after papaverine injection in above-knee prosthetic femoropopliteal bypass
Pedersen G, Laxdal E, Amundsen SR, et al (Haukeland Univ, Bergen, Norway; Univ of Bergen, Norway)
J Vasc Surg 43:729-734, 2006

Objective.—To investigate the value of intraoperative blood flow measurements on early and long-term patency of above-knee prosthetic femoropopliteal bypass.

Methods.—Flow was measured with a transit time flowmeter before (basal flow) and after an intragraft injection of papaverine (papaverine flow) in 87 operations (86 patients) between January 1990 and December 2001. Sixty-one grafts were of polyester, and 26 were of polytetrafluoroethylene. The operations were done under epidural anesthesia. The preoperative angiographic run-off score and clinical risk factors were recorded. Patency rates were analyzed with the product limit method and compared with the log-rank test. Variables found to be near significantly related to patency rates ($P < .1$) were included in a multivariate analysis performed with the Cox proportional hazard model.

Results.—Basal flow measurements were not related to patency. The 2- and 5-year patency rates for grafts with a papaverine flow ≤ 500 mL/min were 48% and 18% compared with 66% and 52% for grafts with a papaverine flow ≥ 500 mL/min. These differences were statistically significant ($P = .012$, hazard ratio, 2.6). Two- and 5-year patency rates for smokers vs nonsmokers were 44% and 18% vs 69% and 54%. The patency rates for patients with poor vs good run-off were 42% and 27% vs 66% and 31%. Smoking ($P = .008$, hazard ratio, 2.75) and poor run-off score ($P = .009$, hazard ratio, 2.38) were found to be independent risk factors for reduced patency rates. Poor run-off score did not correlate with low values of measured basal or papaverine flow.

Conclusions.—Papaverine flow of ≤ 500 mL/min is associated with reduced mid- and long-term patency rates. Additional antithrombotic medication and frequent follow-up for these grafts should be considered. The inferior patency rates of smokers and patients with poor run-off indicate that prosthetic bypass is less suitable for these groups of patients.

▶ Flow was measured distal to new above-knee prosthetic grafts, placed for claudication and critical ischemia, both at baseline and after papaverine injection. Interestingly, the absolute post-papaverine flow, and not the change in flow, predicted eventual graft occlusion. Smoking and poor runoff score also predicted eventual graft occlusion. This information is novel, but is obtained after critical decisions have already been made (ie, the patient has already received the graft!).

G. L. Moneta, MD

Endoscopic versus open saphenous vein harvest for femoral to below the knee arterial bypass using saphenous vein graft
Gazoni LM, Carty R, Skinner J, et al (Univ of Virginia, Charlottesville)
J Vasc Surg 44:282-288, 2006

Background.—Although the use of endoscopic vein harvest (EVH) in coronary artery bypass grafting is accepted, few studies have documented the implementation of EVH in peripheral vascular disease surgery. We hypothesized that EVH improves outcomes compared with open vein harvest (OVH) in patients undergoing femoral to below the knee arterial bypass surgery.

Methods.—The charts of 144 consecutive patients undergoing infrainguinal bypass surgery over the course of 27 months were reviewed. A femoral to below the knee arterial bypass with saphenous vein was done in 88 patients (29 had EVH, 59 had OVH). The preoperative characteristics evaluated were age, gender, renal function, history of diabetes, hypertension, tobacco use, and previous infrainguinal bypass surgery on the affected side. End points included wound complications, length of hospital stay, operative time, angiographic and operative interventions for graft occlusion, patency rates, limb salvage, acute renal failure, myocardial infarction, and death.

Results.—Patient characteristics and demographics were similar in the EVH and OVH groups. No operative intervention for occlusion was required in the EVH group (0/29) compared with 13.4% in the OVH group (8/59) ($P = .03$). At the mean follow-up time of 21 months, primary patency rate was 92.8% in the EVH group and 80.6% in the OVH group ($P = .12$). No significant differences were found between the EVH and OVH groups in

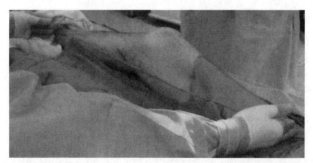

FIGURE 2.—Saphenous vein removed endoscopically from the contralateral leg. The most distal two harvest incisions are seen. (Reprinted by permission of the publisher from Gazoni LM, Carty R, Skinner J, et al. Endoscopic versus open saphenous vein harvest for femoral to below the knee arterial bypass using saphenous vein graft. *J Vasc Surg*. 2006;44:282-288. Copyright 2006 by Elsevier.)

postoperative complications, length of hospital stay, operative time, patency rates, limb salvage, and death.

Conclusion.—Despite our initial concerns of damaging the venous conduit with a minimally invasive approach to saphenous vein harvest, EVH in our experience has resulted in a trend toward improved patency rates and decreased infectious wound complications while affording the benefit of improved cosmesis. An endoscopic approach results in smaller incisions, decreased interventions for occlusion, and improved outcomes compared with OVH. EVH is the procedure of choice for harvesting saphenous vein for femoral to below the knee arterial bypass surgery (Fig 2).

▶ This study and that of Pullatt et al[1] focus on endoscopic harvest of the saphenous vein. Overall, data on this topic is pretty poor and this paper is really no exception. There are too few patients here to derive any conclusions about graft patency. Endovascular vein harvest was performed based on "availability of equipment," and no preoperative vein mapping was performed on any patient. You would think that if you really wanted to do this over the course of 2 years, a major university hospital could have acquired the necessary equipment. Also, in the modern world there is no excuse for not assessing the quality of the saphenous vein preoperatively. Both of these problems suggest a potential lack of dedication to infrainguinal autogenous reconstruction. It is also important to remember endoscopic vein harvest in vascular patients is different than in cardiac surgical patients. A groin incision cannot usually be avoided in an infrainguinal reconstruction. That is the site at most risk for infection. I think endoscopic saphenous vein harvest works best when the saphenous vein is of good quality, when it is reasonably deep in the leg, and when a groin incision can be avoided. You are kidding yourself if you think this technique does not add significant time to the procedure when performed by a single surgeon.

G. L. Moneta, MD

Reference

1. Pullatt R, Brothers TE, Robison JG, Elliott BM. Compromised bypass graft outcomes after minimal-incision vein harvest. *J Vasc Surg.* 2006;44:289-294.

Compromised bypass graft outcomes after minimal-incision vein harvest
Pullatt R, Brothers TE, Robison JG, et al (Med Univ of South Carolina)
J Vasc Surg 44:289-295, 2006

Background.—Minimal incision techniques for vein harvest may lessen wound complications after lower extremity revascularization, but long-term patency and limb salvage data are limited.

Methods.—This retrospective case-control study used a computerized vascular registry set in an academic vascular surgical practice. All patients undergoing lower extremity revascularization using autogenous reversed

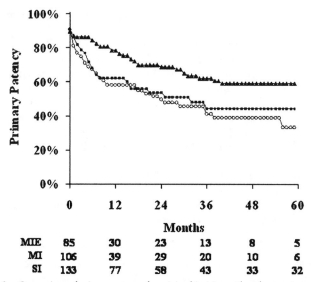

MIE	85	30	23	13	8	5
MI	106	39	29	20	10	6
SI	133	77	58	43	33	32

FIGURE 2.—Comparison of primary patency for minimal incision with endoscopy (*squares*), without endoscopy (*circles*), and single incisions (*triangles*). The standard errors do not exceed 10% at any time point. (Reprinted by permission of the publisher from Pullatt R, Brothers TE, Robison JG, et al. Compromised bypass graft outcomes after minimal-incision vein harvest. *J Vasc Surg.* 2006;44:289-295. Copyright 2006 by Elsevier.)

great saphenous vein by a single vascular surgeon in a 10-year period were reviewed. Harvest of great saphenous vein via long single incision (SI) in 133 patients was compared with minimal incisions with endoscopy (MIE) in 85, or MI without endoscopy in 106. The main outcome measures were primary and secondary graft patency by Kaplan-Meier life-table analysis and cumulative sum failure (CUSUM). Secondary outcomes of interest were limb salvage and wound complications.

Results.—No differences were observed between MIE, MI, and SI patients for demographic data, risk factors, or primary indications, including claudication, rest pain, ischemic ulcer, and gangrene. Endoscopic vein harvest patients were significantly more likely than MI or SI to be women and more likely to use tobacco. Primary patency at 5 years was better after SI vein harvest (59%) than with either MI (33%, $P = .004$) or MIE (44%, $P = .045$) techniques, although both MI groups had a higher proportion of bypass grafts to the popliteal artery. Similarly, cumulative secondary patency was better after SI (66%) than with MI (47%, $P = .045$), but not MIE (58%, $P = .45$). Differences in limb salvage at 5 years in SI (73%) were not statistically superior to either MI (59%, $P = .24$) or MIE (58%, $P = .13$). No learning curve for MI or MIE vein grafts was evident by CUSUM for primary patency at 12 months. No differences in wound complication rates were observed for SI (9%), MI (10%), or MIE (6%) grafts ($P = .54$).

Conclusions.—Graft patency and limb salvage deteriorated during the time when MI or MIE techniques of great saphenous vein harvest were adopted. This observation raises concern about the advisability of limiting the extent of the incision at the potential cost of compromised outcomes without an obvious advantage in limiting wound complications (Fig 2).

▶ The primary conclusions of this paper and the study by Gazoni et al[1] with respect to graft patency are clearly different, but comparison of data is impossible. In Gazoni et al, open harvest is done via skip incisions potentially more traumatic to the vein than an endoscopic harvest. In this paper the saphenous vein is harvested through a continuous incision, which is the preferred open method in my opinion. This paper involved a single primary surgeon for both the open and endoscopic vein harvest. Multiple surgeons and physician's assistants appear to be involved in the study by Gazoni et al. The conclusions of both papers, however, are likely correct for the author's respective institutions and techniques employed for autogenous leg bypass. I do not think the data from either institution can be extrapolated to our practice in Portland, Oregon.

G. L. Moneta, MD

Reference

1. Gazoni LM, Carty R, Skinner J, et al. Endoscopic versus open saphenous vein harvest for femoral to below the knee arterial bypass using saphenous vein graft. *J Vasc Surg.* 2006;44:282-287.

Prognostic Significance of Raised Cardiac Troponin T in Patients Presenting with Acute Limb Ischaemia

Rittoo D, Stahnke M, Lindesay C, et al (Univ Hosp Birmingham NHS Found Trust, England; Worcestershire Acute Hosps NHS Trust, England)
Eur J Vasc Endovasc Surg 32:500-503, 2006

Objective.—To study the relation between serum cardiac troponin T (cTnT) and mortality in patients presenting with acute limb ischaemia secondary to an embolism.

Material and Methods.—A two years prospective study of all patients admitted to the vascular unit with a diagnosis of acute limb ischaemia secondary to an embolism. On admission all patients had an ECG. A blood sample was taken for measurement of cTnT, CRP, serum biochemistry, full blood count and clotting. All embolectomies were performed under local anaesthesia. Patients were followed until discharge from hospital and up to twelve months after surgery.

Results.—There were 37 patients with lower limb and 2 patients with upper limb ischaemia. Twenty four patients were female and fifteen were male, with the mean age of 76 years (50–95) for women and 84 years (77–90) for men. Seventeen patients (44%) had a raised cTnT. The patients with raised cTnT were older than those with normal cTnT [86y (77–92) vs 77y (51–95), $p = 0.01$, t test]. The mean cTnT was 0.20 µg/L (range: 0.11–0.27). Only two patients with raised cTnT gave a history of chest pains. All of the patients with an elevated cTnT had also raised CRP. There was no significant difference in the serum creatinine in the group of patients with elevated cTnT compared to those with normal cTnT [112 μmol/L (range 98–159) vs 119 μmol/L (range: 47–177), p = ns]. The cumulative survival for cTnT+ patients at 7 days was 53% and that of cTnT− patients was 100%. The cumulative survival for cTnT+ and cTnT− patients was statistically different (p = 0.0000, χ^2 = 13.1, Log Rank test). Using regression analysis, an elevated cTnT was found to be an independent predictor of outcome.

Conclusion.—A significant proportion of patients presenting with an acutely ischaemic limb have an elevated cTnT. An elevated cTnT may be an early marker of overall disease severity and a predictor of outcome.

▶ An elevated level of serum troponin T at admission is highly associated with early mortality after treatment for embolism. This makes sense; heart attacks have never been shown to be a good thing.

G. L. Moneta, MD

Clinical outcomes after closed, staged, and open forefoot amputations
Berceli SA, Brown JE, Irwin PB, et al (Malcom Randall Veterans Affairs Med Ctr, Gainesville, Fla; Univ of Florida, Gainesville)
J Vasc Surg 44:347-352, 2006

Background.—Surgical approaches for forefoot osteomyelitis include amputation with immediate wound closure or resection followed by either staged re-resection and wound closure or local care of the open wound for secondary healing. This study evaluated the effectiveness of closed, staged, and open forefoot amputations in preventing major leg amputation and identified those variables that are associated with successful limb preservation.

Methods.—From July 2002 to June 2004, 208 patients with forefoot osteomyelitis or gangrene underwent minor amputation according to a standard treatment algorithm. Wounds with limited cellulitis underwent immediate wound closure (CLOSED), wounds with marginally viable soft tissue underwent open amputation followed by wound closure at 2 to 7 days (STAGED), and wounds with tenosynovitis or extensive necrosis underwent débridement with no attempt at wound closure (OPEN). Patient demographics, need for further operative interventions, time to complete healing, and progression to major amputation were recorded.

Results.—With four subjects lost to follow-up, 204 patients (98%) (94 CLOSED, 56 STAGED, and 54 OPEN) were monitored to complete healing, major amputation, or death. OPEN amputations had a significantly reduced initial healing rate (37%, P < .001) and a frequent need for repeat operative intervention (43%), although successful limb salvage was ultimately achieved in 70% of the cases. Initial healing in the CLOSED and STAGED amputation groups was similar (71% and 78%, respectively), leading to excellent early limb salvage (86% and 91%). The median time to healing for closed, staged, and open amputations was 1.2, 1.6, and 4.6 months, respectively (P < .001). Follow-up evaluation demonstrated the initial improvements in limb salvage with the CLOSED and STAGED groups were lost, resulting in similar amputation rates among the three groups of 30% to 35% over 36 months.

Conclusions.—Although open amputation of extensive forefoot infections frequently requires repeat operative interventions and a prolonged time to complete healing, this approach provides limb salvage rates approaching those observed for less invasive infections amenable to immediate closure. Staged closure offers an improved time to healing without negatively impacting the risk of major limb amputation. Independent of their initial operative approach, these patients frequently progress to early leg amputation.

▶ I believe this report mimics most clinical practices. Obviously, the patients in the closed stage and open groups are not the same. Nevertheless, the important point here is that an open forefoot amputation does not have to remain an open forefoot amputation. If possible, open amputations should be closed, because healing and limb salvage are the same for initial and delayed closure of the forefoot wound. Even though favorable initial healing did not provide improved limb salvage, the decreased need for dressing changes and increased patient discomfort associated with open wounds still makes either initial or stage closure of the forefoot wound preferable to healing by secondary intention.

G. L. Moneta, MD

Predictors for mortality after lower-extremity amputations in geriatric patients
Wong MWN (Chinese Univ of Hong Kong, Shatin)
Am J Surg 191:443-447, 2006

Background.—The identification of independent predictors for operative and long-term mortality after lower-extremity amputations in the geriatric population would allow targeted management for high-risk patients and appropriate allocation of resources.

Methods.—Univariate and multivariate logistic regression analyses were used to identify independent predictors for operative mortality. Life tables and Kaplan-Meier survival curves were generated. Independent predictors for long-term mortality were tested by log-rank test followed by Cox regression analysis.

Results.—Female gender, congestive heart failure, and high-level amputation were identified as independent predictors for operative mortality (odds ratios 4.14, 4.59, and 4.77, respectively). The logistic regression model showed good calibration and discriminative power. Female gender, high-level amputation, cerebrovascular accident, congestive heart failure, noncommunity ambulation, and institutionalization before amputation were associated with an increased risk for long-term mortality. However, only high-level amputation, congestive heart failure, and noncommunity ambulation remained as independent risk factors after Cox regression analysis (relative risks 1.68, 2.08, and 2.10, respectively).

Conclusions.—Extra care should be given to patients identified with independent predictors for operative and long-term mortality.

▶ The article implies more intensive care for patients with the identified predictors of mortality is needed. I am not sure that is a very useful conclusion. Patients should not receive less care because they are less apt to die. In addition, there is so much more to recovery following amputation than simple mortality rates. Such things as potential ambulation, quality of life, and independent living came to mind. This article addressed none of these important issues. The article was selected to emphasize the ominous prognosis of patients with above knee amputation.

G. L. Moneta, MD

Secondary Prevention of Arteriosclerosis in Lower Limb Vascular Amputees: A Missed Opportunity

Bradley L, Kirker SGB (Addenbrooke's Hosp, Cambridge, England)
Eur J Vasc Endovasc Surg 32:491-493, 2006

Objectives.—To determine the numbers of patients with peripheral vascular disease prescribed secondary prevention agents following a lower limb amputation.

Design.—A retrospective cross sectional study.

Methods.—The clinical documentation of 107 vascular amputees (mean age 69.5, 2:1 male:female ratio) referred for prosthesis provision in 2004 and 2005 were analysed to determine levels of prescribing of anti-platelet agents, anti-coagulants and cholesterol lowering drugs.

Results.—Analysis of vascular amputees referred in 2004 and 2005 reveals that 41% were prescribed a statin and 39% were prescribed a statin and 60% an anti-platelet agent. While 39% of these patients were on both drugs, 32% had been prescribed neither.

Conclusions.—The medical management of patients with severe peripheral vascular disease, even where their disease has led to an amputation, is sub-optimal.

▶ This study analyses the use of antiplatelet, anticoagulant, and cholesterol-lowering medications in subjects requiring one lower extremity amputation, and provides further proof that optimal medical therapy is often not employed for patients who need it the most—those with peripheral arterial disease.

G. L. Moneta, MD

Surgical management of popliteal artery aneurysms: Which factors affect outcomes?
Pulli R, Dorigo W, Troisi N, et al (Univ of Florence, Italy)
J Vasc Surg 43:481-487, 2006

Objective.—Popliteal artery aneurysm (PAA) is uncommon. The clinical presentation of PAA includes rupture, embolism, and thrombosis. In this article, we evaluate the results of our 20-year experience with surgical management of PAAs, analyzing the role of anatomic, clinical, and surgical factors that potentially affect early and long-term results.

Methods.—From January 1984 to December 2004, 159 PAAs in 137 patients were operated on at our department. Data from all the patients were retrospectively collected in a database. PAAs were asymptomatic in 67 cases (42%); 5 (3%) PAAs were ruptured. In 51 cases (32%), PAA caused intermittent claudication. The remaining 36 limbs (23%) had threatening ischemia due in 30 cases to acute PAA thrombosis, in 4 cases to chronic PAA thrombosis, and in 2 cases to distal embolization. In selected patients with acute ischemia, preoperative intra-arterial thrombolysis with urokinase was performed. Early results in terms of mortality, graft thrombosis, and limb salvage were assessed. Follow-up consisted of clinical and ultrasonographic examinations at 1, 6, and 12 months and yearly thereafter. Long-term survival, patency, and limb salvage rates were analyzed.

Results.—Forty cases were treated with aneurysmectomy and prosthetic graft interposition; in 39 cases, the aneurysm was opened, and a graft was placed inside the aneurysm. Four patients had aneurysmectomy with end-to-end anastomosis. In 73 cases, ligation of the aneurysm with bypass grafting (39 with a prosthetic graft and 34 with an autologous vein) was performed. The remaining three patients underwent endovascular exclusion of their PAAs. A medial approach was used in 97 patients (61%), and a posterior approach was used in 59 patients (37.1%). The outflow vessel was in most cases (93.7%) the below-knee popliteal artery. Thirty-day amputation and death rates were 4.4% (7/159 limbs) and 2.1% (3/137 patients), respectively. The amputation rate was significantly higher in symptomatic limbs than in asymptomatic ones (6.5% and 1.4%, respectively; $P = .05$). Eight limbs (5%) had an early graft thrombosis that required a reintervention. Follow-up was available in 116 patients (84.7%) and 138 limbs (86%) with a mean follow-up time of 40 months (range, 1-205 months). The cumulative estimated 60-month survival, limb salvage, and primary and secondary patency rates were 84.2%, 86.7%, 66.3%, and 83.6%, respectively. Asymptomatic limbs had significantly better results than symptomatic ones in terms of limb salvage (93.4% and 80.4%, respectively; $P = .03$; log-rank, 4.2) and primary patency (86.5% and 51.6%, respectively; $P = .001$; log-rank, 10.3). Among symptomatic patients, results were better in claudicant limbs than in acutely ischemic ones in terms of limb salvage (90.5% and 58.7%, respectively; $P = .001$; log-rank, 17.5). Univariate analysis showed the absence of symptoms, the presence of two or three tibial vessels, the use

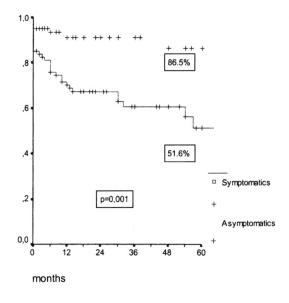

Months	0	12	24	36	48	60
Asymptomatics (n. at risk)	61	41	29	23	19	15
Symptomatics (n. at risk)	79	50	33	24	18	8

FIGURE 2.—Sixty-month estimated primary patency in symptomatic and asymptomatic limbs. (Reprinted by permission of the publisher from Pulli R, Dorigo W, Troisi N, et al. Surgical management of popliteal artery aneurysms: which factors affect outcomes? *J Vasc Surg.* 2006;43:481-487. Copyright 2006 by Elsevier.)

of a posterior approach, the kind of intervention, and the site of distal anastomosis to significantly affect long-term patency. Cox regression for factors affecting 60-month primary patency showed that clinical presentation, runoff status, and the site of distal anastomosis significantly influenced long-term results.

Conclusions.—Results of surgery on asymptomatic PAAs are good—significantly better than those for symptomatic ones. Elective surgical intervention should be performed in patients with a low surgical risk and a long life expectancy when the correct indication exists. In thrombosed aneurysms, intra-arterial thrombolysis may represent an alternative to emergent surgical management. Our data demonstrated that results are similarly good in claudicants, and this fact confirms that only acute ischemia due to PAA thrombosis represents a real surgical challenge. In selected patients with focal lesions, a posterior approach seems to offer better long-term results. The runoff status and the site of distal anastomosis affect long-term patency as well (Fig 2).

▶ A large, single-institution series is presented and emphasizes that outcomes are drastically improved if treatment is performed before the runoff is compromised and symptoms ensue. Mortality was only associated with multiple concomitant surgical interventions being performed in other arterial locations.

G. L. Moneta, MD

12 Upper Extremity and Dialysis Access

Atherosclerotic Renovascular Disease in Older US Patients Starting Dialysis, 1996 to 2001

Guo H, Kalra PA, Gilbertson DT, et al (US Renal Data System Coordinating Ctr, Minneapolis; Hope Hosp, Salford, England; Univ of Minnesota, Minneapolis)
Circulation 115:50-58, 2007

Background.—Temporal trends regarding the epidemiology of atherosclerotic renovascular disease (ARVD) in dialysis populations are poorly defined.

Methods and Results.—United States Renal Data System data were used to identify patients aged 67 years or older at dialysis inception between 1996 and 2001 (n=146,973). Medicare claims in the preceding 2 years were used to identify ARVD and revascularization procedures. Prior ARVD rose from 7.1% to 11.2% between 1996 and 2001 (adjusted odds ratio [AOR], 1.68). Other associations included hypertensive end-stage renal disease (ESRD; AOR, 2.21), ESRD network (AOR, 0.44 in network 17 versus 1.00 in network 1), peripheral vascular disease (AOR, 1.65), black race (AOR, 0.44), urologic cause of ESRD (AOR, 0.57), age >85 years (AOR, 0.58), substance dependency (AOR, 0.62), and inability to ambulate or transfer (AOR, 0.67). The proportion of ARVD patients undergoing revascularization rose from 14.6% to 16.7% between 1996 and 2001 (AOR, 1.27). Other associations included hypertension (AOR, 2.10), ESRD network (AOR, 2.07 for network 13 versus 1.00 in network 1), age >85 years (AOR, 0.53), and black race (AOR, 0.54). The rise in ARVD was not reflected in the proportion of patients with renovascular disease listed as cause of ESRD on the Medical Evidence Report at dialysis inception (5.5% in 1996, 5.0% in 2001).

Conclusions.—ARVD diagnoses have become more common in older patients beginning dialysis therapy. The association of demographic factors including age, race, and geographic residence with utilization patterns suggests possible barriers to care.

▶ This is a complicated article, but several points are worth mentioning. First, it appears that the incidence of atherosclerotic renal vascular disease (ARVD) as a source of end-stage renal disease (ESRD) is increasing. Second, although the proportion of patients with ESRD secondary to ARVD is low in comparison to other causes, it is still a large number of people. Third, it is disturbing that the diagnosis and treatment of ARVD varies by geographic region and with various subgroups of the population. This suggests that there is regional overtreatment, undertreatment, and/or societal barriers to care of patients with ARVD.

G. L. Moneta, MD

Risk Equation Determining Unsuccessful Cannulation Events and Failure to Maturation in Arteriovenous Fistulas (REDUCE FTM I)
Lok CE, Allon M, Moist L, et al (Univ of Toronto; Sunnybrook Health Sciences Ctr, Toronto; Univ of Western Ontario, London, Canada; et al)
J Am Soc Nephrol 17:3204-3212, 2006

Fistulas are the preferred permanent hemodialysis vascular access but a significant obstacle to increasing their prevalence is the fistula's high "failure to mature" (FTM) rate. This study aimed to (1) identify preoperative clinical characteristics that are predictive of fistula FTM and (2) use these predictive factors to develop and validate a scoring system to stratify the patient's risk for FTM. From a derivation set of 422 patients who had a first fistula created, a prediction rule was created using multivariate stepwise logistic regression. The model was internally validated using split-half cross-validation and bootstrapping techniques. A simple scoring system was derived and externally validated on 445 different, prospective patients who received a new fistula at five large North American dialysis centers. The clinical predictors that were associated with FTM were aged ≥65 yr (odds ratio [OR] 2.23; 95% confidence interval [CI] 1.25 to 3.96), peripheral vascular disease (OR 2.97; 95% CI 1.34 to 6.57), coronary artery disease (OR 2.83; 95% CI 1.60 to 5.00), and white race (OR 0.43; 95% CI 0.24 to 0.75). The resulting scoring system, which was externally validated in 445 patients, had four risk categories for fistula FTM: low (24%), moderate (34%), high (50%), and very high (69%; trend $P < 0.0001$). A preoperative, clinical prediction rule to determine fistulas that are likely to fail maturation was created and rigorously validated. It was found to be simple and easily reproducible and applied to predictive risk categories. These categories predicted risk of FTM to be 24, 34, 50, and 69% and are dependent on age, coronary artery disease, peripheral vascular disease, and race. The clinical utility of these risk categories in increasing rates of permanent accesses requires further clinical evaluation.

▶ A scoring system for predicting arteriovenous (AV) fistula "failure to maturation" that is not based on specific factors shown to effect maturation (vein size/quality, obesity, gender, diabetes mellitus, or location) is like trying to have sex with clothes on—it can't be very effective. Although a scoring system that helps select patients for AV fistula creation is a good idea, it must be based on those factors known to be associated with fistula failure.

G. L. Moneta, MD

Inflow Stenoses in Dysfunctional Hemodialysis Access Fistulae and Grafts

Duijm LEM, Liem YS, van der Rijt RHH, et al (Catharina Hosp, Eindhoven, The Netherlands; MC-Univ Med Ctr Rotterdam, The Netherlands)
Am J Kidney Dis 48:98-105, 2006

Background.—The aim of the study is to prospectively determine the incidence of inflow stenoses in dysfunctional hemodialysis access arteriovenous fistulae (AVFs) and grafts (AVGs).

Methods.—Contrast-enhanced magnetic resonance angiography (CE-MRA) was performed of 66 dysfunctional AVFs and 35 AVGs in 56 men and 45 women (mean age, 62 years; age range, 31 to 86 years). Complete inflow (from the subclavian artery), shunt region, and complete outflow (including subclavian vein) were shown at CE-MRA. In addition to standard digital subtraction angiography (DSA) of the shunt region and outflow, DSA of the complete inflow was obtained through access catheterization of all cases in which CE-MRA showed an inflow stenosis. Vascular stenosis is defined as greater than 50% decrease in luminal diameter compared with an uninvolved vascular segment located adjacent to the stenosis. Endovascular intervention of stenoses was performed in connection with DSA.

Results.—CE-MRA showed 19 arterial stenoses in 14 patients (14%). DSA confirmed 18 of these lesions in 13 patients and showed no additional inflow lesions. Of the 13 patients, 7 patients had arterial stenoses only and 6 patients had accompanying stenoses in the shunt region and/or outflow. Referral criteria for the 13 patients to undergo access evaluation had been decreased flow rates (9 patients), steal symptoms (2 patients), and insufficient

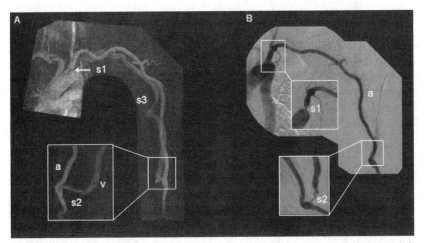

FIGURE 1.—Images obtained with 3-dimensional CE (A) MRA and (B) DSA show a brachiocephalic fistula with 3 stenoses. Abbreviations: a, artery; s1, stenosis at the origin of subclavian artery; s2, stenosis at arteriovenous anastomosis; s3, cephalic vein stenosis; v, vein. (Courtesy of Duijm LEM, Liem YS, van der Rijt RHH, et al. Inflow stenoses in dysfunctional hemodialysis access fistulae and grafts. *Am J Kidney Dis.* 2006;48:98-105. Copyright National Kidney Foundation.)

access maturation (2 patients). Access flow of the 9 patients with a low-flow access improved from 477 ± 74 mL/min to 825 ± 199 mL/min after angioplasty. One patient with steal symptoms became symptom free after angioplasty. Endovascular intervention in 3 patients proved to be unsuccessful.

Conclusion.—Inflow stenoses are not uncommon in dysfunctional hemodialysis access shunts. We suggest that radiological evaluation comprise assessment of the complete arterial inflow (Fig 1).

▶ These authors believe that a complete radiographic evaluation of the arterial inflow should be performed on all dysfunctional arteriovenous accesses and that arterial stenoses, if found, should be treated. Such an approach is costly. Furthermore, given the consequences of an arterial dissection or rupture to the extremity, arterial intervention should not be considered unless it is thought to be causing the access dysfunction. To quote advice from a fortune cookie, "Do not trouble trouble unless trouble troubles you."

G. L. Moneta, MD

Randomized comparison of ultrasound surveillance and clinical monitoring on arteriovenous graft outcomes
Robbin ML, Oser RF, Lee JY, et al (Univ of Alabama at Birmingham)
Kidney Int 69:730-735, 2006

Arteriovenous graft thrombosis is a frequent event in hemodialysis patients, and usually occurs in grafts with significant underlying stenosis. Regular surveillance for graft stenosis, with pre-emptive angioplasty of significant lesions, may improve graft outcomes. This prospective, randomized, clinical trial allocated 126 hemodialysis patients with grafts to either clinical monitoring alone (control group) or to regular ultrasound surveillance for graft stenosis every 4 months in addition to clinical monitoring (ultrasound group). The two randomized groups were closely matched with respect to demographic, clinical, and graft characteristics, with the exception of a lower frequency of diabetes in the ultrasound group. The primary outcome was graft survival, and the secondary outcome was thrombosis-free graft survival. The frequency of pre-emptive graft angioplasty was 64% higher in the ultrasound group than in the control group (1.05 vs 0.64 events per patient-year, $P<0.001$), whereas the frequency of thrombosis was not different (0.67 vs 0.78 per patient-year, $P=0.37$). The median time to permanent graft failure was similar between the two groups (38 vs 37 months, $P=0.93$). Likewise, the median time to graft thrombosis or failure did not differ (22 vs 25 months, $P=0.33$). There was no significant association between diabetes and time to graft failure ($P=0.93$) or time to graft thrombosis or failure ($P=0.88$). In conclusion, the addition of regular ultrasound surveillance for graft stenosis to clinical monitoring increases the frequency of pre-emptive angioplasty, but may not decrease the likelihood of graft failure or thrombosis.

▶ This is one of several prospective randomized studies that should "put a fork" in the notion that a routine program of arteriovenous (AV) graft surveillance with US or fistulography and preemptive angioplasty of asymptomatic stenoses will improve AV graft outcomes. Such programs are costly and do not prevent graft thrombosis or increase graft longevity.

G. L. Moneta, MD

Effect of Change in Vascular Access on Patient Mortality in Hemodialysis Patients
Allon M, for the HEMO Study Group (Univ of Alabama at Birmingham, et al)
Am J Kidney Dis 47:469-477, 2006

Background.—Hemodialysis patients using a catheter have a greater mortality risk than those using an arteriovenous (AV) access (fistula or graft). However, catheter-dependent patients also differ from those with an AV access in several clinical features, and these differences may themselves contribute to their excess mortality.

Methods.—The current study evaluates whether a change in vascular access affects risk for mortality in patients enrolled in the Hemodialysis Study. Time-dependent Cox regression was used to relate mortality risk to current type of access and change in access type during the preceding 1 year.

Results.—Compared with patients who dialyzed using an AV access at both the beginning and end of the preceding 1-year interval, relative risks for mortality were 3.43 (95% confidence interval [CI], 2.42 to 4.86) in patients who dialyzed with a catheter at both times; 2.38 (95% CI, 1.76 to 3.23) in patients switching from an AV access to a catheter, and 1.37 (95% CI, 0.81 to 2.32) in patients switching from a catheter to an AV access. Change from AV access to a catheter was associated with an antecedent decrease in serum albumin level (odds ratio, 1.25; 95% CI, 1.09 to 1.45 per 0.5 g/dL; $P = 0.002$), weight loss (odds ratio, 1.14; 95% CI, 1.06 to 1.22 per 2 kg; $P < 0.001$), and decreases in equilibrated normalized protein catabolic rate (odds ratio, 2.22; 95% CI, 1.41 to 3.57 per 0.25 g/kg/d; $P < 0.001$) and non–access-related hospitalization (odds ratio, 1.19; 95% CI, 1.06 to 1.32 per 1 additional hospitalization over 4 months; $P = 0.002$). Change from a catheter to AV access was predicted by only the antecedent non–access-related hospitalization rate (odds ratio, 0.93; 95% CI, 0.87 to 0.97 per 1 additional hospitalization over 4 months; $P < 0.001$).

Conclusion.—Change from a catheter to AV access is associated with a substantial decrease in mortality risk.

▶ The increased mortality associated with catheter use is due in part to the catheter itself and not just the presence of other factors associated with mortality. The practice of using a catheter to bridge the period of fistula maturation has resulted in a marked increase in catheter use as programs to increase arteriovenous (AV) fistula use have been implemented. It is likely that diminishing benefits will be realized as efforts to further enhance AV fistula use are implemented.

G. L. Moneta, MD

Asymptomatic Central Venous Stenosis in Hemodialysis Patients
Levit RD, Cohen RM, Kwak A, et al (Univ of Pennsylvania, Philadelphia)
Radiology 238:1051-1056, 2006

Purpose.—To retrospectively evaluate the natural history of high-grade (>50%) asymptomatic central venous stenosis (CVS) in hemodialysis patients and the outcome of serial treatment of CVS with percutaneous transluminal angioplasty (PTA).

Materials and Methods.—The institutional review board granted exemption for this retrospective study, the need for informed consent was waived, and all data collection was in compliance with HIPAA. Patients with hemodialysis access requiring maintenance procedures between 1998 and 2004 and incidentally found to have ipsilateral ($\geq$50%) CVS were identified from a departmental database. Thirty-five patients (19 men, 16 women; mean age, 58.7 years) with 38 grafts met inclusion criteria, and 86 venograms were reviewed. CVS was measured by using venograms obtained before and after PTA, if performed. Patients with arm swelling, multiple CVS, indwelling catheters, and stents at the first encounter were excluded. CVS progression was calculated by dividing the change in the degree of stenosis by the time between venographic examinations. Wilcoxon rank sum test was used to evaluate differences in rate of CVS progression between treated and nontreated patients.

Results.—Mean degree of CVS before intervention was 71% (range, 50%–100%). Sixty-two percent (53 of 86) of lesions had associated collateral vessels; 28% (24 of 86) of CVSs were not treated. Mean degree of stenosis in this group was 72% (range, 30%–100%); mean progression was −0.08 percentage point per day. No untreated CVS progressed to symptoms, stent placement, or additional CVS. Seventy-two percent (62 of 86) of CVSs were treated with PTA. Mean degree of stenosis in this group was 74% (range, 50%–100%) before and 40% (range, 0%–75%) after treatment; mean progression was 0.21 percentage point per day after treatment ($P = .03$). Six (8%) of 62 treatments were followed by CVS escalation; one patient developed arm swelling, four required stents, and four developed additional CVS.

Conclusion.—PTA of asymptomatic CVS greater than 50% in the setting of hemodialysis access maintenance procedures was associated with more rapid stenosis progression and escalation of lesions, compared with a nontreatment approach.

▶ In the case where both a distal venous and central venous stenosis is identified during fistulography for a thrombosed arteriovenous (AV) graft, these authors advocate treating only the distal stenosis. The outcome of this approach in terms of AV graft patency was not addressed in this study. Despite this limitation, I tend to agree with their conclusions.

G. L. Moneta, MD

Diagnostic Imaging of and Radiologic Intervention for Bovine Ureter Grafts Used as a Novel Conduit for Hemodialysis Fistulas
Warakaulle DR, Evans AL, Cornall AJ, et al (Churchill Hosp, Oxford, England; John Radcliffe Hosp, Oxford, England)
AJR 188:641-646, 2007

Objective.—The objectives of our study were to review the appearances on diagnostic imaging and amenability to imaging-guided intervention of a novel bovine ureter graft (Syner-Graft 100 [SG 100]) for use as a conduit for hemodialysis fistulas.

Conclusion.—The SG 100 shows initial promise as a conduit for hemodialysis fistulas in patients with difficult vascular access. The SG 100 has characteristic appearances on diagnostic imaging and is prone to similar pathologic processes that affect autogenous venous and synthetic grafts. These grafts are readily amenable to imaging-guided percutaneous intervention, which plays a major role in prolonging graft function.

▶ Although the bovine ureter graft has been on the market since 2002, the worldwide experience with this graft is limited. However, it is comforting to know that the imaging of this graft is remarkably similar to every other graft conduit, just in case the use of this graft catches on.

G. L. Moneta, MD

13 Carotid and Cerebrovascular Disease

Improvement in Stroke Mortality in Canada and the United States, 1990 to 2002
Yang Q, Botto LD, Erickson JD, et al (Ctrs for Disease Control and Prevention, Atlanta, Ga; Univ of Utah, Salt Lake City; Statistics Canada, Ottawa, Ont; et al)
Circulation 113:1335-1343, 2006

Background.—In the United States and Canada, folic acid fortification of enriched grain products was fully implemented by 1998. The resulting population-wide reduction in blood homocysteine concentrations might be expected to reduce stroke mortality if high homocysteine levels are an independent risk factor for stroke.

Methods and Results.—In this population-based cohort study with quasi-experimental intervention, we used segmented log-linear regression to evaluate trends in stroke-related mortality before and after folic acid fortification in the United States and Canada and, as a comparison, during the same period in England and Wales, where fortification is not required. Average blood folate concentrations increased and homocysteine concentrations decreased in the United States after fortification. The ongoing decline in stroke mortality observed in the United States between 1990 and 1997 accelerated in 1998 to 2002 in nearly all population strata, with an overall change from -0.3% (95% CI, -0.7 to 0.08) to -2.9 (95% CI, -3.5 to -2.3) per year ($P=0.0005$). Sensitivity analyses indicate that changes in other major recognized risk factors are unlikely to account for the reduced number of stroke-related deaths in the United States. The fall in stroke mortality in Canada averaged -1.0% (95% CI, -1.4 to -0.6) per year from 1990 to 1997 and accelerated to -5.4% (95% CI, -6.0 to -4.7) per year in 1998 to 2002 ($P\leq0.0001$). In contrast, the decline in stroke mortality in England and Wales did not change significantly between 1990 and 2002.

Conclusions.—The improvement in stroke mortality observed after folic acid fortification in the United States and Canada but not in England and

Wales is consistent with the hypothesis that folic acid fortification helps to reduce deaths from stroke.

▶ The data provide strong, albeit indirect, evidence that stroke mortality can be modified by reducing overall homocysteine levels in the population. The sophisticated statistical method used in this study make it unlikely that the findings represent chance alone. It is, however, unknown whether the reduction in stroke mortality is secondary to a decreased incidence of stroke or a decreased case fatality rate of stroke reflecting better stroke care rather than decreasing stroke incidence.

G. L. Moneta, MD

No evidence that severity of stroke in internal carotid occlusion is related to collateral arteries
Mead GE, for the Lothian Stroke Registry Study Group (Western Gen Hosp, Edinburgh, Scotland; Royal Infirmary of Edinburgh, Scotland)
J Neurol Neurosurg Psychiatry 77:729-733, 2006

Background/Aim.—The neurological effects of internal carotid artery (ICA) occlusion vary between patients. The authors investigated whether the severity of symptoms in a large group of patients with ipsilateral or/and contralateral ICA occlusion at presentation with ocular or cerebral ischaemic symptoms could be explained by patency of other extra or intracranial arteries to act as collateral pathways.

Methods.—The authors prospectively identified all patients (n = 2881) with stroke, cerebral transient ischaemic attack (TIA), retinal artery occlusion (RAO), and amaurosis fugax (AFx) presenting to our hospital over five years, obtained detailed history and examination, and examined the intra and extracranial arteries with carotid and colour-power transcranial Doppler ultrasound. For this analysis, all those with intracranial haemorrhage on brain imaging and cerebral events without brain imaging were excluded.

Results.—Among 2228/2397 patients with brain imaging (1713 ischaemic strokes, 401 cerebral TIAs, 193 AFx, and 90 RAO) who underwent carotid Doppler, 195 (9%) had ICA occlusion. Among those patients with cortical events, disease in potential collateral arteries (contralateral ICA, external carotid, ipsilateral or contralateral vertebral or intracranial arteries) was equally distributed among patients with severe and mild ischaemic presenting symptoms.

Conclusion.—The authors found no evidence that the clinical presentation associated with an ICA occlusion was related to patency of other extra or intracranial arteries to act as collateral pathways. Further work is required to investigate what determines the clinical effects of ICA occlusion (Table 1).

▶ The results of this paper do not make intuitive sense. One would expect collateralization to influence the results of ICA occlusion. Indeed, there are

TABLE 1.—Disease of the Contralateral Internal Carotid Artery, Ipsilateral or Contralateral External Carotid Arteries, and Vertebral Arteries in Patients With Cortical Symptoms and an Ipsilateral ICA Occlusion

	TACI and Ipsilateral ICA Occlusion (n = 22)	PACI and Ipsilateral ICA Occlusion (n = 70)	Cortical TIA and Ipsilateral ICA Occlusion (n = 14)	Other Patients With Any ICA Occlusion (n = 89)
Contralateral ICA disease ≥70% stenosis, n (%)	5 (23%)	20 (29%)	5 (36%)	47 (53%)
Any ipsilateral ECA stenosis, n (%)	10 (45%)	29 (41%)	5 (36%)	42 (47%)
Any contralateral ECA stenosis, n (%)	7 (32%)	18 (26%)	4 (29%)	36 (40%)
Ipsilateral vertebral artery occluded or reduced flow, n (%)	1 (5%)	8 (11%)	0 (0%)	2 (2%)
Contralateral vertebral artery occluded or reduced flow, n (%)	1 (5%)	7 (10%)	0 (0%)	2 (2%)

ICA, internal carotid artery; ECA, external carotid artery.
Ipsilateral vertebral artery is on the same side of the neck as the ipsilaterol ICA.
"Other" includes the contralateral occlusions, and the RAO, Afx, LACI, lacunar TIA, POCI, and posterior circulation TIA with ipsilateral occlusions.
(Courtesy of Mead GE, for the Lothian Stroke Registry Study Group. No evidence that severity of stroke in internal carotid occlusion is related to collateral arteries. *J Neurol Neurosurg Psychiatry.* 2006;77:729-733.Reprinted by permission of the BMJ Publishing Group.)

several limitations to this study. The authors did not include asymptomatic people with ICA occlusion. In addition, patients with very severe symptoms were not studied. Plus the potential extremes of the effects of collateral pathways were not addressed. Finally, US was used to assess collateral pathways. Whereas US may be accurate in detecting patency of collateral pathways, there was no analysis of volume flow or functionality of the collateral pathways. Additional data are required before we can accept that collateral pathways do not influence the clinical outcome of ICA occlusion.

G. L. Moneta, MD

Carotid Intima-Media Thickening Indicates a Higher Vascular Risk Across a Wide Age Range: Prospective Data From the Carotid Atherosclerosis Progression Study (CAPS)

Lorenz MW, von Kegler S, Steinmetz H, et al (Johann Wolfgang Goethe-Univ, Frankfurt am Main Germany; St Georges Univ of London, England)
Stroke 37:87-92, 2006

Background and Purpose.—Carotid intima-media thickness (IMT) is an independent predictor of vascular events in age groups >45 years. However, there is little information about the predictive value of IMT in younger individuals.

Methods.—In the Carotid Atherosclerosis Progression Study (CAPS; n=5056; age range 19 to 90 years; mean age 50.1 years), common carotid artery (CCA) IMT, bifurcation IMT, internal carotid artery IMT and vascular risk factors were evaluated at baseline. The incidence of stroke, myocardial infarction (MI), and death was determined prospectively. Data for younger (<50 years; n=2436) and older subjects (≥50 years; n=2620) were analyzed separately using Cox proportional hazard regression models.

Results.—During a mean follow-up period of 4.2 years, there were 228 cases of MI, 107 strokes, and 50 deaths. IMT at all carotid segments was highly predictive of all end points (eg, hazard rate ratios [HRRs] per 1 SD CCA-IMT increase were 1.43 [95% CI: 1.35 to 1.51] for MI, 1.47 [1.35 to 1.60] for stroke, and 1.45 [1.38 to 1.52] for MI, stroke or death; all $P<0.0001$). Even after adjustment for age, sex, and vascular risk factors, the predictive value of CCA-IMT and bifurcation IMT remained significant for MI and the combined end point. For the latter, the HRRs were considerably higher in the younger than in the older age group (eg, HRR per 0.1 mm CCA-IMT was 1.34 [1.16 to 1.55] vis-à-vis 1.10 [1.05 to 1.15]; $P=0.011$ for age-IMT interaction).

Conclusions.—Carotid IMT independently predicts future vascular events. Its predictive value is at least as high in younger subjects as in older subjects.

▶ Carotid intima-media thickness (IMT) is clearly a marker of vascular risk. This study suggests that the risk associated with increases in IMT may be higher in younger than older individuals. IMT measurements provide extraordinarily interesting epidemiological information. It is, however, time to move forward and determine whether patients with increased IMT can be targeted for modification of atherosclerotic risk factors and a decrease in late vascular event rates.

G. L. Moneta, MD

Elevated Matrix Metalloproteinase-9 Associated With Stroke or Cardiovascular Death in Patients with Carotid Stenosis

Eldrup N, Grønholdt M-LM, Sillesen H, et al (Copenhagen Univ; Univ of Copenhagen)

Circulation 114:1847-1854, 2006

Background.—Matrix metalloproteinase-9 could exhibit an important role in the destabilization of atherosclerotic carotid plaques. We hypothesized that in patients with carotid stenosis, elevated levels of plasma matrix metalloproteinase-9 are associated with ipsilateral stroke or cardiovascular death.

Methods and Results.—We followed up 207 patients with ≥50% carotid stenosis initially for a mean of 4.4 years, during which time 53 patients developed ipsilateral stroke or died of cardiovascular causes. The cumulative incidence of ipsilateral stroke or cardiovascular death was higher in those with matrix metalloproteinase-9 above versus below the median of 41.9 ng/mL (log-rank $P=0.002$). Matrix metalloproteinase-9 above versus below the median had a hazard ratio for ipsilateral stroke or cardiovascular death of 1.9 (95% confidence interval [CI], 1.1 to 3.5); during extended follow-up, this remained significant until 10 years. The absolute risk of ipsilateral stroke or cardiovascular death at 4.4 years was 34% and 17% in those with matrix metalloproteinase-9 above and below the median, respectively. Elevated matrix metalloproteinase-9 and an echolucent plaque on B-mode ultrasound versus a low matrix metalloproteinase-9 and an echorich plaque had a hazard ratio for ipsilateral stroke or cardiovascular death of 4.4 (95% CI, 1.8 to 11.1) and for ipsilateral stroke of 3.3 (95% CI, 1.1 to 9.7).

Conclusions.—Elevated levels of matrix metalloproteinase-9 in patients with ≥50% carotid stenosis were associated with a 2-fold risk of ipsilateral stroke or cardiovascular death. Combining elevated matrix metalloproteinase-9 and plaque echolucency was associated with a 4-fold risk for ipsilateral stroke or cardiovascular death and a 3-fold risk for ipsilateral stroke.

▶ Other studies have also suggested that serum levels of matrix metalloproteinase-9 (MMP-9) may be a marker of cardiovascular risk.[1] It is odd that in this paper symptomatic status or degree of stenosis did not correlate with the risk of stroke. Perhaps this study was underpowered. Nevertheless, it is interesting to speculate how MMP-9 could act as a marker of cardiovascular risk. MMP-9 is released by inflammatory cells and can aid in breaking down extracellular matrix. This could destabilize plaques not only in the neck but in the coronary peripheral circulation as well. So is MMP-9 a link between the inflammatory component of atherosclerosis and the development of clinical events?[1]

G. L. Moneta, MD

Reference

1. Blankenberg S, for the AtheroGene Investigators. Plasma concentrations and genetic variation of matrix metalloproteinase 9 and prognosis of patients with cardiovascular disease. *Circulation.* 2003;107:1579-1585.

High-Dose Atorvastatin after Stroke or Transient Ischemic Attack
Welch KMA, for The Stroke Prevention by Aggressive Reduction in Cholesterol Levels (SPARCL) Investigators (Rosalind Franklin Univ of Medicine and Science, North Chicago; et al)
N Engl J Med 355:549-559, 2006

Background.—Statins reduce the incidence of strokes among patients at increased risk for cardiovascular disease; whether they reduce the risk of stroke after a recent stroke or transient ischemic attack (TIA) remains to be established.

Methods.—We randomly assigned 4731 patients who had had a stroke or TIA within one to six months before study entry, had low-density lipoprotein (LDL) cholesterol levels of 100 to 190 mg per deciliter (2.6 to 4.9 mmol per liter), and had no known coronary heart disease to double-blind treatment with 80 mg of atorvastatin per day or placebo. The primary end point was a first nonfatal or fatal stroke.

Results.—The mean LDL cholesterol level during the trial was 73 mg per deciliter (1.9 mmol per liter) among patients receiving atorvastatin and 129 mg per deciliter (3.3 mmol per liter) among patients receiving placebo. During a median follow-up of 4.9 years, 265 patients (11.2 percent) receiving atorvastatin and 311 patients (13.1 percent) receiving placebo had a fatal or nonfatal stroke (5-year absolute reduction in risk, 2.2 percent; adjusted hazard ratio, 0.84; 95 percent confidence interval, 0.71 to 0.99; P=0.03; unadjusted P=0.05). The atorvastatin group had 218 ischemic strokes and 55 hemorrhagic strokes, whereas the placebo group had 274 ischemic strokes and 33 hemorrhagic strokes. The five-year absolute reduction in the risk of major cardiovascular events was 3.5 percent (hazard ratio, 0.80; 95 percent confidence interval, 0.69 to 0.92; P=0.002). The overall mortality rate was similar, with 216 deaths in the atorvastatin group and 211 deaths in the placebo group (P=0.98), as were the rates of serious adverse events. Elevated liver enzyme values were more common in patients taking atorvastatin.

Conclusions.—In patients with recent stroke or TIA and without known coronary heart disease, 80 mg of atorvastatin per day reduced the overall incidence of strokes and of cardiovascular events, despite a small increase in the incidence of hemorrhagic stroke (Fig 2).

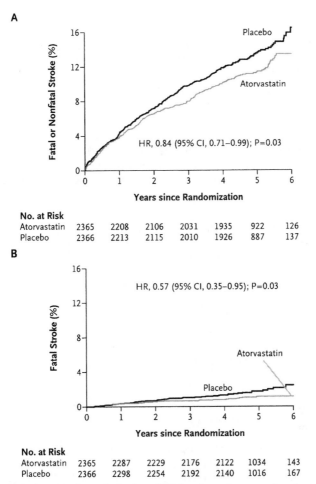

A

B

FIGURE 2.—Kaplan–Meier Curves for Stroke and TIA. Results are shown on an intention-to-treat basis with prespecified adjustments for geographic region, entry event (stroke or TIA), time since entry event, sex, baseline age for first occurrence of a fatal or nonfatal stroke (Panel A) and fatal stroke (Panel B). HR denotes hazard ration, CI confidence interval. (Reprinted by permission of *The New England Journal of Medicine* from Welch KMA, for The Stroke Prevention by Aggressive Reduction in Cholesterol Levels (SPARCL) Investigators. High-dose atorvastatin after stroke or transient ischemic attack. *N Engl J Med.* 2006;355:549-559. Copyright © 2006, Massachusetts Medical Society. All rights reserved.)

▶ We don't really know how statins work. A large meta-analysis has suggested stroke risk reduction parallels decreases in LDL cholesterol level.[1] Favorable pleiotropic effects of statins have also been suggested. Among those pleiotropic effects are favorable effects on plaque inflammation. Perhaps the statins are working to decrease inflammatory selectivity in matrix metalloproteinase-9 (MMP-9) release or somehow counteract the matrix degrading properties of MMP-9? Eldrup et al write about a similar topic.[2]

G. L. Moneta, MD

Reference

1. Amarenco P, Labreuche J, Lavallée P, Touboul PJ. Statins in stroke prevention and carotid atherosclerosis: systematic review and up-to-date meta-analysis. *Stroke.* 2004;35:2902-2909.
2. Eldrup N, Grønholdt M-LM, Sillesen H. Elevated matrix metalloproteinase-9 associated with stroke or cardiovascular death in patients with carotid stenosis. *Circulation.* 2006;114;1847-1854.

Population-Based Study of the Relationship Between Atherosclerotic Aortic Debris and Cerebrovascular Ischemic Events

Petty GW, Khandheria BK, Meissner I, et al (Mayo Clinic, Rochester, Minn)

Mayo Clin Proc 81:609-614, 2006

Objective.—To assess the validity of the suggestion that protruding atheromatous material in the thoracic aorta is an important cause of cerebrovascular ischemic events (CIEs) (ie, transient ischemic attack or ischemic stroke).

Methods.—This case-control study of Olmsted County, Minnesota, residents who underwent transesophageal echocardiography (TEE) from 1993 to 1997 included controls without CIE randomly selected from the population, controls without CIE referred for TEE because of cardiac disease, cases with incident CIE of obvious cause (noncryptogenic), and cases with incident CIE of uncertain cause (cryptogenic).

Results.—Of the 1135 subjects, 520 were randomly selected controls without CIE, 329 were controls without CIE referred for TEE, 159 were noncryptogenic CIE cases, and 127 were cryptogenic CIE cases. Complex atherosclerotic aortic debris in ascending and transverse segments of the arch was detected in 8 randomly selected controls (1.5%), 13 referred controls (4.0%), and 15 noncryptogenic (9.4%) and 4 cryptogenic (3.1%) CIE cases. After adjusting for age, sex, hypertension, smoking, atrial fibrillation, valvular heart disease, congestive heart failure, and atherosclerosis other than in the thoracic aorta, complex atherosclerotic aortic debris was not significantly associated with group status. With randomly selected controls as the referent group, odds ratios (95% confidence intervals) were 1.72 (0.61-4.87) for referred controls, 3.16 (1.18-8.51) for noncryptogenic CIE cases, and 1.39 (0.39-4.88) for cryptogenic CIE cases.

Conclusions.—Complex atherosclerotic aortic debris is not a risk factor for cryptogenic ischemic stroke or transient ischemic attack but is a marker for generalized atherosclerosis and well-established atherosclerotic and cardioembolic mechanisms of cerebral ischemia. Embolization from the aorta is not a common mechanism of ischemic stroke or transient ischemic attack.

▶ This study challenges a generally accepted tenet that atherosclerotic debris in the aortic arch can serve as a cause of ischemic cerebrovascular events. The design of the current study using population-based case controls may have eliminated some selection bias present in earlier studies implicating the aortic arch as a source of stroke. Perhaps we need to rethink the role of aortic arch in cryptogenic stroke. As always, how you look has a lot to do with what you find.

G. L. Moneta, MD

Cerebral emboli as a potential cause of Alzheimer's disease and vascular dementia: case-control study
Purandare N, Burns A, Daly KJ, et al (Univ of Manchester, England; South Manchester Univ, England)
BMJ 332:1119-1122, 2006

Objective.—To compare the occurrence of spontaneous cerebral emboli and venous to arterial circulation shunts in patients with Alzheimer's disease or vascular dementia and controls without dementia.

Design.—Cross sectional case-control study.

Setting.—Secondary care old age psychiatry services, Manchester.

Participants.—170 patients with dementia (85 with Alzheimer's disease, 85 with vascular dementia) and 150 age and sex matched controls. Patients on anticoagulant treatment, patients with severe dementia, and controls with marked cognitive impairment were excluded.

Main Outcome Measures.—Frequencies of detection of spontaneous cerebral emboli during one hour monitoring of the middle cerebral arteries with transcranial Doppler and venous to arterial circulation shunts by a transcranial Doppler technique using intravenous microbubbles as an ultrasound contrast.

Results.—Spontaneous cerebral emboli were detected in 32 (40%) of patients with Alzheimer's disease and 31 (37%) of those with vascular dementia compared with just 12 each (15% and 14%) of their controls, giving significant odds ratios adjusted for vascular risk factors of 2.70 (95% confidence interval 1.18 to 6.21) for Alzheimer's disease and 5.36 (1.24 to 23.18) for vascular dementia. These spontaneous cerebral emboli were not caused by carotid disease, which was equally frequent in dementia patients and their controls. A venous to arterial circulation shunt indicative of patent foramen ovale was found in 27 (32%) Alzheimer's disease patients and 25 (29%) vascular dementia patients compared with 19 (22%) and 17 (20%) controls, giving non-significant odds ratios of 1.57 (0.80 to 3.07) and 1.67 (0.81 to 3.41).

Conclusion.—Spontaneous cerebral emboli were significantly associated with both Alzheimer's disease and vascular dementia. They may represent a potentially preventable or treatable cause of dementia.

▶ Spontaneous cerebral emboli can be detected in more than half of patients with >70% carotid artery stenosis. This study suggests that there are sources of spontaneous cerebral emboli other than carotid artery disease, and that these sources of cerebral emboli may contribute to the development of Alzheimer's disease or vascular dementia. It will be interesting to see if someday long term pharmacologic manipulation can reduce spontaneous cerebral emboli in patients with Alzheimer's disease or vascular dementia as well as patients with carotid stenosis.

G. L. Moneta, MD

Absence of Microemboli on Transcranial Doppler Identifies Low-Risk Patients With Asymptomatic Carotid Stenosis

Spence JD, Tamayo A, Lownie SP, et al (Univ of Western Ontario, London, Canada)
Stroke 36:2373-2378, 2005

Background and Purpose.—Carotid endarterectomy clearly benefits patients with symptomatic severe stenosis (SCS), but the risk of stroke is so low for asymptomatic patients (ACS) that the number needed to treat is very high. We studied transcranial Doppler (TCD) embolus detection as a method for identifying patients at higher risk who would have a lower number needed to treat.

Methods.—Patients with carotid stenosis of $\geq 60\%$ by Doppler ultrasound who had never been symptomatic (81%) or had been asymptomatic for at least 18 months (19%) were studied with TCD embolus detection for up to 1 hour on 2 occasions a week apart; patients were followed for 2 years.

Results.—319 patients were studied, age (standard deviation) 69.68 (9.12) years; 32 (10%) had microemboli at baseline (TCD+). Events were more likely to occur in the first year. Patients with microemboli were much more likely to have microemboli 1 year later (34.4 versus 1.4%; $P<0.0001$) and were more likely to have a stroke during the first year of follow-up (15.6%, 95% CI, 4.1 to 79; versus 1%, 95% CI, 1.01 to 1.36; $P<0.0001$).

Conclusions.—Our findings indicate that TCD− ACS will not benefit from endarterectomy or stenting unless it can be done with a risk <1%; TCD+ may benefit as much as SCS if their surgical risk is not higher. These findings suggest that ACS should be managed medically with delay of surgery or stenting until the occurrence of symptoms or emboli.

▶ This intriguing study suggests there may be a method of stratifying patients with asymptomatic carotid stenosis to those whose risk for stroke is sufficiently high that intervention would seem reasonable to almost everyone. It is noted that the confidence interval for stroke during the first year in patients with microemboli, 4.1%-79%, is quite high. Larger numbers of patients in multiple centers will be needed to confirm the observations in this paper. The data here are sufficiently intriguing and other centers should consider transcranial Doppler studies in their asymptomatic patients with high grade carotid stenosis.

G. L. Moneta, MD

Endarterectomy versus Stenting in Patients with Symptomatic Severe Carotid Stenosis

Mas J-L, for the EVA-3S Investigators (Hôpital Sainte-Anne, Paris; et al)
N Engl J Med 355:1660-1671, 2006

Background.—Carotid stenting is less invasive than endarterectomy, but it is unclear whether it is as safe in patients with symptomatic carotid-artery stenosis.

Methods.—We conducted a multicenter, randomized, noninferiority trial to compare stenting with endarterectomy in patients with a symptomatic carotid stenosis of at least 60%. The primary end point was the incidence of any stroke or death within 30 days after treatment.

Results.—The trial was stopped prematurely after the inclusion of 527 patients for reasons of both safety and futility. The 30-day incidence of any stroke or death was 3.9% after endarterectomy (95% confidence interval [CI], 2.0 to 7.2) and 9.6% after stenting (95% CI, 6.4 to 14.0); the relative risk of any stroke or death after stenting as compared with endarterectomy was 2.5 (95% CI, 1.2 to 5.1). The 30-day incidence of disabling stroke or death was 1.5% after endarterectomy (95% CI, 0.5 to 4.2) and 3.4% after stenting (95% CI, 1.7 to 6.7); the relative risk was 2.2 (95% CI, 0.7 to 7.2). At 6 months, the incidence of any stroke or death was 6.1% after endarterectomy and 11.7% after stenting ($P=0.02$). There were more major local complications after stenting and more systemic complications (mainly pulmonary) after endarterectomy, but the differences were not significant. Cranial-nerve injury was more common after endarterectomy than after stenting.

Conclusions.—In this study of patients with symptomatic carotid stenosis of 60% or more, the rates of death and stroke at 1 and 6 months were lower with endarterectomy than with stenting.

▶ This was a publicly funded, prospective and randomized trial. It has the great benefit of not being tainted by industry sponsorship. There was a lower than predicted stroke and death rate for carotid endarterectomy and a higher than predicted stroke and death rate for carotid artery stenting (CAS). A criticism of the trial will obviously be a possible learning curve effect in the stented patients and a continuing evolving of CAS techniques and devices. The study is far cleaner than the Saffire trial[1] that was used to generate FDA approval of CAS for symptomatic high-risk patients. At the very least, the current trial raises serious concern about the relative safety of CAS in symptomatic patients of standard surgical risk. Given current data, it remains that the only patients who should undergo CAS outside of a clinical trial are very high-risk patients with symptomatic stenosis. Determination of high surgical risk should be by multidisciplinary team that is able to evaluate perioperative systemic and procedure-related risk. It is not acceptable, or ethical, for high surgical risk to be determined by individuals who are only capable of performing carotid stents or who have financial incentives to participate in industry sponsored trials.

G. L. Moneta, MD

Reference

1. Yadav JS, for the Stenting and Angioplasty with Protection in Patients at High Risk for Endarterectomy Investigators. Protected carotid-artery stenting versus endarterectomy in high-risk patients. N Engl J Med. 2004;351:1493-1501.

30 day results from the SPACE trial of stent-protected angioplasty versus carotid endarterectomy in symptomatic patients: a randomised non-inferiority trial

Hacke W, for The SPACE Collaborative Group (Univ of Heidelberg, Germany; et al)
Lancet 368:1239-1247, 2006

Background.—Carotid endarterectomy is effective in stroke prevention for patients with severe symptomatic carotid-artery stenosis, and carotid-artery stenting has been widely used as alternative treatment. Since equivalence or superiority has not been convincingly shown for either treatment, we aimed to compare the two.

Methods.—1200 patients with symptomatic carotid-artery stenosis were randomly assigned within 180 days of transient ischaemic attack or moderate stroke (modified Rankin scale score of ≤3) carotid-artery stenting (n=605) or carotid endarterectomy (n=595). The primary endpoint of this hospital-based study was ipsilateral ischaemic stroke or death from time of

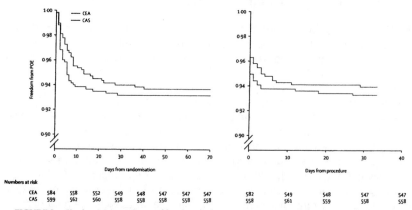

FIGURE 2.—Kaplan-Meier estimate of freedom from primary outcome event per group Left panel shows survival from randomisation to 30 days after treatment. Right panel shows survival from treatment to 30 days after treatment. POE=primary outcome event. CAS=carotid-artery stenting. CEA=carotid endarterectomy. (Courtesy of Hacke W, for The SPACE Collaborative Group. 30 day results from the SPACE trial of stent-protected angioplasty versus carotid endarterectomy in symptomatic patients: a randomised non-inferiority trial. *Lancet*. 2006;368:1239-1247. Copyright 2006 by Elsevier.)

randomisation to 30 days after the procedure. The non-inferiority margin was defined as less than 2.5% on the basis of an expected event rate of 5%. Analyses were on an intention-to-treat basis.

Findings.—1183 patients were included in the analysis. The rate of death or ipsilateral ischaemic stroke from randomisation to 30 days after the procedure was 6.84% with carotid-artery stenting and 6.34% with carotid endarterectomy (absolute difference 0.51%, 90% CI −1.89% to 2.91%). The one-sided p value for non-inferiority is 0.09.

Interpretation.—SPACE failed to prove non-inferiority of carotid-artery stenting compared with carotid endarterectomy for the periprocedural complication rate. The results of this trial do not justify the widespread use in the short-term of carotid-artery stenting for treatment of carotid-artery stenoses. Results at 6–24 months are awaited (Fig 2).

▶ The study was unable to prove carotid stenting was not inferior to carotid endarterectomy. This study does not prove that carotid stenting is inferior to carotid endarterectomy. However, for all outcome analyses, there appeared to be a tendency toward better results with endarterectomy. The authors conclusion that "the results of this trial do not justify the widespread use of carotid stenting for treatment of carotid artery stenosis" is consistent with the recently published trial by the EVA-3S Investigators.[1] In that trial, carotid stenting was found to be inferior to carotid endarterectomy in patients with symptomatic carotid stenosis. The results of the SPACE trial are also consistent with two large meta-analyses.

G. L. Moneta, MD

References

1. Mas JL, and the EVA-3S Investigators. Endarterectomy versus stenting in patients with symptomatic severe carotid stenosis. *N Engl J Med.* 2006;355:1660-1671.
2. Coward LJ, Featherstone RL, Brown MM. Safety and efficacy of endovascular treatment of carotid artery stenosis compared with carotid endarterectomy: a Cochrane systematic review of the randomized evidence. *Stroke.* 2005;36:905-911.
3. Qureshi AI, Kirmani JF, Divani AA, Hobson RW 2nd. Carotid angioplasty with or without stent placement versus carotid endarterectomy for treatment of carotid stenosis: a meta-analysis. *Neurosurgery.* 2005;56:1171-1179.

Protected carotid stenting in high-surgical-risk patients: The ARCHeR results

Gray WA, for the ARCHeR Trial Collaborators (Columbia Univ, New York; et al)
J Vasc Surg 44:258-269, 2006

Background.—Carotid endarterectomy is the standard of care for most patients with severe extracranial carotid bifurcation disease. However, its safety and efficacy in patients with significant surgical risk are unclear. The ARCHeR (ACCULINK for Revascularization of Carotids in High-Risk patients) trial was performed to determine whether carotid artery stenting with embolic protection is a safe and effective alternative to endarterectomy in high-surgical-risk patients.

Methods.—The ARCHeR trial is a series of three sequential, multicenter, nonrandomized, prospective studies. Forty-eight sites enrolled 581 high-surgical-risk patients between May 2000 and September 2003. Patients with severe carotid artery stenosis (angiographically defined, symptomatic ≥50%, or asymptomatic ≥80%) had an ACCULINK nitinol stent implanted. The ACCUNET filter embolic protection system was added to the procedure in the final 2 studies (422 patients). The primary efficacy end point was a composite of periprocedural (≤30 days) death, stroke, and myocardial infarction, plus ipsilateral stroke between days 31 and 365.

Results.—The 30-day rate of death/stroke/myocardial infarction was 8.3% (95% confidence interval [CI], 6.2%-10.8%), and that of stroke/death was 6.9% (95% CI, 5.0%-9.3%). Most (23/32) strokes were minor, of which more than half (12/23) returned to baseline National Institutes of Health Stroke Scale scores within 30 days. The 30-day major/fatal stroke rate was 1.5% (95% CI, 0.7%-2.9%). No hemorrhagic strokes were observed in the study. Ipsilateral cerebrovascular accident occurred in 1.3% between 30 days and 1 year, thus giving a primary composite end point of 30-day death/stroke/myocardial infarction plus ipsilateral stroke at 1 year of 9.6% (95% CI, 7.2%-12.0%), which is below the 14.4% historical control comparator. Target lesion revascularization at 12 months and 2 years was 2.2% and 2.9%, respectively.

Conclusions.—The ARCHeR results demonstrate that extracranial carotid artery stenting with embolic filter protection is not inferior to historical results of endarterectomy and suggest that carotid artery stenting is a safe, durable, and effective alternative in high-surgical-risk patients (Fig 1).

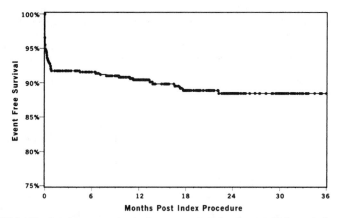

FIGURE 1.—Freedom from any stroke, death, or myocardial infarction up to 30 days or ipsilateral stroke beyond 30 days. The rate of event-free survival was 90.4% (95% confidence interval, 88.0%-92.8%) at 1 year and 88.4% at both 2 and 3 years. (Reprinted by permission of the publisher from Gray WA, for the ARCHeR Trial Collaborators. Protected carotid stenting in high-surgical-risk patients: the ARCHeR results. *J Vasc Surg.* 2006;44:258-269. Copyright 2006 by Elsevier.)

▶ This study tells us what is expected with this particular device. It cannot be used to establish comparitive rates of neurological complications in patients undergoing carotid endarterectomy (CEA) versus those undergoing carotid artery stenting. The study does not really compare anything to anything and was done to gain FDA approval for this particular device. Most coauthors have some link to Guidant. The historical controls used postulated a composite event rate of 14.5% in the CEA group. Patients from combined CEA and coronary artery bypass graft series were also used in the historical control calculations. The combined stroke and death rate in this study in symptomatic patients at 30 days was 11.6%. Too bad some trees had to die for this paper. I suggest reading Dr. William MacKey's invited commentary that accompanies the original article.

G. L. Moneta, MD

Outcome of Carotid Stenting Versus Endarterectomy: A Case-Control Study
Cao P, De Rango P, Verzini F, et al (Univ of Perugia, Italy)
Stroke 37:1221-1226, 2006

Background and Purpose.—To compare perioperative and midterm results of carotid artery stenting (CAS) versus carotid endarterectomy (CEA) in similar cohorts of patients, a retrospectively matched case-control study was performed.

Methods.—Three hundred and one case subjects undergoing CAS with cerebral protection and 301 concurrent matched-controls undergoing CEA were examined. Matching was by sex, age (±2 years), symptoms and coronary disease.

Results.—The 30-day disabling stroke/death rate was 2.6% in the CAS group versus 1.3% in the CEA group (odds ratio [OR] 2; 95% CI, 0.54 to 9.35; P=0.4). CAS patients had a significantly higher risk of periprocedural stroke (7.9% versus 2.3%; OR, 5.2; 95% CI, 1.7 to 18; P=0.001) than CEA patients. However, there was a decreasing trend in 30-day neurological event rates for the last 201 CAS matched cases: 5.4% versus 1.9% (OR 2.8; 95% CI, 0.8 to 10.2; P=0.1). Fifty percent of CAS disabling strokes occurred during cannulation of epiaortic vessels before placement of cerebral protection. Conditional multivariate analysis revealed CAS as a predictor of 30-day stroke (hazard ratios [HR] 3.9; 95% CI, 1.6 to 9.4; P=0.002) but not of 30-day disabling stroke/death (HR 3.6; 95% CI, 0.93 to 13.9; P=0.06). Restenosis free intervals at 36 months were 93.6% versus 92.1% for CAS and CEA, respectively, (P=0.6).

Conclusions.—When comparing CAS with CEA, the risk of any neurological events is still higher, particularly during catheterism and ballooning. The effect of the learning curve related to technical expertise and patient selection may influence the outcome of CAS versus CEA. In the midterm the restenosis rate of CAS compares favorably to CEA.

▶ Another nonrandomized study of carotid endarterectomy (CEA) versus carotid artery stenting (CAS). The case-control study design did not really help much. Risk of any neurolgical event was higher following CAS than CEA, but disabling events were similar. The event rate confidence intervals were relatively wide despite the large number of patients in each group (301). Like the large majority of studies before it, this one gives us a general idea about CAS, but still does not help determine under what circumstances CEA or CAS is preferred. The case-control design did not help much because it is stratified only for very basic clinical risk factors. Case-control methods were also not stratified for angiographic risk factors to CAS, such as plaque length, percent stenosis, internal carotid artery (ICA) or arch tortuosity. This makes the data even less useful.

G. L. Moneta, MD

Carotid angioplasty and stenting for postendarterectomy stenosis: Long-term follow-up
de Borst GJ, Ackerstaff RGA, de Vries J-PPM, et al (Univ Med Ctr Utrecht, The Netherlands; St Antonius Hosp, Nieuwegein, The Netherlands)
J Vasc Surg 45:118-123, 2007

Background.—Carotid angioplasty and stenting (CAS) for recurrent stenosis after carotid endarterectomy (CEA) has been proposed as an alternative to redo CEA. Although early results are encouraging, the extended durability remains unknown. We present the long-term surveillance results of CAS for post-CEA restenosis.

Methods.—Between 1998 and 2004, 57 CAS procedures were performed in 55 patients (36 men) with a mean age of 70 years. The mean interval between CEA and CAS was 83 months (range, 6 to 245). Nine patients (16%) were symptomatic.

Results.—CAS was performed successfully in all patients. No deaths or strokes occurred. A periprocedural transient ischemic attack (TIA) occurred in two patients. During a mean follow-up of 36 months (range, 12 to 72 months), two patients exhibited ipsilateral cerebral symptoms (1 TIA, 1 minor stroke). In 11 patients (19%), in-stent restenosis (≥50%) was detected post-CAS at month 3 (n = 3), 12 (n = 3), 24 (n = 2), 36 (n = 1), 48 (n = 1), and 60 (n = 1). The cumulative rates of in-stent restenosis-free survival at 1, 2, 3, and 4 years were 93%, 85%, 82%, and 76%, respectively. Redo procedures were performed in six patients, three each received repeat angioplasty and repeat CEA with stent removal. The cumulative rates of freedom from reintervention at 1, 2, 3, and 4 years were 96%, 94%, 90%, and 84%, respectively.

Conclusion.—Carotid angioplasty and stenting for recurrent stenosis after CEA can be performed with a low incidence of periprocedural complica-

Freedom from restenosis

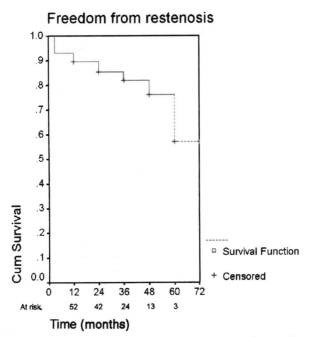

FIGURE 1.—Stenosis-free (<50% diameter reduction) primary patency after carotid angioplasty and stenting for restenosis after carotid endarterectomy. Stenosis-free patency (0-1) vs months. The number of patients included in the analysis at each censored time point were, respectively, 56, 52, 42, 13, and 3 patients at 3, 12, 24, 36, 48, and 60 months. The standard error of cumulative in-stent free survival rate was 0.0338 at 3 months, 0.0406 at 12, 0.0482 at 24, 0.0571 at 36 months, 0.0774 at 48 months, and 0.1746 at 60 months. (Reprinted by permission of the publisher from de Borst GJ, Ackerstaff RGA, de Vries J-PPM, et al. Carotid angioplasty and stenting for postendarterectomy stenosis: long-term follow-up. *J Vasc Surg.* 2007;45:118-123. Copyright 2007 by Elsevier.)

tions with durable protection from stroke. The rate of in-stent recurrent stenosis is high, however, and does not only occur early after CAS but is an ongoing process (Fig 1).

▶ This study says in-stent restenosis following CAS is relatively high and progressive with a 76% freedom from death and in-stent restenosis at 4 years versus the study by Cao et al[1] where restenosis following CAS was described as 6.4% at 3 years. It is likely that neither number is valid. In the study by Cao et al, no criteria for restenosis were given. In this study the criteria for restenotic arteries following CAS was the same as for carotid endarterectomy, but the bulk of the literature suggests different criteria are required for assessing restenosis after CAS.

G. L. Moneta, MD

Reference

1. Cao P, De Rango P, Verzini F, Maselli A, Norgiolini L, Giordano G. Outcome of carotid stenting versus endarterectomy: a case-control study. *Stroke.* 2006;37:1221-1226.

Statin Therapy at Carotid Angioplasty and Stent Placement: Effect on Procedure-related Stroke, Myocardial Infarction, and Death

Gröschel K, Ernemann U, Schulz JB, et al (Univ of Tübingen, Germany; Univ of Göttingen, Germany; Friedrich-Schiller-Univ of Jena, Germany)
Radiology 24:145-151, 2006

Purpose.—To retrospectively determine if preprocedural statin treatment is associated with a reduction of cardiovascular events after carotid angioplasty and stent placement (CAS) in patients with symptomatic carotid stenosis.

Materials and Methods.—A study resulting in a prospective database was approved by the institutional ethics review board; written informed consent was obtained. The approval and informed consent included future retrospective analysis. Consecutive patients ($n = 180$) from the prospective database underwent CAS for high-grade symptomatic carotid disease. The frequency of cardiovascular complications (composite of stroke, myocardial infarction, and death within 30 days after CAS) between 127 patients without preprocedural statin treatment and that of 53 patients with preprocedural statin treatment at CAS were compared with χ^2 and multivariate logistic regression analysis.

Results.—The overall 30-day myocardial infarction rate was two of 180 (1%) patients, the minor stroke rate was 16 of 180 (9%) patients, the major stroke rate was one of 180 (0.5%) patients, and the death rate was two of 180 (1%) patients. The incidence of cardiovascular events (composite of stroke, myocardial infarction, and death within 30 days after CAS) was significantly different between patients with preprocedural treatment (4%) and those without preprocedural statin treatment (15%) ($P < .05$). These higher complication rates among patients without preprocedural statin treatment were not mediated by adjustment for age, sex, other baseline characteristics, degree of carotid stenosis, use of cerebral protection devices, or the year in which CAS was performed.

Conclusion.—Preprocedural statin therapy appears to reduce the incidence of stroke, myocardial infarction, and death within 30 days after CAS. Future prospective randomized trials are warranted to further assess this potential protective effect of statin drugs during carotid interventions.

▶ Stroke and death rates of 10% after 30 days seem relatively common in series of carotid artery stents. The paper suggests that this could be reduced dramatically by at least periprocedural use of statins. Obviously these data are not all that strong, but I am not aware of any data suggesting that statins increase periprocedural vascular complications. It does seem that, when possible, statins should be administered to patients before those patients undergo an arterial procedure of any sort.

G. L. Moneta, MD

Carotid artery stenting in octogenarians is associated with increased adverse outcome
Stanziale SF, Marone LK, Boules TN, et al (Univ of Pittsburgh, Pa; Pittsburgh Vascular Inst, Pa)
J Vasc Surg 43:297-304, 2006

Background.—Carotid artery stenting is an increasingly common endovascular treatment of carotid artery stenosis advocated in high-risk patients despite reports of increased adverse periprocedural outcomes in patients aged >80 years. We sought to evaluate our single institution experience with octogenarians and whether they have an increased incidence of major complications with carotid artery stenting.

Methods.—Three hundred eighty-six patients, including 260 patients from 10 regulatory trials, who underwent carotid artery stenting between June 1996 and March 2004 for symptomatic or asymptomatic carotid stenosis were reviewed from a prospectively maintained database. Periprocedural ($\leq$30 days after carotid artery stenting) cerebrovascular accident, transient ischemic attack, myocardial infarction, and death outcomes were compared between 87 octogenarians and 295 nonoctogenarians. Univariate and multivariate analysis was performed for confounding factors. Kaplan-Meier analysis of stroke and death outcomes was performed for a 1-year follow-up.

Results.—All adverse outcomes were significantly higher in octogenarians compared with younger patients: 30-day stroke rate, 8.0% vs 2.7% ($P = .02$); 30-day stroke, myocardial infarction, or death, 9.2% vs 3.4% ($P = .02$). Cohorts were similar in terms of gender, comorbidities, antiplatelet medications, symptomatic status, and use of cerebral protection. Octogenarians had a greater incidence of contralateral internal carotid artery occlusion (26% vs 12%, $P = .001$), atrial fibrillation (21% vs 8%, $P = .001$), and congestive heart failure (28% vs 15%, $P = .007$), but a lower incidence of hypercholesterolemia (53% vs 72%, $P = .001$) and active smoking (8% vs 24%, $P = .001$). Multivariate analysis of 30-day major adverse outcomes demonstrated an association between age $\geq$80 and adverse outcome (odds ratio, 2.85; $P = .043$) as well as a protective effect of the preprocedural use of aspirin (odds ratio, 0.30, $P = .027$). At 1-year follow-up, only 75% of octogenarians and 87% of nonoctogenarians were free from stroke, myocardial infarction, or death ($P = .005$ Kaplan-Meier analysis).

Conclusions.—Octogenarians undergoing carotid artery stenting are at higher risk than nonoctogenarians for periprocedural complications, including neurologic events and death. Major event-free survival at 1 year is also significantly better in nonoctogenarians. These risks should be weighed when considering carotid stenting in elderly patients.

▶ I believe that data from the lead-in phase of the Carotid Revascularization Endarterectomy vs. Stenting Trial (CREST) first focused attention on higher periprocedural complications in octogenarians undergoing carotid artery stenting (CAS). Findings in this study parallel those of CREST. We are beginning to get a picture of who is at increased risk with CAS: elderly people, those with echolucent plaques, those with symptoms, those not on statin medications.[1] Although these risks are similar to those associated with carotid endarterectomy, angiographic risks associated with CAS are increased with conditions such as adverse arch anatomy, severity of stenosis, lesion length (>10mm), as well as kinks and tortuosity of the internal carotid artery.

G. L. Moneta, MD

Reference

1. Gröschel K, Ernemann U, Schulz JB, Nägele T, Terborg C, Kastrup A. Statin therapy at carotid angioplasty and stent placement: effect on procedure-related stroke, myocardial infarction, and death. *Radiology.* 2006;240:145-151.

Analysis of parameters associated with hypotension requiring vasopressor support after carotid angioplasty and stentin

Trocciola SM, Chaer RA, Lin SC, et al (Cornell Univ, New York; Columbia Univ, New York)
J Vasc Surg 43:714-720, 2006

Introduction.—Systemic hypotension has been observed for up to 36 hours in response to stimulation of the carotid baroreceptor by carotid angioplasty and stenting (CAS). The aim of this study was to identify risk factors and cardiac outcomes for postprocedural hypotension requiring vasopressor support after CAS.

Methods.—Between 2003 and 2005, 143 patients (87 men; mean age, 75 years) with high-grade carotid artery stenosis (mean, 87.3%) were treated with CAS and prospectively entered into a vascular registry. Data were retrospectively analyzed to determine factors predictive of hypotension requiring vasopressor support after CAS. Atropine and appropriate intravenous crystalloid solution were administered during CAS. For the first 30 patients, atropine was only used for symptomatic patients but then became routine and was used for all patients with primary carotid stenosis. Hypotension (systolic blood pressure <90 mm Hg or a mean arterial blood pressure <50 mm Hg) unresponsive to conservative measures was treated with vasopressors (phenylephrine or norepinephrine). Patients were stratified into three groups based on hypotension requiring vasopressors: (1) no vasopressors, (2) vasopressors for ≤24 hours (short duration), and (3) vasopressors for >24 hours (prolonged duration). Risk factors for hypotension requiring vasopressors were analyzed by univariate and multivariate logistic regression analysis.

Results.—Postprocedural hypotension requiring vasopressor treatment was seen in 16 (11%) of 143 of patients, with 6 (4%) requiring vasopressor support for >24 hours. Mean duration of vasopressor administration for all patients was 17 ± 10 hours (range, 6 to 36 hours). By univariate analysis, a history of a previous myocardial infarction ($P = .02$) or use of the PercuSurge occlusion balloon ($P = .05$) were both associated with increased incidence of short duration (≤24 hours) use of vasopressors, and female sex (*P* = .03) and age >80 years old (*P* = .02) were associated with prolonged (>24 hours) vasopressor requirement. On multivariate analysis adjusted for age and sex, a history of myocardial infarction (odds ratio [OR], 4.1; 95% confidence interval [CI], 1.0 to 16.4; *P* = .05) remained an independent predictor of short-duration vasopressors. On multivariate analysis, female sex (OR, 10.9; 95% CI, 1.2 to 100.4; *P* = .04) and age >80 years old (OR, 13.8, 95% CI, 1.5 to 127.2; *P* = .02) remained independent predictors of prolonged vasopressor use. The incidence of periprocedural myocardial infarctions, arrhythmias, or congestive heart failure did not differ between those patients who did not receive vasopressors (5/127) and those who received vasopressors for a short (≤24 hours) duration (1/10, *P* = NS) or prolonged (>24 hours) duration (0/6, *P* = NS).

Conclusion.—Prolonged hypotension requiring vasopressor support occurs in a minority of patients after CAS, with higher incidences in older women. In contrast, hypotension requiring a more limited duration of vasopressor use occurs more commonly in patients who had a prior myocardial infarction, independent of age or sex. In this cohort of patients, vasopressors required for hypotension were not associated with an increased incidence of periprocedural cardiac complications. Despite the increased incidence of prolonged hypotension in older women, this study demonstrates that CAS can be performed without an increase in cardiac morbidity in older women.

▶ I suppose it is of some use to know that older women are at increased risk for need for vasopressor support after carotid angioplasty and stenting. It does not appear, at least based on results of this paper, that this increases cardiac morbidity. However, I would not take the results here as a license to ignore implications of the data. It is likely that the study is underpowered to determine whether or not the increased vasopressor support required by older women will actually serve as a marker for increased cardiac morbidity in a larger cohort of patients.

G. L. Moneta, MD

Cerebral Ischemia after Filter-Protected Carotid Artery Stenting Is Common and Cannot Be Predicted by the Presence of Substantial Amount of Debris Captured by the Filter Devic
Maleux G, Demaerel P, Verbeken E, et al (Univ Hosps Gasthuisberg, Leuven, Belgium)
AJNR Am J Neuroradiol 27:1830-1833, 2006

Purpose.—Protected carotid artery stent placement is currently under clinical evaluation as a potential alternative to carotid endarterectomy. The current study was undertaken to determine the incidence of new ischemic lesions found on diffusion-weighted MR imaging (DWI) in nonselected patients after protected carotid artery stent placement using a filter device and to determine the potential relationship between these new ischemic lesions and the presence or absence of a clear amount of debris captured by the neuroprotection filter device.

Materials and Methods.—A nonrandomized cohort of 52 patients (40 men, 12 women) presenting with carotid occlusive disease underwent protected carotid artery stent placement using a filter device. DWI obtained 1 day before stent placement was compared with that obtained 1 day after stent placement. In addition, the macroscopic and microscopic analysis of debris captured by the filter device during the carotid stent placement procedure was assessed.

Results.—Neuroprotected carotid stent placement was technically successful in all 53 procedures but was complicated by a transient ischemic attack in 3 patients (5.6%). In 22 patients (41.5%), new ischemic lesions were found on DWI, and in 21 filter devices (39.6%), a substantial amount of atheromatous plaque and/or fibrin was found. No clear relationship between the presence of debris captured by the filter device and new lesions detected by DWI was found ($P = .087$; odds ratio 3.067).

Conclusion.—Neuroprotected carotid artery stent placement will not avoid silent cerebral ischemia. Systematic microscopic analysis of debris captured by the filter device has no predictive value for potential cerebral ischemia after carotid artery stent placement.

▶ This abstract and a number of other important abstracts[1-4] focus on the problem of "silent" ischemia following carotid artery stent placement. The papers clearly show that silent ischemia in detectable infarcts after this procedure is common. It may not be influenced all that much by neuroprotective devices. The rate of asymptomatic ischemic infarcts in this study is especially high, as was the portion of neuroprotective devices that captured "substantial debris." These researchers are probably very honest. They may also be clumsy, but the actual clinical infarction rate was low. I am guessing there is a lot more debris ending up in the brain following carotid artery stent placement than has been widely appreciated.

G. L. Moneta, MD

References

1. Kastrup A, Nägele T, Gröschel K, et al. Incidence of new brain lesions after carotid stenting with and without cerebral protection. *Stroke.* 2006;37:2312-2316.
2. McDonnell CO, Fearn SJ, Baker SR, Goodman MA, Price D, Lawrence-Brown MMD. Value of diffusion-weighted MRI during carotid angioplasty and stenting. *Eur J Vasc Endovasc Surg.* 2006;32:46-50.
3. Ihara K, Murao K, Sakai N, Yamada N, Nagata, Miyamoto S. Outcome of carotid endarterectomy and stent insertion based on grading of carotid endarterectomy risk: a 7-year prospective study. *J Neurosurg.* 2006;105:546-554.
4. Protack CD, Bakken AM, Saad WA, Illig KA, Waldman DL, Davies MG. Radiation arteritis: a contraindication to carotid stenting? *J Vasc Surg.* 2007;45:110-117.

Incidence of New Brain Lesions After Carotid Stenting With and Without Cerebral Protection
Kastrup A, Nägele T, Gröschel K, et al (Univ of Göttingen, Germany; Univ of Tübingen, Germany)
Stroke 37:2312-2316, 2006

Background and Purpose.—Diffusion-weighted imaging (DWI) may be a useful tool to evaluate the efficacy of cerebral protection devices in preventing thromboembolic complications during carotid angioplasty and stenting (CAS). The goals of this study were (1) to compare the frequency, number, and size of new DWI lesions after unprotected and protected CAS; and (2) to determine the clinical significance of these lesions.

Methods.—DWI was performed immediately before and within 48 hours after unprotected or protected CAS. Clinical outcome measures were stroke and death within 30 days.

Results.—The proportion of patients with any new ipsilateral DWI lesion (49% versus 67%; $P<0.05$) as well as the number of new ipsilateral DWI lesions (median=0; interquartile range [IQR]=0 to 3 versus median=1; IQR=0 to 4; $P<0.05$) were significantly lower after protected (n=139) than unprotected (n=67) CAS. The great majority of these lesions were asymptomatic and less than 10 mm in diameter. Although there were no significant differences in clinical outcome between patients treated and not treated with protection devices (7.5% versus 4.3%, not significant), the number of new DWI lesions was significantly higher in patients who developed a stroke (median=7.5; IQR=1.5 to 17) than in patients who did not (median=0; IQR=1 to 3.25; $P<0.01$).

Conclusions.—The use of cerebral protection devices significantly reduces the incidence of new DWI lesions after CAS of which the majority are asymptomatic and less than 10 mm in diameter. The frequent occurrence of these lesions and their close correlation with the clinical outcome indicates that DWI could become a sensitive surrogate end point in future randomized trials of unprotected versus protected CAS.

▶ Carotid artery stenting results in a large number of silent cerebral infarcts. Most are asymptomatic. However, the number of DWI infarcts correlates with clinical stroke. This suggests that detection of DWI infarcts may be a reasonable surrogate end point for comparison of cerebral protection devices used in carotid artery stenting.

G. L. Moneta, MD

Value of Diffusion-weighted MRI During Carotid Angioplasty and Stentin
McDonnell CO, Fearn SJ, Baker SR, et al (Mount Hosp, Perth, WA, Australia)
Eur J Vasc Endovasc Surg 32:46-50, 2006

Introduction.—The incidence of neurological injury following carotid angioplasty and stenting is of great interest to those advocating it as an alternative to endarterectomy in the management of critical carotid stenosis. A significant inter-observer variation exists in determining the presence or absence of a neurological deficit following the procedure objective imaging would be advantageous. In this study, we sought to assess diffusion weighted MRI as a diagnostic tool in evaluating the incidence of neurological injury following carotid angioplasty and stenting (CAS).

Patients and Methods.—The first 110 cases of CAS in our unit were included in this series. The procedure was abandoned in three patients. Patients underwent intracranial and extracranial MR angiography, together with diffusion-weighted MRI (DWI) prior to and following CAS and had a formal neurological assessment in the intensive care unit after the procedure.

Results.—One hundred and ten Procedures were attempted in 98 patients. Twenty-eight percent were asymptomatic. Following CAS, 7.2% of patients had a positive neurological exam (two major strokes with one fatality) and 21% had positive DWI scans, equating to a sensitivity of 86% and a specificity of 85% for DWI in detecting cerebral infarction following CAS. The positive predictive value of the test was 0.3 and negative predictive value 0.99. The major stroke and death rate was 1.8%. While the use of a cerebral

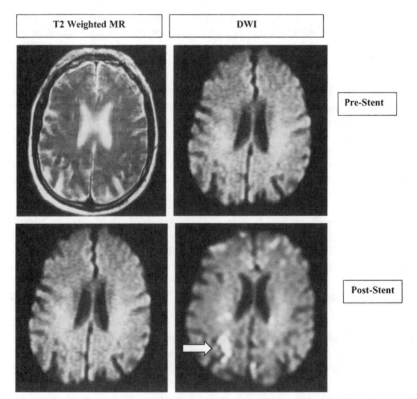

FIGURE 1.—Cerebral infarct (arrowed) seen on DWI but not on standard T2 weighted MR. (Courtesy of McDonnell CO, Fearn SJ, Baker SR, et al. Value of diffusion-weighted MRI during carotid angioplasty and stenting. *Eur J Vasc Endovasc Surg.* 2006;32:46-50.

protection device appeared to significantly reduce the incidence of cerebral infarction (5% vs. 25%, $p=0.031$) this may be a reflection of the learning curve encountered during the study.

Conclusion.—The incidence of subclinical DWI detected neurological injury was significantly higher than clinical neurological deficit following CAS. Conventional methods of neurological assessment of patients undergoing CAS may be too crude to detect subtle changes and more sensitive tests of cerebral function are required to establish whether these subclinical lesions are relevant (Fig 1).

▶ The article emphasizes that DWI lesions present post CAS imperfectly predict a clinical neurologic event in that the positive predictive value of DWI imaging was only 0.3%. However, the negative predictive value was 99%, suggesting that development of techniques of CAS and neuroprotective devices that eliminate DWI lesions will effectively minimize clinically evident neurologic events as well. As mentioned in the previous abstract commentary DWI lesions may, therefore, serve as an effective end point in assessment of new neuroprotective devices for CAS.

G. L. Moneta, MD

Reference

1. Kastrup A, Nägele, Gröschel K, et al. Incidence of new brain lesions after carotid stenting with and without cerebral protection. *Stroke.* 2006;37:2312-2316.

Outcome of carotid endarterectomy and stent insertion based on grading of carotid endarterectomy risk: a 7-year prospective Study
Iihara K, Murao K, Sakai N, et al (Natl Cardiovascular Ctr, Osaka, Japan)
J Neurosurg 105:546-554, 2006

Object.—The authors of this study prospectively compared periprocedural neurological morbidity and the appearance of lesions on diffusion-weighted (DW) magnetic resonance (MR) imaging in patients who had undergone carotid endarterectomy (CEA) or carotid artery stent placement (CASP) with distal balloon protection, based on a CEA risk grading scale.

Methods.—Patients undergoing CEA (139 patients) and CASP (92 patients) were classified into Grades I to IV, based on the presence of angiographic (Grade II), medical (Grade III), and neurological (Grade IV) risks. Although not randomized, the CEA and CASP groups were well matched in terms of the graded risk factors except for a greater proportion of neurologically unstable patients in the CEA group (11 compared with 3%, p = 0.037). There were greater proportions of asymptomatic (64 compared with 34%, p = 0.006) and North American Symptomatic Carotid Endarterectomy Trial-ineligible patients (29 compared with 14%, p < 0.0001) in the CASP group. The overall rates of neurological morbidity with ischemic origin and the appearance of lesions on DW MR imaging after CEA were 2.2 and 9.3%, and those after CASP were 7.6 and 35.9% (nondisabling stroke only), respectively. The only disabling stroke was caused by an intracerebral hemorrhage attributable to hyperperfusion in one case (0.7%) of CEA. There were no deaths. There was no significant association between neurological morbidity and the risk grade in patients who had undergone CEA, although the incidence of lesions on DW imaging was significantly greater in the Grade IV risk group compared with that in the other risk groups combined (42.1 compared with 4.2%, p < 0.0001). After CASP, a higher incidence of neurological morbidity and lesions on DW imaging was noted for the Grade II and III risk groups combined as compared with that in the Grade I risk group, regardless of a symptomatic or an asymptomatic presentation (neurological morbidity: 10.5 compared with 3.1%, respectively, p = 0.41; and DW imaging lesions: 47.4 compared with 19.4%, p = 0.01). The incidence of lesions on DW imaging after CEA was significantly lower than that after CASP except for the Grade IV risk groups.

Conclusions.—Despite a higher incidence of DW imaging-demonstrated lesions in the Grade IV risk group, there was no significant association between the risk group and neurological morbidity rates after CEA. The presence of vascular and medical risk profiles conferred higher rates of neurological morbidity and an increased incidence of lesions on DW imaging after CASP. Considering that no serious nonneurological complications were noted, CEA and CASP appear to be complementary methods of revascularization for carotid artery stenosis with various risk profiles.

▶ Because the study was not randomized, the comparison of new DW imaging lesions in patients undergoing CEA versus CASP doesn't mean much. All we can say is that this is another study documenting high rates of DW imaging lesions post CASP (35.9%). In this study we learn that CASP also is associated with a surprising number of new DW imaging lesions (9.3%).

G. L. Moneta, MD

Radiation arteritis: A contraindication to carotid stenting
Protack CD, Bakken AM, Saad WA, et al (Univ of Rochester, NY)
J Vasc Surg 45:110-117, 2007

Background.—Carotid artery stenting (CAS) for high-risk anatomic lesions is accepted practice. Neck irradiation and radiotherapy-induced arteritis are common indications. The clinical outcomes of CAS for radiation arteritis have been poorly defined.

Methods.—A prospective database of patients undergoing CAS at a tertiary referral academic medical center was maintained from 1999 to 2006. Patients undergoing primary carotid artery stenting for significant atherosclerotic (ASOD) and radiotherapy (XRT)-induced occlusive disease were analyzed. Life-table analyses were performed to assess time-dependent outcomes. Cox proportional hazard analysis or Fisher's exact test was performed to identify factors associated with outcomes. Data are presented as the mean ± SEM unless otherwise indicated.

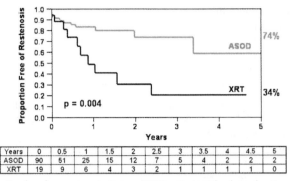

FIGURE 1.—Freedom from restenosis. Sixteen (13%) patients with atherosclerotic occlusive disease (*ASOD*) and 10 patients (43%) with radiotherapy-induced (*XRT*) arteritis restenosed (*P* < .05). The 3-year rates for freedom from restenosis were 74% for ASOD and 20% for XRT. Error bars are omitted for clarity. The number of procedures at risk at each time interval is shown below the figure. The standard error did not exceed 10% at all time intervals that were analyzed. (Reprinted by permission of the publisher from Protack CD, Bakken AM, Saad WA. Radiation arteritis: a contraindication to carotid stenting. *J Vasc Surg.* 2007;45:110-117. Copyright 2007 by Elsevier.)

Results.—During the study period, 150 patients underwent primary CAS, 75% with embolic protection. Fifty-eight percent were symptomatic. One hundred twenty-seven (85%) were treated for ASOD, and 23 (15%) had XRT. The 30-day all-cause mortality rate was 1% for ASOD and 0% for XRT (*P* = NS); overall survival at 3 years was equivalent. There was no significant difference in major adverse event rates as defined by the Stenting and Angioplasty with Protection in Patients at High Risk for Endarterectomy (SAPPHIRE) trial between the groups. The 3-year neurologic event-free rate was 85% for ASOD and 87% for XRT (*P* = NS). Late asymptomatic occlusions were seen only in XRT patients. The 3-year freedom from restenosis rate was significantly worse for the XRT group, at 20%, vs 74% for the ASOD group (*P* < .05). Likewise, the 3-year patency rate was also worse for the XRT group, at 91%, vs 100% for ASOD by Kaplan-Meier analysis (*P* < .05). No factor was predictive of occlusion or stenosis by Cox proportional hazards analysis.

Conclusion.—CAS for radiation arteritis has poor long-term anatomic outcome and can present with late asymptomatic occlusions. These findings suggest that these patients require closer postoperative surveillance and raise the question of whether CAS is appropriate for carotid occlusive lesions caused by radiation arteritis (Fig 1).

▶ Nothing works all that well to treat stenosis in an irradiated artery. The results of this review should, therefore, not be very surprising. There is enough uncertainty about the results of management of irradiated carotid arteries either with CAS or carotid endarterectomy that it may be prudent to restrict it to those with associated symptoms.

G. L. Moneta, MD

Mechanisms and Predictors of Carotid Artery Stent Restenosis: A Serial Intravascular Ultrasound Study

Clark DJ, Lessio S, O'Donoghue M, et al (St Elizabeth's Med Ctr of Boston; Austin Hosp, Melbourne)
J Am Coll Cardiol 47:2390-2396, 2006

Objectives.—The aim of this study was to determine the mechanisms and predictors of carotid artery restenosis after carotid artery stenting (CAS) using serial intravascular ultrasound (IVUS) imaging.

Background.—Carotid artery stenting is increasingly used to treat high-grade obstructive carotid disease, but our knowledge of carotid in-stent restenosis and remodeling remains limited.

Methods.—Post-procedural and 6-month (median 6 months) follow-up quantitative carotid angiography and IVUS were performed after self-expanding stent deployment in 50 internal carotid arteries (ICA). The IVUS measurements at multiple designated sites included minimal luminal diameter, lumen area, stent area (SA), and neointimal hyperplasia area (NIH).

Results.—Late stent enlargement at follow-up was found at all segments, and the percentage increase was greatest at the ICA lesion site (mean ± SD, 48.9 ± 35.3%). The NIH, expressed as a percentage of SA, was seen within all segments of the stent and was greatest at the ICA lesion site (37.3 ± 23.3%). There was a strong positive correlation between the amount of NIH and late stent enlargement (r = 0.64; p < 0.001). Immediate post-procedural minimum ICA SA (r = −0.37; p < 0.01) and stent expansion (r = −0.44; p = 0.001) correlated negatively with the percentage restenotic area at follow-up.

Conclusions.—Although self-expanding carotid stents generate considerable neointimal hyperplasia, the process is balanced by marked late stent en-

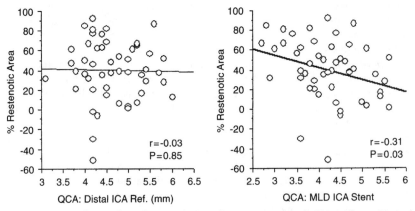

FIGURE 4.—(Left) Correlation between the immediate post-procedure distal internal carotid artery (ICA) reference vessel diameter (mm) measured by quantitative carotid angiography (QCA) and percentage restenotic area after six months. (Right) Correlation between the immediate post-procedure ICA stent minimal lumen diameter (MLD) (mm) measured by QCA and percentage restenotic area after six months. (Courtesy of Clark DJ, Lessio S, O'Donoghue M, et al. Mechanisms and predictors of carotid artery stent restenosis: a serial intravascular ultrasound study. 2006;47:2390-2396.)

largement. Small stent dimensions immediately post-procedure were associated with a higher risk of restenosis (Fig 4).

▶ At first it appeared that restenosis following carotid artery stenting was not going to be a significant problem. Indeed, symptomatic restenosis is uncommon, but anatomic restenosis rates with longer follow-up appear to be increasing with some subgroups of patients, such as women and the elderly, who have restenosis rates up to 20%.[1] The previous paper also suggested that diabetes and previous irradiation increased the risk of restenosis following CAS. This paper suggests that stent oversizing and self-expanding stents may decrease the rates of restenosis. Neointimal hyperplasia, however, is greater and one wonders with longer follow-up if stent restenosis will "catch up" with the greater initial lumen diameter provided by self-expanding stents.

G. L. Moneta, MD

Reference

1. Khan MA, Liu MW, Chio FL, Roubin GS, Iyer SS, Vitek JJ. Predictors of restenosis after successful carotid artery stenting. *Am J Cardiol.* 2003;92:895-897.

Stenting of vertebrobasilar arteries in symptomatic atherosclerotic disease and acute occlusion: Case series and review of the Literature
Eberhardt O, Naegele T, Raygrotzki S, et al (Univ of Tübingen, Germany)
J Vasc Surg 43:1145-1154, 2006

Purpose.—Two of three patients with vertebrobasilar stroke harbor a stenosis of the vertebral or basilar arteries. The best treatment for secondary prophylaxis in vertebrobasilar occlusive disease has not been defined. In patients with high-grade stenoses, and especially those refractory to medication, stenting offers the chance to restore normal flow and prevent major strokes.

Methods.—We provide data regarding outcome and complications on 20 consecutive patients who underwent vertebrobasilar stenting at our institution (9 V0, 2 V3, 5 V4, and 4 basilar artery lesions). Furthermore, we provide a comprehensive overview of the literature on >600 cases of vertebrobasilar stenting, including all published cases up to 2005.

Results.—Primary interventional success was achieved in all cases, with a mean residual stenosis of 3% ± 4% in V0, 5% ± 4% in V3/4, and 7% ± 3% in basilar artery lesions. No peri-interventional neurologic complications and no transient ischemic attack or stroke at follow-up were noted in patients with vertebral ostial lesions, whereas two transient and three permanent clinical deteriorations occurred in patients with V4 or basilar artery lesions, some of which had presented with acute stroke. Patency rate was 100% at the last examination. According to published data on proximal vertebral artery stenting, mortality is 0.3%, the rate of neurologic complications is 5.5%, and the risk of posterior stroke at follow-up is 0.7%. Interventions for distal vertebral or basilar artery disease carry a 3.2% mortality risk,

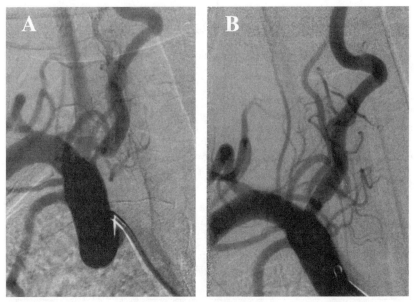

FIGURE 1.—A, Angiography of the right subclavian artery in frontal oblique view shows a high-grade ostial stenosis of the right vertebral artery with poststenotic dilatation. B, Control angiography after primary stenting with a balloon-mounted stent confirms adequate restoration of vessel lumen. (Reprinted by permission of the publisher from Eberhardt O, Naegele T, Raygrotzki S, et al. Stenting of vertebrobasilar arteries in symptomatic atherosclerotic disease and acute occlusion: case series and review of the literature. *J Vasc Surg.* 2006;43:1145-1154. Copyright 2006 by Elsevier.)

a 17.3% risk for neurologic complications and a 2% risk for stroke at follow-up.

Conclusions.—Stenting of the vertebral origin can be performed safely and with a low rate of cerebral ischemic events at follow-up, although restenosis may occur. Larger comparative trials are needed. Treatment decisions in distal vertebrobasilar disease have been made on an individual basis (Fig 1).

▶ This article provides an excellent overview of the role of stenting in management of vertebrobasilar atherosclerotic lesions. The main points are that vertebral origin lesions are amenable to stenting with low complication rates and that interventions for distal vertebral and basilar artery lesions have a significantly higher complication rate. Restenosis may be up to 30% at 30 months of follow-up, although symptomatic restenosis is infrequent. Overall, stenting for proximal vertebral artery lesions is likely to become more common, especially in patients with questionable neurologic symptoms.

G. L. Moneta, MD

Has evidence changed practice? Appropriateness of carotid endarterectomy after the clinical trial
Halm EA, Tuhrim S, Wang JJ, et al (Mount Sinai School of Medicine, New York; Univ at Albany, Rensselaer, NY)
Neurology 68:187-194, 2007

Objective.—To assess how appropriateness of and indications for carotid endarterectomy (CEA) have changed following the publication of several large international randomized controlled trials (RCTs) designed to rationalize use of CEA.

Methods.—The New York Carotid Artery Surgery Study (NYCAS) is a population-based cohort study of all CEAs performed on elderly patients from January 1998 through June 1999 in New York State. Detailed clinical data were abstracted from medical charts to assess indications for and appropriateness of surgery using a list of 1,557 indications for CEA developed by national experts using RAND appropriateness methods. Deaths and strokes within 30 days of surgery were ascertained and confirmed by two physicians.

Results.—Among the 9,588 patients, the mean age was 74.6 years and 93.6% had 70 to 99% carotid stenosis. Nearly three-quarters of patients (72.3%) underwent CEA for asymptomatic stenosis, 18.6% for TIA, and 9.1% for stroke. Overall, 87.1% of operations were done for appropriate reasons, 4.3% for uncertain reasons, and 8.6% for inappropriate reasons (vs 32% inappropriate before the RCTs, $p < 0.0001$). Among procedures judged inappropriate, the most common reasons were high comorbidity in asymptomatic patients (62.2%), operating after a major stroke (14.2%), or for minimal stenosis (10.5%). Among asymptomatic patients, those with high comorbidity had over twice the risk of death or stroke compared to those without high comorbidity (7.13% vs 2.69%, $p < 0.0001$).

Conclusions.—Since publication of the randomized controlled trials, there has been a reduction in the proportion of patients undergoing carotid endarterectomy (CEA) for inappropriate reasons. The shift toward many asymptomatic patients undergoing CEA is concerning because the net benefit from surgery for these patients is low and is reduced further for patients with high comorbidity.

▶ The paper indicates that surgeons pay attention to good scientific evidence and incorporate that evidence into their practices. Our European colleagues, however, must be amazed at the high proportion of CEAs performed in the United States for asymptomatic stenosis. Given that there is a low therapeutic margin for carotid intervention for asymptomatic stenosis, it is difficult to understand why high-risk patients should undergo any type of carotid intervention.

G. L. Moneta, MD

Trends in the in-hospital stroke rate following carotid endarterectomy in California and Maryland

Matsen SL, Chang DC, Perler BA, et al (Johns Hopkins Dept of Surgery, Baltimore, Md)
J Vasc Surg 44:488-495, 2006

Objective.—We examined the outcome of carotid endarterectomy (CEA) in the state of Maryland during the last decade to identify any trends in the incidence of in-hospital stroke and mortality and compared these results with the outcome of the operation throughout the state of California as a control population.

Method.—We performed a retrospective analysis of 10 years (1994 to 2003) of the Maryland and 5 years (1999 to 2003) of the California hospital discharge databases. The following patients were included in the analysis: (1) International Classification of Diseases, 9th Revision, Clinical Modification (ICD-9-CM) procedure code 38.12 (endarterectomy of the vessels of the head and neck other than intracranial vessels) in the primary coding position but not in any secondary position, or (2) the diagnosis code 433.00 to 433.91 (occlusion/stenosis, precerebral artery), or (3) the diagnosis-related group (DRG) 5 (extracranial vascular procedure). Symptomatic patients were identified by history of previous stroke (ICD-9 codes 342 or 438), transient ischemic attack (435 or 781.4), or amaurosis fugax (362.34 or 368.12). In-hospital strokes were identified by ICD-9 codes 997.0, 997.00, 997.01, and 997.09. Low-, moderate-, and high-volume surgeons were defined as performing <15, 15 to 74 and ≥75 CEAs annually. Hospital volumes were similarly classified as low for those performing ≤20 CEAs, moderate for 21 to 100, and high for >100 annually.

Results.—In the Maryland data, 23,237 CEA cases were identified with 169 in-hospital strokes over 10 years (0.73%), whereas the 51,331 California CEAs had 232 in-hospital strokes over 5 years (0.45%). The stroke rate in Maryland was 2.12% in 1994, 1.47% in 1995, and 0.29% to 0.65% from 1996 to 2003. The decrease in strokes was more pronounced among symptomatic patients, where the rate was 3.82% in 1994, 4.44% in 1995, and 0.90% to 2.29% from 1996 to 2003. A similar decrease was identified in the asymptomatic patient population but was less pronounced: 1.64% in 1994, 0.81% in 1995, and 0.15% to 0.44% from 1996 to 2003. The low recent stroke rates were confirmed by the California data (0.44% to 0.48% from 1999 to 2003). Changes in the death rate for CEA during this time frame have not been as pronounced, from 0.33% to 0.58% for Maryland and 0.78% to 0.91% for California.

Conclusions.—A dramatic decrease in the in-hospital stroke rates in Maryland occurred around 1995. The stroke rates in Maryland in the past 5 years are similar to those in California during the same period. An analysis of data from the two states shows that the in-hospital stroke rate now for carotid endarterectomy is approximately 0.54%.

▶ I would really like to believe that statewide stroke rates for CEA are under 0.6%, but I don't. I do think we are getting better at carotid endarterectomy, but we have not gotten 10 times better than the results of the randomized trials. Perhaps part of the improvement in statistics for CEA is that 85% of CEAs were performed for asymptomatic lesions. This is a staggering proportion of endarterectomies performed for asymptomatic disease. I am sure the authors of Asymptomatic Carotid Atherosclerosis Study and North American Symptomatic Carotid Endarterectomy Trial never expected such a dramatic transformation in the indication for carotid endarterectomy.[1]

G. L. Moneta, MD

Reference

1. Perler BA. Has evidence changed practice? Appropriateness of carotid endarterectomy after the clinical trials. *Perspect Vasc Surg Endovasc Ther.* 2007;19: 409-410.

Defining the high-risk patient for carotid endarterectomy: An analysis of the prospective National Surgical Quality Improvement Program database
Stoner MC, Abbott WM, Wong DR, et al (Massachusetts Gen Hosp, Boston; Univ of Colorado Health Outcomes Program, Aurora; Veterans Affairs Boston Healthcare System, West Roxbury, Mass)
J Vasc Surg 43:285-296, 2006

Background.—Carotid endarterectomy (CEA) is the gold standard for the treatment of carotid stenosis, but carotid angioplasty and stenting has been advocated in high-risk patients. The definition of such a population has been elusive, particularly because the data are largely retrospective. Our study examined results for CEA in the National Surgical Quality Improvement Program database (both Veterans Affairs and private sector).

Methods.—National Surgical Quality Improvement Program data were gathered prospectively for all patients undergoing primary isolated CEA during the interval 2000 to 2003 at 123 Veterans Affairs and 14 private sector academic medical centers. Study end points included the 30-day occurrence of any stroke, death, or cardiac event. A variety of clinical, demographic, and operative variables were assessed with multivariate models to identify risk factors associated with the composite (stroke, death, or cardiac event) end point. Adjudication of end points was by trained nurse reviewers (previously validated).

Results.—A total of 13,622 CEAs were performed during the study period; 95% were on male patients, and 91% of cases were conducted within the Veterans Affairs sector. The average age was 68.6 ± 0.1 years, and 42.1% of the population had no prior neurologic event. The composite stroke, death, or cardiac event rate was 4.0%; the stroke/death rate was 3.4%. Multivariate correlates of the composite outcome were (odds ratio, *P* value) as follows: deciles of age (1.13, .018), insulin-requiring diabetes (1.73, <.001), oral agent–controlled diabetes (1.39, .003), decade of pack-years smoking (1.04, >.001), history of transient ischemic attack (1.41, >.001), history of stroke (1.51, >.001), creatinine >1.5 mg/dL (1.48, >.001), hypoalbuminemia (1.49, >.001), and fourth quartile of operative time (1.44, >.001). Cardiopulmonary comorbid features did not affect the composite outcome in this model. Regional anesthesia was used in 2437 (18%) cases, with a resultant relative risk reduction for stroke (17%), death (24%), cardiac event (33%), and the composite outcome (31%; odds ratio, 0.69; $P = .008$).

Conclusions.—Carotid endarterectomy results across a spectrum of Veterans Affairs and private sector hospitals compare favorably to contemporary studies. These data will assist in selecting patients who are at an increased risk for adverse outcomes. Use of regional anesthetic significantly reduced perioperative complications in a risk-adjusted model, thus suggesting that it is the anesthetic of choice when CEA is performed in high-risk patients.

▶ There are two primary points to take home from this study: (1) Carotid endarterectomy can be performed across a wide spectrum of hospitals with results equal to those of the random trials of carotid endarterectomy, and (2) In high-risk patients' regional anesthesia is associated with better results than is general anesthesia. This is one of the best pieces of evidence seen supporting the use of regional anesthesia for carotid endarterectomy.

G. L. Moneta, MD

Early carotid endarterectomy in symptomatic patients is associated with poorer perioperative outcome

Rockman CB, Maldonado TS, Jacobowitz GR, et al (New York Univ)
J Vasc Surg 44:480-487, 2006

Objective.—The optimal timing of carotid endarterectomy (CEA) after ipsilateral hemispheric stroke is controversial. Although early studies suggested that an interval of about 6 weeks after a completed stroke was preferred, more recent data have suggested that delaying CEA for this period of time is not necessary. With these issues in mind, we reviewed our experience to examine perioperative outcome with respect to the timing of CEA in previously symptomatic patients.

Methods.—A retrospective review of a prospectively maintained database of all CEAs performed at our institution from 1992 to 2003 showed that 2537 CEA were performed, of which 1158 (45.6%) were in symptomatic patients. Patients who were operated on emergently ≤48 hours of symptoms for crescendo transient ischemic attacks (TIAs) or stroke-in-evolution were excluded from analysis (n = 25). CEA was considered "early" if performed ≤4 weeks of symptoms, and "delayed" if performed after a minimum of a 4-week interval following the most recent symptom.

Results.—Of nonurgent CEAs in symptomatic patients, in 87 instances the exact time interval from symptoms to surgery could not be precisely de-

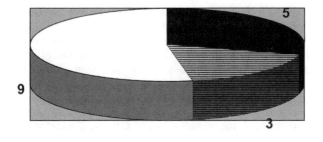

■ ICH ▤ Hyperperfusion □ TE / other

FIGURE 3.—Causes of the perioperative strokes in patients with preoperative strokes operated on in an early time period. *ICH,* Intracerebral hemorrhage; *TE,* thromboembolic. (Reprinted by permission of the publisher from Rockman CB, Maldonado TS, Jacobowitz GR, et al. Early carotid endarterectomy in symptomatic patients is associated with poorer perioperative outcomes. *J Vasc Surg.* 2006;44:480-487. Copyright 2006 by Elsevier.)

termined secondary to the remoteness of the symptoms (>18 months), and these were excluded from further analysis. Of the remaining 1046 cases, 62.7% had TIAs and 37.3% had completed strokes as their indication for surgery. Among the entire cohort, patients who underwent early CEA were significantly more likely to experience a perioperative stroke than patients who underwent delayed CEA (5.1% vs 1.6%, *P* = .002). Patients with TIAs alone were more likely to be operated on early rather than in a delayed fashion (64.3% vs 46.7%, *P* < .0001), likely reflecting institutional bias in selecting delayed CEA for stroke patients. However, even when examined as two separate groups, both TIA patients (n = 656) and CVA patients (n = 390) were significantly more likely to experience a perioperative stroke when operated upon early rather than in a delayed fashion (TIA patients, 3.3% vs 0.9%, *P* = .05; CVA patients, 9.4% vs 2.4%, *P* = .003). There were no significant differences in demographics or other meaningful variables between patients who underwent early CEA and those who underwent delayed CEA.

Conclusions.—In a large institutional experience, patients who underwent CEA ≤4 weeks of ipsilateral TIA or stroke experienced a significantly increased rate of perioperative stroke compared with patients who underwent CEA in a more delayed fashion. This was true for both TIA and stroke patients, although the results were more impressive among stroke patients. On the basis of these results, we continue to recommend that waiting period of 4 weeks be considered in stroke patients who are candidates for CEA (Fig 3).

► This study stands at odds with the recent and well-accepted trend to perform CEA early in patients with small stable neurologic deficits. Why do the authors' results differ from the bulk of the current literature? Undoubtedly patient selection, stroke severity, and innumerable intangible factors present in a retrospective study account for the differences. Perhaps the authors can conclude that at New York University, overall, a policy of waiting 4 weeks following a TIA or stroke to perform CEA is best. However, as much as I respect the New York University surgeons, and their long interest in CEA, I don't think this type of analysis from a single institution should change practice patterns. It tells us, at most, to be careful in selection of symptomatic patients for early CEA.

G. L. Moneta, MD

Routine Completion Angiography during Carotid Endarterectomy is not Mandatory
Pratesi C, Dorigo W, Troisi N, et al (Univ of Florence, Italy)
Eur J Vasc Endovasc Surg 32:369-373, 2006

Objective.—Intraoperative quality control after carotid endarterectomy (CEA) has been advocated to improve the results of surgical treatment of extracranial carotid artery disease. The aim of this study was to evaluate the

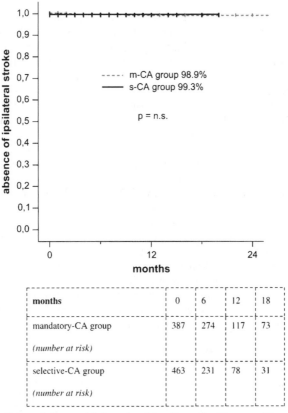

months	0	6	12	18
mandatory-CA group (number at risk)	387	274	117	73
selective-CA group (number at risk)	463	231	78	31

FIGURE 1.—Estimated absence of ipsilateral stroke at 18 months. (Courtesy of Pratesi C, Dorigo W, Troisi A, et al. Routine completion angiography during carotid endarterectomy is not mandatory. *Eur J Vasc Endovasc Surg.* 2006;32:369-373. Reprinted by permission of the publisher.)

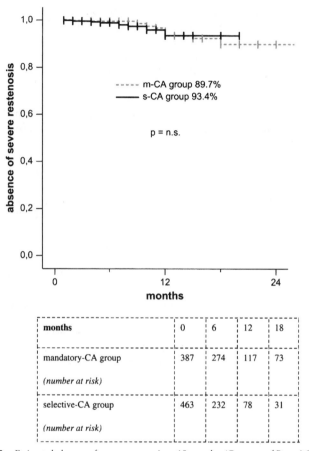

FIGURE 2.—Estimated absence of severe restenosis at 18 months. (Courtesy of Pratesi C, Dorigo W, Troisi A, et al. Routine completion angiography during carotid endarterectomy is not mandatory. *Eur J Vasc Endovasc Surg.* 2006;32:369-373. Reprinted by permission of the publisher.)

usefulness of completion angiography (CA) in prevention of stroke and restenosis after CEA in a single center experience.

Materials and Methods.—Data concerning 914 consecutive CEAs performed in 3 years (2000–2002) were prospectively collected in a dedicated database. Patients were divided into two groups: in the first group (mandatory-CA group; 430 cases) CA was routinely carried out, except in presence of contraindications to iodinate contrast agents; in the second group (selective-CA group, 484 cases) CA was performed only in selected cases, at surgeon's discretion.

Results.—There were no significant differences between the two groups in terms of neurological complications at awakening (0.5% in mandatory-CA group and 0.4% in selective-CA group; p=n.s.) and in 30-day stroke and death rate (1.9% and 1.4%, respectively; p=n.s.). A surgical revision on the basis of CA findings was performed in 5 cases in mandatory-CA group and in 2 cases in selective-CA group (1.2% and 0.4%, respectively; p=n.s.). In the second group, the conditions significantly associated with the need for CA examination were internal carotid near-occlusion, preoperative symptoms, shunt insertion, kind of surgical reconstruction, redo surgery. Estimated absence of ipsilateral stroke and absence of restenosis at 18 months was 98.9% and 89.7% in mandatory-CA group and 99.3% and 93.4% in selective-CA group (p=n.s.) respectively.

Conclusions.—Based on our experience, routine CA following CEA is not suggested. A policy of selected CA at the surgeon's discretion seems to make the intervention safe and durable as well (Figs 1 and 2).

▶ I agree completely with the authors' findings. Intraoperative assessment of the carotid artery, whether it be with angiography or duplex scanner, has been given more press than it is worth. If one has a policy of routine tacking of the distal end point and routine patching, the results should be excellent in the absence of confounding variables such as common carotid artery stenosis or internal carotid artery tortuosity. The question is not whether intraoperative assessment is routinely needed, but whether it should be done routinely to maintain skills and performance and interpretation when there is a real question of the adequacy of the technical result.

G. L. Moneta, MD

Combined carotid endarterectomy and coronary artery bypass grafting in patients with asymptomatic high-grade stenoses: An analysis of 758 procedures
Byrne J, Darling RC III; Roddy SP, et al (Albany Med College, NY)
J Vasc Surg 44:67-72, 2006

Purpose.—Surgical treatment of hemodynamically significant carotid artery stenoses has been well documented, especially in the asymptomatic patient. However, in those patients presenting with hemodynamically significant asymptomatic carotid artery disease who are to undergo cardiac surgery, optimal treatment remains controversial. In this study, we analyze our experience with patients who underwent synchronous carotid endarterectomy (CEA) and coronary artery bypass graft procedures (CABG) for hemodynamically significant (>70%) asymptomatic carotid artery stenosis and coronary artery disease (CAD).

Methods.—Demographics and outcomes of all patients undergoing synchronous CEA/CABG for asymptomatic carotid stenosis between April 1980 and January 2005 were reviewed from our vascular registry and patient charts. We included patients who underwent standard patching of their carotid artery and those undergoing eversion CEA. All neurologic events within the first 30 days that persisted >24 hours were considered a stroke. For purposes of comparison, we also reviewed outcomes for patients undergoing synchronous CEA/CABG for symptomatic carotid stenosis.

Results.—Asymptomatic carotid artery stenosis (>70%) was the indication in 702 patients (276 women and 426 men) undergoing 758 CEAs. In the asymptomatic group, 22 patients, of which 21 succumbed to cardiac dysfunction, and one died from a hemorrhagic stroke. The overall mortality rate was 3.1%. Seven permanent nonfatal neurologic deficits occurred in this series (1 woman, 6 men). The combined stroke mortality was 4.3%. This compares to a 30-day stroke mortality of 6.1% in 132 symptomatic combined CEA/CABG patients. The difference in stroke mortality in women compared with men was not significant.

Conclusion.—In this experience, patients presenting with hemodynamically significant (>70%) asymptomatic carotid artery stenosis can undergo synchronous CEA/CABG with low morbidity and mortality.

▶ It is important to read carefully the conclusion of this abstract. Although it is clear CABG and CEA for asymptomatic carotid disease can be performed simultaneously with a low incidence of adverse neurologic outcomes, it is not clear that this should be done. Many large centers are now reporting permanent neurologic deficit rates following CEA for asymptomatic lesions of 1% or less. This is a rate one fourth of that reported here. At best, combined carotid endarterectomy for asymptomatic stenosis with CABG is a "wash." My guess, however, is that in most centers, probably including Albany, you will be better off by staging the procedures.

G. L. Moneta, MD

Is There Any Benefit From Staged Carotid and Coronary Revascularization Using Carotid Stents? A Single-Center Experience Highlights the Need for a Randomized Controlled Trial
Randall MS, McKevitt FM, Cleveland TJ, et al (Sheffield Teaching Hosps NHS Found Trust, England)
Stroke 37:435-439, 2006

Background and Purpose.—To assess the benefits of carotid artery stenting before coronary artery bypass surgery to reduce the risk of stroke occurring during the cardiac procedure.

Methods.—A prospective cohort study was performed in patients undergoing carotid artery stenting before coronary artery bypass surgery, or combined bypass and valve replacement procedures, to assess the procedures effectiveness in stroke prevention. Outcome measures including 30-day post stenting and cardiac surgery neurological complication and all-cause mortality rates were assessed.

Results.—A total of 52 patients were included. Two patients underwent aortic valve replacements at the same time as coronary revascularization. No neurological complications occurred because of the stenting procedure. One cardiac death not related to coronary artery bypass surgery occurred in the 30-day follow-up period for the stent procedure. An additional 6 (11.5%) outcome events (3 strokes and 3 deaths) occurred in the 30-day follow-up period after the cardiac procedure. Three patients died of cardiac causes while awaiting their cardiac bypass procedure.

Conclusions.—Our results are comparable to those in patients that undergo staged or combined carotid endarterectomy before cardiac surgery. Our small cohort study adds to the limited world literature on the subject but is not sufficiently powered to recommend alterations in practice.

▶ This article by Randall et al and another article by Ziada et al[1] evaluate carotid stents placed immediately before open heart surgery. The pictures gleamed from these articles are somewhat different. In this article, the 30-day stroke/death rate with the staged approach was 19.2% (10 of 52). This is too high and suggests a problem with a concept, with technical performance of the operators, or with patient selection. It certainly suggests that this approach is not likely a viable one at the author's institution.

G. L. Moneta, MD

Reference

1. Ziada KM, Yadav JS, Mukherjee D, et al. Comparison of results of carotid stenting followed by open heart surgery versus combined carotid endarterectomy and open heart surgery (coronary bypass with or without another procedure). *Am J Cardiol.* 2005;96:519-523.

Comparison of Results of Carotid Stenting Followed by Open Heart Surgery Versus Combined Carotid Endarterectomy and Open Heart Surgery (Coronary Bypass With or Without Another Procedure)

Ziada KM, Yadav JS, Mukherjee D, et al (Cleveland Clinic Found, Ohio; Univ of Kentucky, Lexington; Univ Hosp, Zurich, Switzerland)
Am J Cardiol 96:519-523, 2005

We compared a novel strategy of carotid stenting (CS) followed by open heart surgery (OHS) to the combined carotid endarterectomy (CEA) and the OHS approach in patients requiring coronary and carotid revascularization. Between 1997 and 2002, CS as a prelude to OHS was performed in 56 patients, and 111 patients underwent combined CEA+OHS. Adverse events included stroke, myocardial infarction (MI), death, and their combinations. At baseline, the CS+OHS group had more unstable/severe angina (52% vs 27%, p = 0.002), severe left ventricular dysfunction (20% vs 9%, p = 0.05), symptomatic carotid disease (46% vs 23%, p = 0.002), and the need for repeat OHS (32% vs 9%, p = 0.0002). Severe contralateral carotid disease was more prevalent in the CEA+OHS group (28% vs 11%, p = 0.01). At 30 days, CS+OHS patients had a significantly lower incidence of stroke or MI (5% vs 19%, p = 0.02). A propensity score was created for each patient to account for baseline differences. In a final logistic regression model that included the propensity score, CS+OHS was associated with a trend toward reduced stroke or MI (odds ratio 0.26, 95% confidence interval 0.06 to 1.09, p = 0.06) and reduced death, stroke, or MI (odds ratio 0.40, 95% confidence interval 0.12 to 1.27, p = 0.12). In conclusion, despite a higher baseline risk profile, patients who underwent CS+OHS had significantly fewer adverse events than those undergoing CEA+OHS. CS may be a safer carotid revascularization option for this challenging patient population.

▶ Compared with the abstract by Randall et al,[1] this paper presents an entirely different picture of the use of carotid stents before OHS, with a 30-day stroke and myocardial infarction rate of 5% in these patients. This fourfold difference in morbidity and mortality rates between this and the previous abstract demands an explanation. The explanation may be the small number of patients in each series, but patient selection, technical expertise, and the retrospective nature of both studies are probably also involved. It seems intuitive that the 30-day results of combining CAS and OHS ought to be worse than either alone. Both subject the patient to a fixed risk of myocardial infarction and death. This is clearly a controversial field. The question was never settled for the combined use of CEA and OHS, and now we have moved on with the same silly retrospective analysis for CAS before OHS. Sometimes I wonder if we will ever learn.

G. L. Moneta, MD

Reference

1. Randall MS, McKevitt FM, Cleveland TJ, Gaines PA, Venables GS. Is there any benefit from staged carotid and coronary revascularization using carotid stents? A single-center experience highlights the need for a randomized controlled trial. 2006;37:435-439.

Familial Cervical Artery Dissections: Clinical, Morphologic, and Genetic Studies
Martin JJ, Hausser I, Lyrer P, et al (Sanatorio Allende, Cordoba, Argentina; Univ of Heidelberg, Germany; Univ Hosp Basel, Switzerland; et al)
Stroke 37:2924-2929, 2006

Background and Purpose.—Genetic risk factors are thought to play a role in the etiology of spontaneous cervical artery dissections (CAD). However, familial CAD is extremely rare. In this study we analyzed patients with familial CAD and asked the question whether familial CAD has particular features.
Methods.—Seven families with 15 CAD patients were recruited. All patients were carefully investigated by a neurologist, a neuroradiologist, and a dermatologist for clinical characteristics. From 11 patients a skin biopsy was performed to study the morphology of the connective tissue and to analyze the coding sequences of COL3A1, COL5A1, COL5A2, and part of COL1A1.
Results.—The mean age of the patients (n=15, 9 women) at their first dissection was 36.2 years (median age 32 years, range 18 to 59). Two patients had bilateral CAD. One patient had a right and a left internal carotid artery

dissection in successive weeks, another patient had 5 dissections over a period of 8 years. A high intrafamilial correlation was found between the affected vessels (ie, the carotid and the vertebral arteries) and between ages at the first dissection. In 1 patient we found clear and reproducible ultrastructural abnormalities in the skin biopsy, but the second patient from the family was not studied, because he died as a result of CAD before this study. The dermal connective tissue aberrations in the examined patient were similar to mild findings in patients with vascular Ehlers-Danlos syndrome (EDS type IV), but might be iatrogenic and related to long-term corticosteroid inhalation therapy. All other analyzed patients showed normal connective tissue morphology. In patients from 6 families we analyzed the whole coding sequence of COL3A1, COL5A1, and COL5A2, and from part of COL1A1. A missense mutation in the COL3A1 gene (leading to a G157S substitution in type III procollagen) was detected in both patients from 1e family. Two patients from another family carried a rare nonsynonymous coding polymorphism in COL5A1 (D192N); 1 of them carried also a rare variant in COL5A2 (T12337).

Conclusions.—Familial CAD patients are young and probably are at high risk for recurrent or multiple CAD. Ultrastructural alterations of the dermal connective tissue might not be an important risk factor for familial CAD. However, the finding of a COL3A1 mutation revealed the presence of an inherited connective tissue disorder in 1 family.

▶ Patients with familial spontaneous CAD are younger than the general quota of patients with spontaneous CAD. Microscopic analysis of skin biopsy specimens is essentially unrevealing. Younger patients with spontaneous CAD should perhaps be counseled as to the familial tendency for this disease, but it does not appear that genetic testing, at least as we currently understand it, is helpful.

G. L. Moneta, MD

Subclinical Carotid Atherosclerosis in HIV-Infected Patients: Role of Combination Antiretroviral Therapy

Jericó C, Knobel H, Calvo N, et al (Hosp del Mar, Barcelona; Universidad Autónoma de Barcelona)
Stroke 37:812-817, 2006

Background and Purpose.—Whether or not combination antiretroviral therapy (CART) alone directly contributes to accelerating atherosclerosis in HIV-infected patients has not been studied in depth. This study aimed to ascertain the relationship between this therapy and subclinical carotid atherosclerosis according to cardiovascular risk.

Methods.—Sixty-eight HIV-infected patients with ≤1 cardiovascular risk factors and 64 with ≥2 risk factors completed the study protocol consisting of clinical, laboratory, and vascular evaluation by carotid high-resolution B-mode ultrasonography. Univariate and multivariate logistic regression analyses were performed with the presence of subclinical carotid atherosclerosis, defined by carotid intima-media thickness >0.8 mm or the presence of plaque being the dependent variable.

Results.—Among the 132 enrolled patients, 93 (70.5%) were on CART and 39 (29.5%) had never been on antiretroviral therapy. In accordance with cardiovascular risk stratification, subclinical carotid atherosclerosis was found in 26.6% (17 of 64 patients) of the very low–risk group (10-year coronary risk <5%), 35.3% (12 of 34 patients) of the low-risk group (10-year coronary risk between 5% and 9%) and 76.5% (26 of 34 patients) of the moderate/high-risk group (10-year coronary risk ≤10%). Thus, 55 (41.7%) of the 132 HIV-infected patients had subclinical carotid atherosclerosis, and independent variables associated with carotid atherosclerosis (odds ratio; 95% CI) were: CART exposure (10.5; 2.8 to 39) and 10-year coronary risk ≤10% (4.2; 1.5 to 12). In very low coronary risk patients (<5%), age (per 10-year increment: 4.01; 1.12 to 14.38), systolic blood pressure (per unit mm Hg 1.07; 1.01 to 1.14), and CART exposure (8.65; 1.54 to 48.54) were independently associated with subclinical carotid atherosclerosis.

Conclusions.—CART should be considered a strong, independent predictor for the development of subclinical atherosclerosis in HIV-infected patients, regardless of known major cardiovascular risk factors and atherogenic metabolic abnormalities induced by this therapy.

▶ The HIV-infected population appears to be at increased risk of atherosclerosis. Combination antiretroviral therapy (CART) has dramatically decreased morbidity and mortality in the HIV infected population. However, the adverse effects of CART, including dyslipidemia and insulin resistance, appear to increase the risk of subclinial atherosclerosis in the HIV-infected population. However, I feel that most HIV-infected patients will regard this as an acceptable price for their antiretroviral therapy.

G. L. Moneta, MD

Silent Ischemia after Neuroprotected Percutaneous Carotid Stenting: A Diffusion-Weighted MRI Study
Piñero P, González A, Mayol A, et al (Hospitales Universitarios Virgen del Rocio, Sevilla, Spain)
AJNR Am J Neuroradiol 27:1338-1345, 2006

Background and Purpose.—To assess by diffusion-weighted MR imaging (DWI) the efficacy of cerebral protection devices in avoiding embolization and new ischemic lesions in patients with severe internal carotid artery (ICA) stenosis undergoing carotid artery stent placement (CAS).

Methods.—One hundred sixty-two CASs in the extracranial ICA were performed with the use of distal filters. Mean age of the patients was 68.5 years (range, 33–86) and 122 patients (75.3%) were symptomatic. MR imaging was performed in all patients during the 3-day period before CAS, and

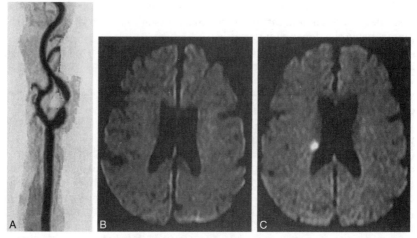

FIGURE 1.—A, MR angiography of the right common carotid artery before carotid artery stent (CAS) placement, showing a severe stenosis of the proximal internal carotid artery. B, Diffusion-weighted image (DWI) obtained at the same time shows no abnormalities. C, DWI after CAS with a new ipsilateral lesion in the deep territory of the ipsilateral middle cerebral artery. (Courtesy of Piñero P, González A, Mayol A, et al. Silent ischemia after neuroprotected percutaneous carotid stenting: a diffusion-weighted MRI study. *AJNR Am J Neuroradiol.* 2006;27:1338-1345. Copyright by American Society of Neurodiology.)

DWI was obtained within 24 hours after the procedure. Ninety-five patients (58.6%) were monitored by transcranial Doppler ultrasonography for microemboli detection in the territory of the middle cerebral artery (MCA), ipsilateral to the vessel being treated.

Results.—Twenty-eight patients (17.3%) showed 58 new ischemic foci in DWI (Fig 1), and 13 patients (46.4%) had multiple foci. Location of new lesions was mainly in the vascular territory supplied by the treated vessel (19 patients; 67.9%), but also in the contralateral MCA (1 patient; 3.6%), and the posterior fossa (4 patients; 14.3%). A significant relationship ($P < .03$) was found between occurrence of transient ischemic attack (TIA) and appearance of new lesions. Microembolic signals (MES) were detected in 88 patients (92.6%), with no relationship between number of MES and the appearance of new ischemic foci.

Conclusion.—New ischemic foci were observed in 17.3% of the patients undergoing neuroprotected CAS. Appearance of new ischemic lesions were only significantly related to the occurrence of TIA but not to the number of MES registered or other variables. Despite the encouraging results, the incidence of new ischemic lesions should promote research for safer techniques and devices.

▶ Another article documenting a high incidence of new ischemic foci after CAS even with neuroprotective devices. Clearly, there is room for improvement in the design of neuroprotection devices as adjuncts to CAS.

G. L. Moneta, MD

14 Vascular Trauma

Traumatic Arterial Injuries of the Extremities: Initial Evaluation with MDCT Angiography
Rieger M, Mallouhi A, Tauscher T, et al (Innsbruck Univ, Austria)
AJR 186:656-664, 2006

Objective.—The purpose of this study was to retrospectively assess the accuracy of MDCT angiography as the initial diagnostic technique to depict arterial injury in patients with extremity trauma.

Materials and Methods.—Over 36 months, 87 patients (16 females and 71 males; age range, 16–87 years) with clinically suspected arterial injury after extremity trauma underwent 4-MDCT angiography and 67 ultimately underwent surgery. Eighty patients had blunt injuries, and seven had penetrating injuries. The presence of arterial involvement was investigated prospectively by the radiologist in charge and retrospectively by two independent radiologists. Each detected arterial lesion was then characterized as a spasm, stenosis, occlusion, or rupture. The standard of reference was surgery in 67 patients, angiography in two patients, and clinical and radiologic follow-up findings in 18 patients. MDCT angiography was assessed by means of receiver operating characteristic (ROC) curve analysis for lesion detection and Spearman's rank correlation test for lesion characterization. Image quality, lesion depiction, and artifacts were subjectively assessed.

Results.—Sixty-two traumatic arterial lesions were confirmed at surgery in 55 patients. Multidetector-row computed tomography, or MDCT, angiography yielded high accuracy in detection (area under the ROC curve [A_z] = 0.96; $p < 0.001$) and characterization ($r = 0.94$; $p < 0.001$) of traumatic arterial injuries and in recognizing an underlying dissection ($A_z = 0.82$; $p < 0.001$). Prospective sensitivity and specificity were 95% and 87%, respectively, and retrospective sensitivity and specificity were 99% and 87%, respectively. MDCT angiography was considered to be sufficient for a reliable diagnosis in 83 patients ($p < 0.001$). Image quality and lesion depiction on MDCT angiograms were considered to be good and artifacts were considered mild with substantial interobserver agreement (κ, 0.62–0.69).

Conclusion.—MDCT angiography provides significant and reproducible technique for the detection and characterization of arterial injuries to the extremities with high image quality and vascular delineation.

▶ I believe this study targets the wrong population. Most patients with clinically suspected injury to an extremity can be treated by exploration without preoperative imaging. Although it is certainly easy to image suspected arterial injuries with MDCTA, the test is unnecessary if one is going to operate based on strong clinical findings of arterial injury. What would be more interesting is to evaluate patients with possible arterial injury based on mechanism but who had no sign of actual arterial insufficiency.

G. L. Moneta, MD

Operative and nonoperative management of children aged 13 years or younger with arterial trauma of the extremities
Lazarides MK, Georgiadis GS, Papas TT, et al (Demokritos Univ, Alexandroupolis, Greece; Athens Gen Hosp "G Gennimatas," Greece)
J Vasc Surg 43:72-76, 2006

Background.—Previous studies have suggested that open repair of arterial injuries in very young children often leads to less satisfactory outcomes. The aim of this study is to describe a decade's experience in the management of pediatric arterial trauma of the limbs, with an additional specific objective to evaluate the long-term outcome of arterial traumas in preschool children treated conservatively.

Methods.—Hospital charts were reviewed for all children aged ≤13 years with arterial trauma of the extremities who underwent operative or nonoperative treatment. Twenty-three children were located who had arterial traumas equally divided between the upper extremity (13) and lower extremity (10).

Results.—The method of treatment was either open surgical repair or medical treatment consisting of systematic heparin administration. In 11 of 12 school-aged children (>6 years; mean age, 10 years), open surgical repair was performed. In six of 11 preschool children (≤6 years; mean, 3.2 years) medical treatment was offered. Open repair was deferred in all children <2.5 years. Autologous vein interposition grafting was the most common surgical procedure and was performed in 10 patients. There were no deaths, and 87% limb salvage (21/23) was achieved. Two patients, both in the surgical arm, underwent lower limb amputation. The long-term outcome of those treated conservatively was excellent in all but one child, in whom minor limb-length discrepancy was detected.

Conclusion.—Surgical repair can be performed in school-aged children as in adults. Surgical treatment of arterial injuries in neonates, infants, and those children <2.5 years old might best be deferred in ischemic but nonthreatened limbs. In a nonthreatened ischemic extremity in this age group, systemic heparinization is an alternative safe method of management. Limb loss is rare if distal Doppler signals are present; but as children grow, limb shortening is a threat. In preschool children, the risks of an open surgical repair must be weighed against any potential benefits.

▶ I agree with the authors' approach to arterial injury in children. My bias is that although there are certainly technical problems when dealing with arterial injuries in children (the vessels may be small, have a tendency to spasm, and are thin walled), successful repair usually is possible if the arteries are of reasonable caliber, such as is the case in children who have reached school age. I also think that very small children with many extremity injuries can frequently, but obviously not always, be managed conservatively. Although limb length discrepancy later in life is possible, it is remarkably infrequent.[1]

G. L. Moneta, MD

Reference

1. Taylor LM Jr, Troutman R, Feliciano P, Menashe V, Sunderland C, Porter JM. Late complications after femoral artery catheterization in children less than five years of age. *J Vasc Surg.* 1990;11:297-304.

Limb salvage and outcomes among patients with traumatic popliteal vascular injury: An analysis of the National Trauma Data Bank
Mullenix PS, Steele SR, Andersen CA, et al (Madigan Army Med Ctr, Tacoma, Wash; Los Angeles County Hosp/USC Med Ctr)
J Vasc Surg 44:94-100, 2006

Purpose.—Popliteal arterial trauma carries the greatest risk of limb loss of any peripheral vascular injury. The purpose of this study was to analyze outcomes after popliteal arterial injuries and identify factors contributing to disability.

Methods.—A retrospective analysis was conducted of prospectively collected trauma data from the National Trauma Data Bank (NTDB). We studied all patients with popliteal arterial injury in terms of demographics, injury patterns, interventions, limb salvage, resource utilization, and outcomes.

Results.—We identified 1395 popliteal arterial injuries among the 1,130,000 patients in the NTDB, for an incidence <0.2%. The patients were 82% male, with a mean age of 33 years, and they presented with a mean initial systolic blood pressure of 124 mm Hg, base deficit −4.6, injury severity score of 11.8, and an extremity abbreviated injury score of 2.6. The mechanism was blunt in 61% and penetrating in 39%, and significant baseline demographic differences existed between the two groups. Associated ipsilateral lower-extremity trauma included combined popliteal arterial and venous (AV) injuries, fractures and dislocations, and major nerve disruptions. Fasciotomies were performed in 49%, complex soft tissue repairs in 24%, and amputations in 14.5%. The overall mean hospital and intensive care unit lengths of stay were 16.9 and 5.9 days. The mean functional independence measure for locomotion was 2.8, but was significantly lower for patients with blunt trauma. In-hospital mortality was 4.5% and did not significantly differ by mechanism. Amputation rates were 15% with combined AV injuries, 21% for associated nerve injuries, 12% for major soft tissue disruptions, and 21% for femur, 12% for knee, and 20% for tibia-fibula fractures or dislocations. Among the 312 patients with combined AV injuries, those with blunt mechanism had a significantly higher amputation rate than those with penetrating injury (27% vs 9%, $P < .001$). Adjusting for age, gender, mechanism, and overall physiologic impact of injuries sustained, independent predictors of amputation in logistic regression analysis of the entire cohort included fracture (odds ratio [OR], 2.4; 95% confidence interval [CI], 1.4 to 4.1), complex soft tissue injury (OR, 1.9; 95% CI, 1.2 to 3.0), nerve injury (OR, 1.7; 95% CI, 1.1 to 2.8), and extremity abbreviated injury score (OR, 1.6; 95% CI, 1.2 to 2.2).

Conclusions.—Popliteal vascular injury remains an uncommon but challenging clinical entity associated with significant rates of limb loss, functional disability, and mortality. Blunt vs penetrating mechanism and associated musculoskeletal injuries generally involve longer hospital stays, worse functional outcomes, and twice the amputation rate.

▶ The only group more interested in popliteal artery injuries than surgeons is attorneys. This particular injury has proclivity to produce lawsuits, and it's easy to see why with such high disability and amputation rates. In a leg with a significant popliteal injury, everything has to work well for the limb to be salvaged. First and foremost, a high index of suspicion is required when treating the patient with appropriate mechanism of injury.

G. L. Moneta, MD

Femoral Vessel Injuries: Analysis of Factors Predictive of Outcomes
Asensio JA, Kuncir EJ, García-Núñez LM, et al (Los Angeles County and Univ of Southern California)
J Am Coll Surg 203:512-520, 2006

Background.—Femoral vessel injuries are the most common vascular injuries treated in a Level I trauma center. No studies have identified risk factors for survival and complications.

Study Design.—We performed a retrospective, 132-month study that included univariate and multivariate analyses.

Results.—We studied 204 patients with 298 vessel injuries: 204 were arterial, 94 were venous. Mean age (±SD) was 29±13 years and mean Injury Severity Score (±SD) was 17±8. There were 176 (86%) penetrating injuries and 28 (14%) blunt injuries. Arterial repairs included: reverse saphenous vein graft bypass, 108 (53%); primary repair, 53 (26%); PTFE, 21 (10.2%); ligation, 13 (6.4%); and vein patch, 9 (4.4%). Venous repairs included: ligation, 49 (52%); primary repair, 41 (44%); and bypass, 4 (4%). Fasciotomies included: calf, 56 (27%); thigh, 25 (12%); traumatic amputations, 6 (3%); and delayed amputations, 0. Overall survival rate was 91% (186 of 204), and adjusted survival was 95% (excluding emergency department thoracotomy deaths). There were 1 or more complications in 47 (23%), including wound infection, 31 (15%); venous thrombosis, 6 (3%); bleeding, 5 (2.5%); ARDS, 4 (2%); and arterial thrombosis, 1 (0.5%). Predictors of mortality were age > 45 years, Injury Severity Score > 25, common femoral artery injury, associated venous and abdominal injury, hypotension, hypothermia, and acidosis; coagulopathy in the operating room and the need for PTFE repair also predicted outcomes. Predictors of postoperative complications were intraoperative hypotension, arterial intimal injury, bony fracture, and thoracic injury.

Conclusions.—Although survival and limb salvage rates are high for femoral vessel injuries, these injuries incur high complication rates. Independent predictors for mortality are: Injury Severity Score > 25, Glasgow Coma Scale 28, presence of coagulopathy in the operating room, presence of two or more vascular signs, and age > 45 years.

▶ Papers such as this do not provide much in the way of new insights. Predictors of mortality, complications, and types of complications are what one would expect. However, it is interesting to note the very high survival rate in patients with such injuries that were managed in a Level I trauma center.

G. L. Moneta, MD

The Belfast Approach to Managing Complex Lower Limb Vascular Injuries
Barros D'Sa AAB, Harkin DW, Blair PHB, et al (Royal Victoria Hosp, Belfast, Ireland)
Eur J Vasc Endovasc Surg 32:246-256, 2006

Introduction.—Complex lower limb vascular injuries (CLVIs) in high-energy penetrating or blunt trauma are associated with an unacceptably high incidence of complications including amputation. Traumatic ischaemia and ischaemia-reperfusion injury (IRI) of skeletal muscle often lead to limb loss, the systemic inflammatory response syndrome (SIRS) which affects remote organs and even the potentially fatal multiple organ dysfunction syndrome (MODS). Surgical care of CLVIs everywhere, including Northern Ireland until 1978, was governed by an anxiety to restore arterial flow quickly often using expedient and flawed repair techniques while a damaged major vein was frequently ligated.

Materials and Methods.—A new policy centred on early intraluminal shunting of both artery and vein, restoring arterial inflow and venous outflow, respectively, was introduced at the Regional Vascular Surgery Unit of The Royal Victoria Hospital, Belfast in 1979. It imposed a disciplined one-stage comprehensive approach to treatment involving a sequence of operative manoeuvres in which all damaged anatomical elements receive meticulous and optimal attention unshackled by time constraints.

Results.—Comparisons drawn between the pre-shunt period of unplanned treatment (1969–1978) and the post-shunt period centred on the

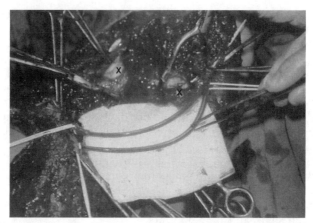

FIGURE 2.—A virtually dismembered leg at mid-thigh showing the bone ends (XX) of a fractured femur, a Javid shunt bridging a lengthy gap in femoral artery and perfusing the distal limb; another such shunt bridging adjoining femoral vein and draining the limb. (Reproduced with permission from Barros D'Sa AAB, Moorehead RJ. Combined arterial and venous intraluminal shunting in major trauma of the lower limb. *Eur J Vasc Surg.* 1989;3:577-581. Courtesy of Barros D'Sa AAB, Harkin DW, Blair PHB, et al. The Belfast approach to managing complex lower limb vascular injuries. *Eur J Vasc Endovasc Surg.* 2006;32:246-256. Reprinted by permission of the publisher.)

use of shunts (1979–2000) showed that early shunting of both artery and vein in both penetrating (P) and blunt (B) injuries significantly reduced the necessity for fasciotomy (*P:* p = 0.016, *B:* p = 0.02) and caused a significant fall in the incidence of contracture (*P:* p = 0.018, *B:* p = 0.02) and of amputation (*P:* p = 0.009, *P:* p = 0.012).

Conclusions.—The policy of early shunting of artery and vein in CLVIs has proved to be of great benefit in terms of significantly improved outcomes, better operative discipline and harmonious collaboration among the specialists involved (Fig 2).

▶ We are all aware of the terrorist violence that engulfed Northern Ireland for the last 30 years of the twentieth century. Despite the level of violence, the authors report relatively few major lower extremity vascular injuries. This paper uses somewhat flowery prose and is essentially a review of management of extremity vascular injury. The authors' main point is that the use of intravascular shunts can buy some time in the repair of vascular injuries. They also discuss panel and spiral vein grafts but present no new information.

G. L. Moneta, MD

Predictors of Mortality and Management of Patients with Traumatic Inferior Vena Cava Injuries

Huerta S, Bui TD, Nguyen TH, et al (Univ of Texas, Dallas; UCI Med Ctr, Orange, Calif)
Am Surg 72:290-296, 2006

The aim of this study was to determine factors that predict mortality in patients with traumatic inferior vena cava (IVC) injuries and to review the current management of this lethal injury. A 7-year retrospective review of all trauma patients with IVC injuries was performed. Factors associated with mortality were assessed by univariate analysis. Significant variables were included in a multivariate regression analysis model to determine independent predictors of mortality. Statistical significance was determined at $P \leq 0.05$. A literature review of traumatic IVC injuries was performed and compared with our institutional experience. Thirty-six IVC injuries were identified (mortality, 56%; mechanisms of injury, 28% blunt and 72% penetrating). There was no difference in mortality based on mechanism of injury. Injuries with closer proximity to the heart were associated with increased mortality ($P < 0.001$). Univariate analysis demonstrated that nonsurvivors had a higher injury severity scale, a lower systolic blood pressure in the emergency department, a lower Glasgow coma score (GCS), and were more likely to have thoracotomies performed in the emergency department or operating room. Multivariate analysis revealed that only GCS ($P = 0.03$) was an independent predictor of mortality. Typical factors predicting mortality were identified in our cohort of patients, including GCS. The mechanism of injury is not associated with survival outcome, although mortality is higher with injuries more proximal to the heart. The form of management by IVC level is reviewed in our patient population and compared with the literature.

▶ Mortality from vena cava injuries remains high and has not changed in 30 years. Albert Einstein once said that to keep doing something that doesn't work is a sign of insanity. We can't do much about the associated injuries in patients with vena cava injury. Perhaps, however, a new technical approach to the injury itself is needed. It seems that pressure control of hemorrhage and placement of a covered stent should at least be considered in some cases. Clearly, we are not making a lot of progress with continued attempts at suture ligation.

G. L. Moneta, MD

The effect of changing presentation and management on the outcome of blunt rupture of the thoracic aorta

Cook J, Salerno C, Krishnadasan B, et al (Univ of Washington, Seattle)
J Thorac Cardiovasc Surg 131:594-600, 2006

Background.—The management of traumatic aortic rupture has evolved from emergency surgery for all to incorporating nonoperative and endovascular approaches. In addition, the greater emphasis on restraint systems over the past decade might result in lower immediate mortality.

Methods.—We reviewed our contemporary experience with reference to a previous report from the same institution to determine whether there has been improvement in outcome related to these factors.

Results.—In 1990, a review of 104 patients admitted to our center over a 15-year period (1975-1990) noted an overall mortality of 65%. Forty-two patients died before they could reach the operating room, including 15 who were declared dead on arrival and 27 who died before reaching the operating room. All patients underwent angiography, followed by immediate operation. The mortality rate of those who reached the operating room was 34%, and paralysis-paraplegia occurred in 26% of survivors. A review of 53 patients admitted between January 1, 2000, and April 2005 documented an overall mortality of 26% and a paralysis rate of 4.5% in operative survivors. Only 3 patients died during initial evaluation, 2 who were in arrest on arrival. Eight patients were managed nonoperatively, and 13 were managed by means of deliberate delay before intervention to improve physiologic status. Finally, 19 patients were managed with endografts.

Conclusion.—The improved outcome over the decade since the initial experience reflects both a reduced severity of injury attributable to restraint systems and a more flexible approach to the acute management, which can modify the effect of associated injuries.

▶ It is always hard to derive specific recommendations from papers such as this which use historic controls and many different surgeons over almost 30 years. Nevertheless, improved mortality is likely multifactorial. I doubt that it is related to improved surgical operative skill but rather improved restraint devices, better patient selection for urgent repair, and new endograft techniques to decrease operative trauma. Probably the best way to reduce death from blunt injury of the thoracic aorta will come from more clever innovations by automotive engineers and hopefully by more responsible social behavior in the population.

G. L. Moneta, MD

Management and Hospital Outcomes of Blunt Renal Artery Injuries: Analysis of 517 Patients from the National Trauma Data Bank
Sangthong B, Demetriades D, Martin M, et al (Univ of Southern California, Los Angeles)
J Am Coll Surg 203:612-617, 2006

Background.—Blunt renal artery injuries are rare and no single trauma center can accumulate substantial experience for meaningful conclusions about optimal therapeutic strategies. The purpose of this study was to assess the incidence of renal artery injuries after different types of blunt trauma, and evaluate the current therapeutic approaches practiced by American trauma surgeons and the effect of various therapeutic modalities on hospital outcomes.

Study Design.—This was a National Trauma Data Bank study including all blunt trauma admissions with renal artery injuries. Demographics, mechanism of injury, Injury Severity Score, Abbreviated Injury Score for each body area (head, chest, abdomen, extremities) injuries, type of management (nephrectomy, arterial reconstruction, or observation), time from admission to definitive treatment, and hospital outcomes (mortality, ICU, and hospital stay) were analyzed. Multiple and logistic regression analyses were used to examine the relationship between type of management and hospital outcomes.

Results.—Of a total of 945,326 blunt trauma admissions, 517 patients (0.05%) had injuries to the renal artery. Of the 517 patients, the kidney was not explored in 376 (73%), 95 (18%) patients had immediate nephrectomy, and 45 (9%) patients underwent surgical revascularization. In 87 of 517 (17%) patients, renal artery injury was the only intraabdominal injury. Of the 87 patients with isolated renal artery injuries, 73 (84%) were observed, 7 (8%) underwent surgical revascularization, and 7 (8%) had early nephrectomy. Multiple regression analysis demonstrated that patients who had surgical revascularization had a considerably longer ICU and hospital stay than observed patients. Patients who had nephrectomy had a considerably longer hospital stay than observed patients.

Conclusions.—Blunt renal artery injury is rare. Nonoperative management should be considered as an acceptable therapeutic option.

▶ The rarity of blunt renal artery injury, time constraints, complexity of repair, and reported poor outcomes[1] all combine to make repair of the blunt renal artery injury a rare event. Nevertheless, in appropriately stable patients, a renal artery injury to a single functioning kidney or bilateral renal artery occlusion following blunt trauma should be considered for repair in an attempt to avoid permanent dialysis.

Reference

1. Haas CA, Spirnak JP. Traumatic renal artery occlusion: a review of the literature. *Tech Urol.* 1998;4:1-11.

G. L. Moneta, MD

15 Nonatherosclerotic Conditions

Aneurysm Syndromes Caused by Mutations in the TGF-β Receptor
Loeys BL, Schwarze U, Holm T, et al (Johns Hopkins Univ, Baltimore, Md; Kennedy Krieger Inst, Baltimore, Md; Univ of Washington, Seattle; et al)
N Engl J Med 355:788-798, 2006

Background.—The Loeys–Dietz syndrome is a recently described autosomal dominant aortic-aneurysm syndrome with widespread systemic involvement. The disease is characterized by the triad of arterial tortuosity and aneurysms, hypertelorism, and bifid uvula or cleft palate and is caused by heterozygous mutations in the genes encoding transforming growth factor β receptors 1 and 2 (*TGFBR1* and *TGFBR2*, respectively).

Methods.—We undertook the clinical and molecular characterization of 52 affected families. Forty probands presented with typical manifestations of the Loeys–Dietz syndrome. In view of the phenotypic overlap between this syndrome and vascular Ehlers–Danlos syndrome, we screened an additional cohort of 40 patients who had vascular Ehlers–Danlos syndrome without the characteristic type III collagen abnormalities or the craniofacial features of the Loeys–Dietz syndrome.

Results.—We found a mutation in *TGFBR1* or *TGFBR2* in all probands with typical Loeys–Dietz syndrome (type I) and in 12 probands presenting with vascular Ehlers–Danlos syndrome (Loeys–Dietz syndrome type II). The natural history of both types was characterized by aggressive arterial aneurysms (mean age at death, 26.0 years) and a high incidence of pregnancy-related complications (in 6 of 12 women). Patients with Loeys–Dietz syndrome type I, as compared with those with type II, underwent cardiovascular surgery earlier (mean age, 16.9 years vs. 26.9 years) and died earlier (22.6 years vs. 31.8 years). There were 59 vascular surgeries in the cohort, with one death during the procedure. This low rate of intraoperative mortality distinguishes the Loeys–Dietz syndrome from vascular Ehlers–Danlos syndrome.

Conclusions.—Mutations in either *TGFBR1* or *TGFBR2* predispose patients to aggressive and widespread vascular disease. The severity of the clinical presentation is predictive of the outcome. Genotyping of patients presenting with symptoms like those of vascular Ehlers–Danlos syndrome may be used to guide therapy, including the use and timing of prophylactic vascular surgery.

▶ Mutations of genes encoding for transforming growth factor β (TGF-β) receptors 1 and 2 are associated with a continuum of clinical features, including mutations that result in Marfan's syndrome, those associated with the Loweys-Deitz syndrome, and those associated with vascular Ehlers-Danlos syndrome. Given the different phenotypic characteristics of patients with TGF-β receptor mutations and the potential for pharmacologic manipulation of the TGF-β receptor, a study such as this that correlates phenotype with genotype is crucial to more precisely targeting therapy in patients with genetically based disorders.

G. L. Moneta, MD

Evolution from axillofemoral to *in situ* prosthetic reconstruction for the treatment of aortic graft infections at a single center
Oderich GS, Bower TC, Cherry KJ Jr, et al (Mayo Clinic, Rochester, Minn)
J Vasc Surg 43:1166-1174, 2006

Objective.—The primary purpose of this study was to analyze the clinical outcome in patients treated for aortic graft infections with *in situ* reconstruction (ISR). As a secondary aim, the outcomes were compared between patients who had similar clinical characteristics and extent of infection, needed total graft excision, and had either ISR or axillofemoral reconstruction (AXFR).

Methods.—117 consecutive patients treated for aortic graft infection over a 20 year period from January 1981 to December 2001 were identified. 52 patients had prosthetic ISR, 49 had AXFR, and 16 had other reconstructions. The ISR patients treated with total (n = 35) or partial (n = 17) graft excision comprised the primary analysis. A second analysis was done between 34 ISR and 43 AXFR patients (non-concurrent groups), as stated above. Primary outcome measures were early and late procedure-related death, primary graft patency and limb loss. Secondary outcomes were operative morbidity, patient survival, and graft reinfection rates.

Results.—There were 40 males and 12 females with a mean age of 69 years treated with ISR. 43 patients had Rifampin-soaked grafts and 39 had omental flap or other autogenous coverage. Operative morbidity occurred in 23 patients (44%). There were 4 early and no late procedure-related deaths after a median follow up of 3.4 years (range, 2 months to 9.6 years). Primary patency and limb salvage rates at 5 years were 89% and 100%, respectively. Graft reinfection occurred in 6 patients (11.5%) and was not associated with procedure-related death. In the comparative analysis, the procedure-related death rate for patients treated with ISR was not different than those treated with AXFR (9% versus 23%; P = 0.11). There was a significant improvement in primary patency between ISR and AXFR at 5 years (89% versus 48%; P = .01). Limb salvage was 100% for ISR and 89% for

AXFR at 5 years (P = .06). The incidence of graft reinfection was similar in both groups: 11% for ISR and 17% for AXFR (P = .28). Major complications or procedure-related deaths occurred in 12 patients after ISR (30%) and 26 patients (60%) after AXFR (P < .04).

Conclusion.—ISR is a safe and effective alternative in the treatment of select patients with aortic graft infection. Graft reinfection occurred in 11.5% of the patients. The graft patency and limb salvages rates are excellent.

▶ There are now many accepted and no perfect techniques for treatment of aortic graft infection. When the infected graft is entirely interabdominal an axillobifemoral graft makes sense; reinfection rates will be low and significantly better patency rates than presented here are to be expected. When infection involves the groins and/or there is significant interabdominal infection, femoral vein reconstruction is preferred. For minimal interabdominal infection, an in situ replacement with prosthetic is reasonable. Reinfection, if it occurs, is a real problem and graft-related deaths will occur. There were none in this series, but that is more a matter of luck than what is to be expected long term.

G. L. Moneta, MD

Diagnosis and management of primary chylous ascites
Campisi C, Bellini C, Eretta C, et al (Univ of Genoa, Italy)
J Vasc Surg 43:1244-1248, 2006

Background.—Chylous ascites is the accumulation of triglyceride-rich, free, milk-like peritoneal fluid caused by the presence of intestinal lymph in the abdominal cavity. Primary chylous ascites is uncommon. We present our experience in the diagnosis and treatment of this condition.

Methods.—Twelve patients (7 adults, 5 children) affected by primary chylous ascites were studied. Diagnostic investigations included abdominal sonography scans, lymphoscintigraphy, and lymphography combined with computed tomography (CT) with intravenous and intralymphatic lipid-soluble contrast, and laparoscopy. Magnetic resonance imaging was used when lymphography and lymphatic CT were not able to define the dysplasia well, or in the presence of lymphatic dilatation. Surgical treatment included laparoscopy (12/12), drainage of ascites (12/12), the search for and treatment of abdominal and retroperitoneal chylous leaks (12/12), exeresis of lymphodysplastic tissues (12/12), ligation of incompetent lymph vessels (9/12), carbon dioxide laser treatment (cut and welding effects) of the dilated lymph vessels using an operating microscope for magnification (9/12), and chylovenous and lymphovenous microsurgical shunts (7/12).

Results.—Eight patients did not have a relapse of the ascites, and three patients had a persistence of a small quantity of ascites with no protein imbalance. Postoperative lymphoscintigraphy in seven patients confirmed better lymph flow and less lymph reflux. Median follow-up was 5 years (range, 3 to

7 years). We observed early relapse of chylous ascites in only one case that required a peritoneal-jugular shunt and led to good outcome.

Conclusion.—Primary chylous ascites is closely correlated to lymphatic-lymphonodal dysplasia that does not involve a single visceral district alone. Medical preoperative treatment played an essential role in the global management of this complex pathology. We demonstrated that the use of laparoscopy is remarkably advantageous for confirming diagnosis, for draining the ascites, and for evaluating the extension of the dysplasia. Our diagnostic work-up provided us with an exact diagnostic assessment and allowed us to plan a precise surgical approach.

▶ Primary chylous ascites is very uncommon and treatment is, therefore, institution specific. The treatment algorithm outlined here makes good sense. Preoperative medical control of the chyle leak is obtained, followed by precise characterization of the lymphatic anatomy using lymphography, CT lymphography, and laparoscopy. A combination of surgical and chemical lymphatic obliteration and lymphovenous anastomosis to drain congested intra-abdominal lymphatics is then employed to correct as much as possible of the abnormal lymphatic anatomy.

G. L. Moneta, MD

Hemodynamic and morphologic evaluation of sequelae of primary upper extremity deep venous thromboses treated with anticoagulation

Persson LM, Arnhjort T, Lärfars G, et al (Karolinska Institutet, Stockholm)
J Vasc Surg 43:1230-1235, 2006

Objectives.—This study was performed to describe venous function, residual morphologic abnormalities, and the occurrence of post-thrombotic syndrome in patients with conservatively treated primary upper-extremity deep venous thromboses (UEDVT).

Method.—This was a retrospective follow-up study of 31 patients with previous primary UEDVT treated with anticoagulation only, identified by a search of medical records. The mean follow-up time was 5 years. The patients were evaluated by interview, clinical examination, computerized strain-gauge plethysmography, and color duplex ultrasound imaging. The grade of post-thrombotic syndrome was rated according to the Villalta score (0 to 3 on each of four subjective and five clinically assessed features).

Results.—The rate of venous emptying was significantly lower in the arms with DVTs than in the contralateral arms ($P < .001$). Eleven of the patients (35%) had a remaining outflow obstruction in the affected arm (venous emptying <68 mL/100 mL per min). Eighteen (58%) had a residual thrombus according to color duplex ultrasound scans, with four remaining occluded subclavian veins. None of the patients had deep or superficial venous reflux. There was no statistically significant relationship between plethysmographic and duplex findings. Most (77%) of the patients reported remaining symptoms in the affected arm, and there was a significant side difference in upper arm circumference (*P* < .001). Approximately one third had developed a moderate grade of post-thrombotic syndrome according to the Villalta score (total, 5 to 9). No significant relation was evident between the post-thrombotic syndrome score and duplex findings. Patients with post-thrombotic syndrome had a lower venous emptying value than those without (69 vs 84 mL/100 mL per min), but this difference was not statistically significant.

Conclusions.—Patients with conservatively treated previous primary UEDVT had significantly reduced venous outflow capacity and a residual thrombus was common. Swelling of the arm was the most common symptom, and one third had a moderate grade of post-thrombotic syndrome. However, there was no clear relation between hemodynamic and morphologic factors and the development of post-thrombotic syndrome in these 31 patients, examined at a mean of 5 years after an acute DVT episode.

▶ Patients with primary upper extremity venous thrombosis treated with anticoagulation only often have mild swelling and mild symptoms but seldom are severely symptomatic over the long term. One has to ask if the current approach to primary upper extremity venous thrombosis with aggressive resection of the first rib following thrombolysis is actually really worth the effort. After all, aggressive treatment also does not have perfect results. It is not surprising that physiologic and duplex assessments of the upper extremity veins in this study did not correlate. They do not correlate well in the lower extremity veins either.

G. L. Moneta, MD

Prosthetic Replacement of the Infrahepatic Inferior Vena Cava for Leiomyosarcoma
Illuminati G, Calio' FG, D'Urso A, et al (Univ of Rome; Sant'Anna Hosp, Catanzaro, Italy)
Arch Surg 141:919-924, 2006

Hypothesis.—Resection of the infrahepatic inferior vena cava associated with prosthetic graft replacement for caval leiomyosarcoma is an acceptable procedure to obtain prolonged and good-quality survival.

Design.—A consecutive sample clinical study with a mean follow-up of 40 months.

Setting.—The surgical department of an academic tertiary center and an affiliated secondary care center.

Patients.—Eleven patients, with a mean age of 51 years, who have primary leiomyosarcoma of the infrahepatic inferior vena cava.

Interventions.—All of the patients underwent radical resection of the tumor en bloc with the affected segment of the vena cava. Reconstruction consisted of 10 cavocaval polytetrafluoroethylene grafts and 1 cavobiliac graft. An associated right nephrectomy was performed in 2 cases. The left renal vein was reimplanted in the graft in 3 cases.

Main Outcome Measures.—Cumulative disease-specific survival, disease-free survival, and graft patency rates expressed by standard life-table analysis.

Results.—No patients died in the postoperative period. The cumulative (SE) disease-specific survival rate was 53% (21%) at 5 years. The cumulative (SE) disease-free survival rate was 44% (19%) at 5 years. The cumulative (SE) graft patency rate was 67% (22%) at 5 years.

Conclusion.—Radical resection followed by prosthetic graft reconstruction is a valuable method for treating primary leiomyosarcoma of the infrahepatic inferior vena cava.

▶ The patients in this series did well in the perioperative period with no early deaths or perioperative graft thromboses. Technical details not included in the abstract include use of 14- to 18-mm diameter grafts, no long-term anticoagulation unless the graft thrombosed, no use of arteriovenous fistulas, and frequent coverage of the graft with omentum. Clearly, this is an operation that can be done. I do think, however, in many cases the infrarenal vena cava can be removed and not reconstructed without significant morbidity as long as there is no proximal deep venous thrombosis in the legs.

G. L. Moneta, MD

Leiomyosarcoma of the Inferior Vena Cava: Experience in 22 Cases
Kieffer E, Alaoui M, Piette J-C, et al (Pitié-Salpêtrière Univ, Paris)
Ann Surg 244:289-295, 2006

From 1979 to 2004, 22 patients were seen with leiomyosarcomas of the inferior vena cava (IVC). Twenty were treated surgically. Involvement of the IVC included the infrarenal segment in 3 cases, the suprarenal and/or retrohepatic segment in 13, and the suprahepatic segment in 4. Nineteen patients underwent wide tumor resection followed by ligation of the IVC in 5 cases, replacement with a PTFE prosthesis in 13, and cavoplasty in 1. An intracardiac tumor extension was resected during hypothermic circulatory arrest in 1 patient. Vascular exclusion of the liver was used in 5 cases and simple clamping of the IVC in 13 cases. There were 1 intraoperative death due to cardiac failure and 3 postoperative deaths due to multiple organ failure, liver failure, and duodenal fistula after treatment of a bleeding ulcer. Fifteen of the 16 surviving patients underwent adjuvant chemotherapy associated with radiation therapy in 4 cases. One patient was lost from follow-up at 10 months. Four patients including one with metastasis are still alive with a mean follow-up of 18.3 months. Eleven patients died after a mean follow-up period of 43.7 months due to local recurrence and/or distant metastasis in 9 cases and complications of chemotherapy in 2. The 3- and 5-year mean actuarial survival rates in patients who underwent resection were 52.0% and 34.8%, respectively. Leiomyosarcoma of the IVC is a serious disease. Although surgical resection combined with chemotherapy is usually not curative, it can achieve reasonably long-term survival. We recommend aggressive operative management using the latest vascular surgery and oncology techniques.

▶ This is a more complex series of patients than that presented in the previous abstract[1] More complex surgical techniques were, therefore, required. The paper reflects Dr. Kieffer's referral pattern. In addition to the data in the abstract, Dr. Kieffer points out that most of these tumors do not obstruct the vena cava lumen and, therefore, there is no lower extremity edema at presentation. Most patients with leiomyosarcoma are female and present with abdominal pain rather than swelling. Budd-Chiari syndrome and intracardiac extension of the tumors are possible.

G. L. Moneta, MD

Reference

1. Illuminati G, Calio' FG, D'Urso A, Giacobbi D, Papaspyropoulos V, Ceccanei G. Prosthetic replacement of the infrahepatic inferior vena cava for Leiomyosarcoma. *Arch Surg.* 2006;141:919-924.

Correction of Extrahepatic Portal Vein Thrombosis by the Mesenteric to Left Portal Vein Bypass
Superina R, Bambini DA, Lokar J, et al (Northwestern Univ, Chicago)
Ann Surg 243:515-521, 2006

Objective.—The goal of this study was to determine the effectiveness of mesenteric vein to left portal vein bypass operation (MLPVB) in correcting extrahepatic portal vein thrombosis (EHPVT) in children. The treatment of idiopathic EHPVT has been primarily palliative, whereas MLPVB restores hepatic portal flow in patients with EHPVT.
Methods.—Thirty-four children with symptomatic EHPVT underwent surgery with intent to perform MLPVB and were followed for up to 7 years. MLPVB was successful in 31 patients (91%), all of whom maintain patent vein grafts and have symptomatic relief of EHPVT in follow-up. All patients had complete relief from gastrointestinal bleeding. Patients with hypersplenism had significant increases in platelet and leukocyte counts and reduction in spleen size. Superior mesenteric vein flow increased from 119 ± 66 mL/min before bypass to 447 ± 225 mL/min ($P < 0.0001$) after surgery. Postoperative blood flow in the bypass graft expressed as a fraction of calculated ideal portal flow for size correlated inversely with age ($P < 0.001$). Left-portal vein diameter increased from 2.6 ± 1.6 mm to 7.3 ± 2.4 mm 2 years after surgery ($P < 0.002$). Liver volume increased from 703 ± 349 cm^3 to 799 ± 351 cm^3 1 week after surgery ($P < 0.001$). Prothrombin time improved to normal in all patients 1 year after surgery.
Conclusions.—MLPVB provides excellent relief of symptoms in children with idiopathic EHPVT and results in liver growth and normalization of co-

agulation parameters. This surgery is corrective and should be done at as early an age as possible.

▶ It should be noted that younger patients in this series were more likely to eventually achieve bypass blood flows that approximated ideal portal venous blood flow. In addition, the fraction of ideal flow achieved was inversely proportional to age. This suggests mesenteric to left portal vein bypass is effective treatment for extrahepatic portal vein thrombosis but should be performed at as young an age as possible.

G. L. Moneta, MD

Surgical treatment of jugular vein phlebectasia in children
Jianhong L, Xuewu J, Tingze H (Shantou Univ, Shantou City, People's Republic of China)
Am J Surg 192:286-290, 2006

Background.—Jugular vein phlebectasia (JVP) is a cervical mass that occurs relatively infrequently and usually presents in children as a soft cystic swelling in the neck during straining. It is liable to be misdiagnosed or managed inappropriately. This report elucidates the clinical presentation, diagnosis, treatment choices, and postoperative complications of JVP, and diagnostic methods and treatment choices are recommended.

Methods.—Fifty-one cases of JVP were reviewed (right vein in 38 patients, left in 7 patients, and bilateral in 6 patients). The internal jugular vein was involved the most frequently. The main complaint was a soft and compressible mass in the neck, becoming more prominent with the Valsalva maneuver. All of the children except 2 had an ultrasound or color Doppler flow imaging (CDFI) performed in combination with the Valsalva's breathing test. Surgical intervention was performed in 46 patients and the other 5 patients were followed-up conservatively for 2 to 15 years.

Results.—Ultrasound or CDFI showed local dilatation of unilateral or bilateral veins in all patients except 2, and confirmed the diagnosis in combination with the Valsalva's breathing test. Surgical intervention included ligation of the involved jugular vein in 32 patients, and longitudinal constriction suture venoplasty plus encapsulation with medical Dacron cloth or PTFE in 14 patients. All of the children who had surgery recovered uneventfully, except 3 patients undergoing ligation of the right internal jugular vein.

Conclusions.—The Valsalva maneuver was most important for establishing the diagnosis. Ultrasound or CDFI, or in combination with the Valsalva's breathing test, was the diagnostic procedure of choice to confirm the diagnosis of JVP because of its clarity, safety, and low cost. Surgical intervention was recommended for cosmetic and psychologic purposes. Ligation or excision of the involved jugular vein was very safe, simple, and effective for most patients. However, in cases of lesions of the right and bilateral internal jugular veins, longitudinal constriction suture venoplasty plus encapsulation might be more preferable and safer, and should be recommended. Otherwise, treatment should be conservative (follow-up evaluation).

▶ Local dilatation of neck veins in children treated with surgery appears reasonably common in this part of China—who knows why. Nevertheless, the authors' point of performing ligation of the external jugular and anterior jugular veins for phlebectasia and plication of the internal jugular vein for phlebectasia makes some sense. This may avoid the rare case of intracranial venous hypertension secondary to jugular vein ligation.

G. L. Moneta, MD

Incidence and natural history of Raynaud phenomenon: a long-term follow-up (14 years) of a random sample from the general population
Carpentier PH, Satger B, Poensin D, et al (Centre de Recherche Universitaire, La Léchère, France; Centre Hosptalier Universitaire, Grenoble, France, Med Univ of South Carolina, Charleston)
J Vasc Surg 44:1023-1028, 2006

Background.—Because the natural history of primary Raynaud phenomenon (RP) is unclear, we undertook this long-term (14 years) follow-up of an epidemiologic study on RP to investigate the incidence, remittance rate, and transition rate toward systemic sclerosis and other scleroderma spectrum disorders in a population-based sample of subjects.

Methods.—In 1988 and 1989, 296 subjects obtained from a random sample of the general population of the Alpine valley of Tarentaise (southeast France) completed a cross-sectional study on RP. Of these, 78 met the diagnostic criteria for RP (RP$^+$). From April 2002 to March 2003, we were able to get follow-up information on 292 people (dropout rate, 1.4%). Eighteen subjects (6.1%) had died, and the remaining 274 were successfully contacted. They were first evaluated by a standardized phone interview regarding their cold sensitivity, digital color changes, and RP. If any significant medical changes related to RP and/or suggesting scleroderma were reported, these subjects were invited for a medical evaluation.

Results.—Mortality was similar in RP$^+$ and RP$^-$ subjects, and no death was due to an RP-related condition. Seven cases of new RP were diagnosed in the RP$^-$ group, which corresponds to an annual incidence rate of 0.25%. Among the 72 RP$^+$ subjects and the 7 subjects with a new RP available for follow-up, none developed clinical features of scleroderma. A disappearance of RP attacks for 2 winters or more was reported by 24 RP$^+$ subjects (33%).

Conclusions.—These results show that, in the general population, RP is most often a benign condition and may disappear in a substantial proportion of subjects.

▶ This article and the following abstract[1] reach different conclusions about the frequency of development of a systemic disorder in patients presenting with what appears to be primary Raynaud's syndrome. The next paper is more sophisticated, but patients had presented to the physician with Raynaud's syndrome. In this article patients were randomly sampled from the population. For those who work outside academic centers, the data in this article are more likely to apply to their practice than to that in the following article. Note that in this abstract many patients have resolution of Raynaud's symptoms over time. This is consistent with observations from our Raynaud's clinic in Oregon, where over 1,000 patients have been evaluated.

G. L. Moneta, MD

Reference

1. Hirschl M, Hirschl K, Lenz M, Katzenschlager R, Hutter HP, Kundi M. Transition from primary Raynaud's phenomenon to secondary Raynaud's phenomenon identified by diagnosis by an associated disease: results of ten years of prospective surveillance. *Arthritis Rheum.* 2006;54:1974-1981.

Transition From Primary Raynaud's Phenomenon to Secondary Raynaud's Phenomenon Identified by Diagnosis by an Associated Disease: Results of Ten Years of Prospective Surveillance
Hirschl M, Hirschl K, Lenz M, et al (Hanuschkrankenhaus, Vienna; Med Univ of Vienna)
Arthritis Rheum 54:1974-1981, 2006

Objective.—To assess the early signs, risk factors, and rate of transition from primary Raynaud's phenomenon (primary RP) to secondary RP.

Methods.—A clinical sample of 307 consecutive patients with RP was included in a prospective followup study. After an initial screening, 244 patients were classified as having primary RP, of whom 236 were followed up for a mean SD of 11.2 ± 3.9 years. Patients classified according to the screening as having suspected secondary RP underwent an extended screening program annually until transition to secondary RP occurred.

Results.—The initial prevalence of secondary RP was 11%. The annual incidence of transition to suspected secondary RP was 2%, and the annual incidence of transition to secondary RP was 1%. Overall, 46 patients were classified as having suspected secondary RP, and 23 of these later were classified as having secondary RP. Older age at onset of RP (hazard ratio 2.59, 95% confidence interval [95% CI] 1.40–4.80), shorter duration of RP at enrollment (hazard ratio 0.87, 95% CI 0.81–0.94), and abnormal findings on thoracic outlet test (hazard ratio 2.69, 95% CI 1.12–6.48) were associated with an increased risk for transition to secondary RP. Compared with patients with suspected secondary RP, those diagnosed as having secondary RP had a higher number and earlier occurrence of pathologic findings. Furthermore, antinuclear antibodies at a titer of ≥1:320 and positive findings in specific serologic subsets were associated with a significantly increased risk for developing a connective tissue disease.

Conclusion.—Patients diagnosed initially as having primary RP may actually comprise 1 of 3 groups: those with idiopathic RP, those with a rather benign disease course, and those with a more severe course of the disease.

▶ It is widely believed that some patients present with Raynaud's syndrome as their initial manifestation of a systemic disorder such as scleroderma. However, the systemic disorder may be independent of the much more common primary Raynaud's syndrome. If that is the case, one wonders if the extensive screening procedures outlined in this article are really effective in reducing overall morbidity of a Raynaud's-associated disease. The answer is probably no. The most effective variables identified in this article for predicting a possible eventual diagnosable systemic disorder were relatively simple ones such as age at presentation, duration of symptoms and the presence of an antinuclear antibody (ANA) titer of greater than 1:320. Such patients should have a rheumatologic evaluation. Patients with normal finger photoplethysmographic studies and negative ANA titers, even if they present at an older age, should be reassured. Further evaluation is only necessary for development of additional symptoms.

G. L. Moneta, MD

Thoracoscopic sympathectomy for Raynaud's phenomenon: A long term follow-up study

Thune TH, Ladegaard L, Licht PB (Odense Univ, Denmark)
Eur J Vasc Endovasc Surg 32:198-202, 2006

Objectives.—To assess the long term results of thoracoscopic sympathectomy for Raynaud's phenomenon.

Design, materials and methods.—A retrospective study of 34 consecutive patients who were treated for Raynaud's phenomenon by thoracoscopic sympathectomy from 1996 to 2005. Eight patients presented with ulcerations of the digits and 10 had severe ischaemia without ulcerations. The hospital records were retrieved and questionnaires were mailed to the patients for follow-up.

Results.—The questionnaire was answered by 91% of patients after a median follow-up time of 40 months. An immediate effect was seen in 83% of the patients but symptoms recurred in 60% during the follow-up period. Compensatory sweating occurred in 63 and 30% reported gustatory sweating. Thirteen patients (43%) regretted having the operation.

Conclusion.—The majority of patients with Raynaud's phenomenon have an excellent immediate effect from thoracoscopic sympathectomy and one third achieve a long lasting effect. Side effects are frequent. We now only use thoracoscopic sympathectomy in severe cases of Raynaud's phenomenon.

▶ History repeats itself again: open sympathectomy has never been an effective treatment for Raynaud's syndrome. It is not surprising that thoracoscopic approaches to sympathectomy are also not effective. There is a very limited, if nonexistent, role for sympathectomy in the long-term management of Raynaud's syndrome.

G. L. Moneta, MD

A randomized trial of T3-T4 versus T4 sympathectomy for isolated axillary hyperhidrosis

Munia MAS, Wolosker N, Kauffman P, et al (Univ of São Paulo, Brazil)
J Vasc Surg 45:130-133, 2007

Introduction.—Video-assisted thoracic sympathectomy (VATS) is one minimally invasive definitive treatment for axillary hyperhidrosis. Different techniques exist for controlling axillary sudoresis, but they are temporary and have high cost. This study was conducted to compare the initial results from sympathectomy using two distinct levels for treating axillary sudoresis: T3-T4 vs T4.

Methods.—Sixty-two patients with axillary hyperhidrosis were prospectively randomized for denervation of T3-T4 or T4 alone. All patients were examined preoperatively and were followed-up at 1 and 6 months postoperatively. Evaluated were the axillary hyperhidrosis treatment, the presence, location, and severity of compensatory hyperhidrosis, and the quality of life.

Results.—All the patients said that their axillary hyperhidrosis was successfully treated by the surgery after 6 months. There was no treatment failure. Compensatory hyperhidrosis was present in 29 patients (90.6%) of the T3-T4 group and in 17 T4 patients (56.7%) after 1 month. After 6 months, all the T3-T4 patients presented some degree of compensatory hyperhidrosis vs 13 T4 patients (43.3%). The severity of the compensatory hyperhidrosis was also lower in the T4 patients ($P < .01$). The quality of life was poor in both groups before the surgery, and was equally improved in both groups after 1 and 6 months of follow-up. There were no deaths or significant postoperative complications nor a need for conversion to thoracotomy.

Conclusion.—Both techniques are effective for treating axillary hyperhidrosis, but the T4 group presented milder compensatory hyperhidrosis and had a greater satisfaction rate.

▶ Taken together this abstract and an article by Panhofer et al[1] indicate that denervation at the T4 level is an acceptable procedure for axillary hyperhidrosis. Quality of life is improved and complications minimized with the denervation at the T4 level rather than the T3-T4 level. In this case, less is better.

G. L. Moneta, MD

Reference

1. Panhofer P, Zacheri J, Jakesz R, Bischof G, Neumayer C. Improved quality of life after sympathetic block for upper limb hyperhidrosis. *Br J Surg.* 2006;93:582-586.

Improved quality of life after sympathetic block for upper limb hyperhidrosis

Panhofer P, Zacheri J, Jakesz R, et al (Med Univ of Vienna; St Josef Hosp, Vienna)
Br J Surg 93:582-586, 2006

Background.—The aim of the study was to assess two disease-specific quality of life (QoL) instruments after limited endoscopic thoracic sympathetic block (TS) at T4 for upper limb hyperhidrosis.

Methods.—Between 2001 and 2005, 112 patients underwent 223 TS procedures in a prospective study. Some 103 patients (92.0 per cent) had palmar, 87 (77.7 per cent) had axillary and 75 (67.0 per cent) had combined hyperhidrosis. QoL questionnaires devised by Keller et al and Milanez de Campos et al were employed before and after treatment. Mean(s.d.) follow-up was 21.9(10.1) months.

Results.—A total of 106 patients (94.6 per cent) were evaluated. All patients with palmar hyperhidrosis were completely or almost dry after surgery. Side-effects of compensatory sweating and gustatory sweating were observed in 17.0 and 28.3 per cent of patients respectively. QoL improved after TS in 100 per cent (Keller) and 97.3 per cent (Milanez de Campos) of patients illustrated by ameliorated scores of 78.7 and 67.8 per cent, respectively (both $P < 0.001$). Both questionnaires showed that compensatory sweating resulted in reduced postoperative QoL ($P = 0.011$, Keller; $P = 0.032$, Milanez de Campos).

Conclusion.—Endoscopic sympathetic block at T4 leads to improved QoL. Both current questionnaires fulfilled validation criteria for disease-specific QoL instruments in upper limb hyperhidrosis.

▶ This study serves to remind us that hyperhydrosis, while not life threatening or life limiting or painful, can severely adversely affect quality of life and that complications of surgery can be quantified from the patient's perspective. The authors are to be congratulated for their willingness to move beyond investigation of surgical technique and focus on outcome variables that matter to patients. We need more studies like this comparing disease-specific and generic quality of life instruments in surgical patients.

G. L. Moneta, MD

Antiplatelet and Anticoagulant Therapy in Patients With Giant Cell Arteritis

Lee MS, Smith SD, Galor A, et al (Univ of Minnesota, Minneapolis; Cleveland Clinic Found, Ohio)
Arthritis Rheum 54:3306-3309, 2006

Objective.—Vision loss and cerebrovascular accidents often complicate giant cell arteritis (GCA). Antiplatelet and anticoagulant therapy reduce the risk of stroke in other populations. We sought to determine whether antiplatelet or anticoagulant therapy reduces ischemic complications in patients with GCA.

Methods.—A retrospective chart review for patients with GCA was conducted. Included patients fulfilled modified 1990 American College of Rheumatology criteria for GCA. Collected information included demographic data, dates of antiplatelet or anticoagulant use, vision loss or stroke, and presence of bleeding complications and cerebrovascular risk factors.

Results.—A total of 143 patients were included with a mean followup period of 4 years. The cohort included 109 women (76%) and 34 men (24%) with a mean age of 71.8 years. A total of 104 patients (73%) had a biopsy-proven diagnosis. Eighty-six patients (60.1%) had received long-term antiplatelet or anticoagulant therapy, including 18 (12.6%) who did not start therapy until after an ischemic event had occurred. Antiplatelet agents or anticoagulants were not used in 57 patients (39.9%). Overall, 11 of 68 patients (16.2%) had an ischemic event while receiving antiplatelet or anticoagulant therapy, compared with 36 of 75 patients (48.0%) not receiving such therapy ($P < 0.0005$). Univariate analysis failed to show a statistical difference between groups in regard to cerebrovascular risk factors, age, sex, or biopsy-proven diagnosis. Bleeding complications occurred in 2 patients receiving aspirin, 1 patient receiving warfarin, and 5 patients who did not receive anticoagulant or antiplatelet therapy.

Conclusion.—Antiplatelet or anticoagulant therapy may reduce the risk of ischemic events in patients with GCA. An increased risk of bleeding complications was not observed.

▶ There may be some reluctance to use antiplatelet medication in patients with giant cell arteritis since giant cell arteritis is generally treated with steroids and bleeding complications may be increased with the combination of steroids and antiplatelet agents. The dose and type of antiplatelet agent were not specifically defined in this report. No recommendation for dosage or specific antiplatelet agent can, therefore, be made. I would recommend initially using a low dose of aspirin unless there are other reasons to use higher doses or clopidogrel. However, this recommendation is clearly only a guess.

G. L. Moneta, MD

Role of C–C chemokines in Takayasu's arteritis disease

Dhawan V, Mahajan N, Jain S (Postgraduate Inst of Med Education and Research, Chandigarh, India)
Int J Cardiol 112:105-111, 2006

Background.—Takayasu's arteritis (TA) is a chronic obliterative inflammatory disease. Inflammatory cell infiltration and destruction of the vessel wall in TA strongly suggest that cell mediated immunological mechanisms play an important role in the pathogenesis of this disease. Therefore, in the present study our aim was to focus on the role of chemokines and adhesion molecules in patients with Takayasu's disease.

Methods.—Twenty-one patients with clinically defined TA and 21 healthy control volunteers were recruited by using the standard criteria. Patients with TA were divided into those with clear-cut clinically active or inactive disease based on vasculitis activity score.

Results.—MCP-1 and hRANTES were significantly increased in patients with TA as compared to controls. MCP-1 and hRANTES values were reliably able to distinguish between patients with active disease vs. subjects in remission. sVCAM-1 levels remained unaltered between patients and controls.

Conclusions.—C–C chemokines can be used as reliable markers/diagnostic tools in determining the activity of Takayasu's arteritis.

▶ Mononuclear cell infiltration into the arterial wall characterizes both giant cell arteritis and Takayasu's arteritis. The elevated chemokines (MCP-1 and hRANTES) found in patients with Takayasu's arteritis may be the signal that leads to infiltration of the arterial wall with inflammatory mononuclear cells. The article, therefore, suggests a possible mechanism for more direct treatment of Takayasu's arteritis through direct inhibition of chemokines promoting inflammation.

G. L. Moneta, MD

Randomized Trial of Pulsed Corticosteroid Therapy for Primary Treatment of Kawasaki Disease

Newburger JW, for the Pediatric Heart Network Investigators (Harvard Med School; et al)
N Engl J Med 356:663-675, 2007

Background.—Treatment of acute Kawasaki disease with intravenous immune globulin and aspirin reduces the risk of coronary-artery abnormalities and systemic inflammation, but despite intravenous immune globulin therapy, coronary-artery abnormalities develop in some children. Studies have suggested that primary corticosteroid therapy might be beneficial and that adverse events are infrequent with short-term use.

Methods.—We conducted a multicenter, randomized, double-blind, placebo-controlled trial to determine whether the addition of intravenous methylprednisolone to conventional primary therapy for Kawasaki disease reduces the risk of coronary-artery abnormalities. Patients with 10 or fewer days of fever were randomly assigned to receive intravenous methylprednisolone, 30 mg per kilogram of body weight (101 patients), or placebo (98 patients). All patients then received conventional therapy with intravenous immune globulin, 2 g per kilogram, as well as aspirin, 80 to 100 mg per kilogram per day until they were afebrile for 48 hours and 3 to 5 mg per kilogram per day thereafter.

Results.—At week 1 and week 5 after randomization, patients in the two study groups had similar coronary dimensions, expressed as z scores adjusted for body-surface area, absolute dimensions, and changes in dimensions. As compared with patients receiving placebo, patients receiving intravenous methylprednisolone had a somewhat shorter initial period of hospitalization (P=0.05) and, at week 1, a lower erythrocyte sedimentation rate (P=0.02) and a tendency toward a lower C-reactive protein level (P=0.07). However, the two groups had similar numbers of days spent in the hospital, numbers of days of fever, rates of retreatment with intravenous immune globulin, and numbers of adverse events.

Conclusions.—Our data do not provide support for the addition of a single pulsed dose of intravenous methylprednisolone to conventional intravenous immune globulin therapy for the routine primary treatment of children with Kawasaki disease.

▶ Another therapy, when actually investigated objectively, does not prove to work.

G. L. Moneta, MD

One of the most frequent vascular diseases in northeastern of Turkey: Thromboangiitis obliterans or Buerger's disease (experience with 344 cases)
Ates A, Yekeler I, Ceviz M, et al (Atatürk Univ, Erzurum, Turkey; Siyami Ersek Thoracic and Cardiovascular Surgery Research and Training Hosp, Istanbul, Turkey; Yüksek Ihtisas Hosp, Ankara, Turkey; et al)
Int J Cardiol 111:147-153, 2006

Purpose.—This is a retrospective clinical study on adult patients treated surgically for Buerger's disease in our region.

Methods.—In our clinic, 344 patients with Buerger's disease were surgically treated between 1980 and 2004. The major complaints included foot coldness in 312 (90.6%) patients, color changes in 290 (84.3%), rest pain in 160 (46.5%), claudication in 166 (48.2%) and necrotic ulcers in 185 (53.1%). Lumbar sympathectomy was made in 278 (80.2%) patients, thoracic sympathectomy in 7 (2.2%), thoracic and lumbar sympathectomy in 12 (3.6%), lumbar sympathectomy and femoropopliteal or femorotibial bypass in 30 (9%), and femoropopliteal or femorotibial bypass in 17 (5%).

Results.—Color changes were improved in 230 (79.3%) patients, food coldness were decreased in 288 (92.3%) and rest pains were improved in 43 (26.8%). Intermittent claudications decreased in 132 of 166 patients. Necrotic ulcers healed in 30 of 185 patients. Amputation was made totally in 155 (53%) patients in 10 years.

Conclusions.—As a nonatherosclerotic, segmental, inflammatory disease, Buerger's disease is causally related to tobacco use. The main goal is to discontinue the use of tobacco. Sympathectomy may be helpful in healing the ulcers and decreasing the symptoms. Vascular reconstruction is rarely possible for patients with Buerger's disease due to segmental involvement and distal nature of the disease.

▶ The authors used sympathectomy liberally in their patients. The data analysis was relatively simple and the results were not controlled for smoking status. I do not think we can use this paper to advocate almost routine use of sympathectomy in patients with Buerger's disease. Smoking cessation should be the mainstay of therapy for Buerger's patients. When avoidance of tobacco is sustained, 94% of patients can expect to avoid amputation.[1]

G. L. Moneta, MD

Reference

1. Olin JW. Current concepts: thromboangiitis obliteran's (Buerger's Disease). *N Engl J Med.* 2000;343:864-869.

An implantable carotid sinus stimulator for drug-resistant hypertension: Surgical technique and short-term outcome from the multicenter phase II Rheos feasibility trial
Illig KA, Levy M, Sanchez L, et al (Univ of Rochester, NY; Virginia Commonwealth Univ, Richmond; Washington Univ, St Louis; et al)
J Vasc Surg 44:1213-1218, 2006

Background.—A large number of patients have hypertension that is resistant to currently available pharmacologic therapy. Electrical stimulation of the carotid sinus baroreflex system has been shown to produce significant chronic blood pressure decreases in animals. The phase II Rheos Feasibility Trial was performed to assess the response of patients with multidrug-resistant hypertension to such stimulation.

Methods.—The system consists of an implantable pulse generator with bilateral perivascular carotid sinus leads. Implantation is performed bilaterally with patients under narcotic anesthesia (to preserve the reflex for assessment of optimal lead placement). Dose-response testing at 0 to 6 V is assessed before discharge and at monthly intervals thereafter; the device is activated after 1 month's recovery time. This was a Food and Drug Administration–monitored phase II trial performed at five centers in the United States.

Results.—Ten patients with resistant hypertension (taking a median of six antihypertensive medications) underwent implantation. All 10 were successful, with no significant morbidity. The mean procedure time was 198 minutes. There were no adverse events attributable to the device. Predischarge dose-response testing revealed consistent ($r = .88$) reductions in systolic blood pressure of 41 mm Hg (mean fall is from 180-139 mm Hg), with a peak response at 4.8 V ($P < .001$) and without significant bradycardia or bothersome symptoms.

Conclusions.—A surgically implantable device for electrical stimulation of the carotid baroreflex system can be placed safely and produces a significant acute decrease in blood pressure without significant side effects.

▶ The electrical baroreflux stimulation achieved by this device appears to dramatically reduce blood pressure probably through a combination of decreased sympathetic nervous system activity and inhibition of the renin-angiotension system. When one considers that decreases in blood pressure of 10 to 15 mm Hg over the long term can have huge cardiovascular benefits, the potential of this device to have substantial clinical impact is huge if reductions in blood pressure can be maintained over time.

G. L. Moneta, MD

16 Venous Thrombosis & Pulmonary Embolism

Effect of Hypobaric Hypoxia, Simulating Conditions During Long-Haul Air Travel, on Coagulation, Fibrinolysis, Platelet Function, and Endothelial Activation
Toff WD, Jones CI, Ford I, et al (Univ of Leicester, England; Univ of Aberdeen, Scotland; Royal Air Force Centre of Aviation Medicine, Henlow, Bedfordshire, England; et al)
JAMA 295:2251-2261, 2006

Context.—The link between long-haul air travel and venous thromboembolism is the subject of continuing debate. It remains unclear whether the reduced cabin pressure and oxygen tension in the airplane cabin create an increased risk compared with seated immobility at ground level.

Objective.—To determine whether hypobaric hypoxia, which may be encountered during air travel, activates hemostasis.

Design, Setting, and Participants.—A single-blind, crossover study, performed in a hypobaric chamber, to assess the effect of an 8-hour seated exposure to hypobaric hypoxia on hemostasis in 73 healthy volunteers, which was conducted in the United Kingdom from September 2003 to November 2005. Participants were screened for factor V Leiden G1691A and prothrombin G20210A mutation and were excluded if they tested positive. Blood was drawn before and after exposure to assess activation of hemostasis.

Interventions.—Individuals were exposed alternately (≥ 1 week apart) to hypobaric hypoxia, similar to the conditions of reduced cabin pressure during commercial air travel (equivalent to atmospheric pressure at an altitude of 2438 m), and normobaric normoxia (control condition; equivalent to atmospheric conditions at ground level, circa 70 m above sea level).

Main Outcome Measures.—Comparative changes in markers of coagulation activation, fibrinolysis, platelet activation, and endothelial cell activation.

Results.—Changes were observed in some hemostatic markers during the normobaric exposure, attributed to prolonged sitting and circadian variation. However, there were no significant differences between the changes in the hypobaric and the normobaric exposures. For example, the median difference in change between the hypobaric and normobaric exposure was 0 ng/mL for thrombin-antithrombin complex (95% CI, -0.30 to 0.30 ng/ mL); -0.02 [corrected] nmol/L for prothrombin fragment 1 + 2 (95% CI, -0.03 to 0.01 nmol/L); 1.38 ng/mL for D-dimer (95% CI, -3.63 to 9.72 ng/mL); and -2.00% for endogenous thrombin potential (95% CI, -4.00% to 1.00%).

Conclusion.—Our findings do not support the hypothesis that hypobaric hypoxia, of the degree that might be encountered during long-haul air travel, is associated with prothrombotic alterations in the hemostatic system in healthy individuals at low risk of venous thromboembolism.

▶ It is important to recognize who was studied and who was not studied in this investigation. Patients taking oral contraceptive pills were included, as were patients older than 50 years of age. However, individuals with factor V Leiden and prothrombin gene mutation were excluded as were those with a history of venous thromboembolism (VTE). Thus, the patients at highest risk for VTE associated with long-haul air travel were not studied. The study addresses potential changes in coagulation induced by hypobaric hypoxia. It does not address the clinical question of potential coagulation changes in individuals at most risk for long-haul air travel associated VTE.

G. L. Moneta, MD

The Pathogenesis of Venous Thromboembolism: Evidence for Multiple Interrelated Causes

Brouwer J-LP, Veeger NJGM, Kluin-Nelemans HC, et al (Univ Med Ctr Groningen, the Netherlands)
Ann Intern Med 145:807-815, 2006

Background.—Venous thromboembolism (VTE) is thought to result from interactions between multiple genetic and environmental risk factors.

Objective.—To assess the contribution of multiple thrombophilic defects and exogenous risk factors to the absolute risk for VTE.

Design.—Retrospective family cohort study.

Setting.—Single university hospital.

Participants.—468 relatives of 91 probands with a symptomatic hereditary deficiency of protein S, protein C, or antithrombin.

Measurements.—All relatives were tested for 10 thrombophilic deficiencies and defects in addition to the index deficiency and were assessed for exogenous risk factors (surgery, trauma, immobilization, use of oral contraceptives, and pregnancy). The authors compared annual incidences and relative risks for VTE in deficient and nondeficient relatives.

Results.—Annual incidences of VTE in relatives with 0, 1, and 2 or more additional thrombophilic deficiencies or defects were 1.16 (95% CI, 0.60 to 2.03), 1.75 (CI, 1.17 to 2.53), and 2.64 (CI, 1.67 to 3.96) per 100 person-years, respectively, compared with 0.06 (CI, 0.002 to 0.33) per 100 person-years in nondeficient relatives without additional deficiencies or defects. Adjusted relative risks were 16.3 (CI, 2.0 to 131.0), 50.3 (6.5 to 389.7), and 102.8 (12.5 to 843.4). Of deficient relatives, 38% with no additional defect, 57% with 1 additional defect, and 81% with 2 or more additional defects had VTE at age 65 years compared with 5% of nondeficient relatives (*P* < 0.001). In deficient relatives with additional deficiencies or defects, exogenous risk factors increased the risk for VTE from 1.20% to 2.51% per year (relative risk, 2.1 [CI, 1.1 to 4.2]).

Limitations.—This was a retrospective study without the ability to distinguish interactions between specific thrombophilic deficiencies and defects.

Conclusion.—Additional thrombophilic defects and exogenous risk factors increase the risk for VTE in persons with hereditary deficiencies of protein S, protein C, or antithrombin and provide evidence that multiple genetic and environmental risk factors contribute to VTE.

▶ The basic message is simple—in individuals who already have a thrombophilic defect (protein C, protein S, or antithrombin deficiencies in this study), the risk of VTE increases further with additional thrombophilic defects or environmental risk factors. This, of course, is not the first time such an observation has been made. The magnitude of increased risk for relatives of probands with symptomatic protein C, protein S, or antithrombin deficiency is, however, sufficiently great that one wonders if prophylactic anticoagulation may be indicated in such patients.

G. L. Moneta, MD

Polymorphism in the β$_2$-Adrenergic Receptor and Lipoprotein Lipase Genes as Risk Determinants for Idiopathic Venous Thromboembolism: A Multilocus, Population-Based, Prospective Genetic Analysis
Zee RYL, Cook NR, Cheng S, et al (Harvard Med School; Roche Molecular Systems, Alameda, Calif; Roche Ctr for Med Genomics, Basel, Switzerland)
Circulation 113:2193-2200, 2006

Background.—Candidate genes in inflammation, thrombosis, coagulation, and lipid metabolism pathways have been implicated in venous thromboembolism (VTE).

Method and Results.—Using DNA samples collected at baseline in the Physicians' Health Study cohort, we genotyped 92 polymorphisms from 56 candidate genes among 304 individuals who subsequently developed VTE (144 idiopathic, 156 secondary cases) and among 2070 individuals who remained free of reported vascular disease over a mean follow-up of 13.2 years to prospectively determine whether these gene polymorphisms contribute to the risk of VTE. For idiopathic VTE, in addition to the factor V (Leiden) mutation (odds ratio [OR], 5.13; 95% confidence interval [CI], 3.24 to 8.14; *P*<0.0001; false discovery rate [FDR], *P*<0.0001), an N291S lipoprotein lipase gene polymorphism (OR, 3.09; 95% CI, 1.56 to 6.09; *P*=0.001; FDR, *P*=0.036) and a Q27E β$_2$-adrenergic receptor gene polymorphism (OR, 1.40; 95% CI, 1.09 to 1.79; *P*=0.006; FDR, *P*=0.036) were found to be significantly associated with increased risk. For secondary VTE, a Q360H apo-lipoprotein A4 gene polymorphism (OR, 0.34; 95% CI, 0.18 to 0.65; $P=0.001$; FDR, $P=0.07$) and an I50V interleukin-4 receptor polymorphism (OR, 0.66; 95% CI, 0.52 to 0.84; $P=0.0009$; FDR, $P=0.07$) were moderately, but not statistically and significantly, associated with reduced risk after adjustment for multiple comparisons.

Conclusions.—These present findings are hypothesis generating and require replication and confirmation in an independent investigation.

▶ Blood clots for a reason, and idiopathic VTE occurs for a reason. I suspect, in addition to the major hypercoagulable abnormalities that have been identified, such as factor V Leiden and the prothrombin gene mutation, there are going to be dozens of genetic polymorphisms that alone, or in combination with relatively mild clinical risk factors for VTE, result in increased risk for VTE.

G. L. Moneta, MD

Risk of deep vein thrombosis and pulmonary embolism after acute infection in a community setting
Smeeth L, Cook C, Thomas S, et al (London School of Hygiene and Tropical Medicine, London; Univ of Nottingham, England; Univ College London)
Lancet 367:1075-1079, 2006

Background.—Acute infection increases the risk of arterial cardiovascular events, but effects on venous thromboembolic disease are less well established. Our aim was to investigate whether acute infections transiently increase the risk of venous thromboembolism.

Methods.—We used the self-controlled case-series method to study the risk of first deep vein thrombosis (DVT) (n=7278) and first pulmonary embolism (PE) (n=3755) after acute respiratory and urinary tract infections. Data were obtained from records from general practices who had registered patients with the UK's Health Improvement Network database between 1987 and 2004.

Findings.—The risks of DVT and PE were significantly raised, and were highest in the first two weeks, after urinary tract infection. The incidence ratio for DVT was 2.10 (95% CI 1.56–2.82), and that for PE 2.11 (1.38–3.23). The risk gradually fell over the subsequent months, returning to the baseline value after 1 year. The risk of DVT was also higher after respiratory tract infection, but possible diagnostic misclassification precluded a reliable estimate of the risk of PE after respiratory infection.

Interpretation.—Acute infections are associated with a transient increased risk of venous thromboembolic events in a community setting. Our results confirm that infection should be added to the list of precipitants for venous thromboembolism, and suggest a causal relation.

▶ There are obviously limitations to this study. The data apply only to patients whose infections were severe enough to report to the physician. In addition, only routine clinical data, and not specifically acquired for the purposes of the study, were employed. Also, patients may have had some period of immobility induced by their infection and data were not corrected for this either. Nevertheless, the data are well analyzed and it's a large study. It appears that we should consider adding acute infection to a growing list of risk factors for VTE.

G. L. Moneta, MD

Comparison of Fixed-Dose Weight-Adjusted Unfractionated Heparin and Low-Molecular-Weight Heparin for Acute Treatment of Venous Thromboembolism

Kearon C, for the Fixed-Dose Heparin (FIDO) Investigators (McMaster Univ, Hamilton, Ont, Canada; et al)
JAMA 296:935-942, 2006

Context.—When unfractionated heparin is used to treat acute venous thromboembolism, it is usually administered by intravenous infusion with coagulation monitoring, which requires hospitalization. However, subcutaneous administration of fixed-dose, weight-adjusted, unfractionated heparin may be suitable for inpatient and outpatient treatment of venous thromboembolism.

Objective.—To determine if fixed-dose, weight-adjusted, subcutaneous unfractionated heparin is as effective and safe as low-molecular-weight heparin for treatment of venous thromboembolism.

Design, Setting, and Patients.—Randomized, open-label, adjudicator-blinded, noninferiority trial of 708 patients aged 18 years or older with acute venous thromboembolism from 6 university-affiliated clinical centers in Canada and New Zealand conducted from September 1998 through February 2004. Of the randomized patients, 11 were subsequently excluded from the analysis of efficacy and 8 from the analysis of safety.

Interventions.—Unfractionated heparin was administered subcutaneously as an initial dose of 333 U/kg, followed by a fixed dose of 250 U/kg every 12 hours (n=345). Low-molecular-weight heparin (dalteparin or enoxaparin) was administered subcutaneously at a dose of 100 IU/kg every 12 hours (n=352). Both treatments could be administered out of hospital and both were overlapped with 3 months of warfarin therapy.

Main Outcome Measures.—Recurrent venous thromboembolism within 3 months and major bleeding within 10 days of randomization.

Results.—Recurrent venous thromboembolism occurred in 13 patients in the unfractionated heparin group (3.8%) compared with 12 patients in the low-molecular-weight heparin group (3.4%; absolute difference, 0.4%; 95% confidence interval, −2.6% to 3.3%). Major bleeding during the first 10 days of treatment occurred in 4 patients in the unfractionated heparin group (1.1%) compared with 5 patients in the low-molecular-weight heparin group (1.4%; absolute difference, −0.3%; 95% confidence interval, −2.3% to 1.7%). Treatment was administered entirely out of hospital in

72% of the unfractionated heparin group and 68% of the low-molecular-weight heparin group.

Conclusion.—Fixed-dose subcutaneous unfractionated heparin is as effective and safe as low-molecular-weight heparin in patients with acute venous thromboembolism and is suitable for outpatient treatment.

▶ The data suggest both unfractionated heparin administered subcutaneously on a weight-based dosage regimen and low-molecular-weight heparin can provide equal protection against recurrent venous thromboembolism (VTE) in patients with acute VTE. This study has significant implications for all patients who are unable to afford the cost of low-molecular-weight heparin as an outpatient. Perhaps such patients can be treated at home with weight-based, fixed doses of unfractionated heparin. This would remove a potential barrier to outpatient treatment of acute VTE in patients who cannot afford the cost of low-molecular-weight heparin as an outpatient.

G. L. Moneta, MD

Long-term Low-Molecular-Weight Heparin versus Usual Care in Proximal-Vein Thrombosis Patients with Cancer
Hull RD, for the LITE Trial Investigators (Univ of Calgary, Alta, Canada; et al)
Am J Med 119:1062-1072, 2006

Purpose.—A substantial clinical need exists for an alternative to vitamin K antagonists for treating deep-vein thrombosis in cancer patients who are at high risk of both recurrent venous thromboembolism and bleeding. Low-molecular-weight heparin, body-weight adjusted, avoids anticoagulant monitoring and has been shown to be more effective than vitamin-K-antagonist therapy.

Subjects and Methods.—Subjects were patients with cancer and acute symptomatic proximal-vein thrombosis. We performed a multi-centre randomized, open-label clinical trial using objective outcome measures comparing long-term therapeutic tinzaparin subcutaneously once daily with usual-care long-term vitamin-K-antagonist therapy for 3 months. Outcomes were assessed at 3 and 12 months.

Results.—Of 200 patients, 100 received tinzaparin and 100 received usual care. At 12 months, the usual-care group had an excess of recurrent venous thromboembolism; 16 of 100 (16%) versus 7 of 100 (7%) receiving low-molecular-weight heparin ($P=.044$; risk ratio=.44; absolute difference −9.0; 95% confidence interval [CI], −21.7 to −0.7). Bleeding, largely minor, occurred in 27 patients (27%) receiving tinzaparin and 24 patients (24%) receiving usual care (absolute difference −3.0; 95% CI, −9.1 to 15.1). In patients without additional risk factors for bleeding at the time of randomization, major bleeding occurred in 0 of 51 patients (0%) receiving tinzaparin and 1 of 48 patients (2.1%) receiving usual care. Mortality at 1 year was high, reflecting the severity of the cancers; 47% in each group died.

Conclusion.—Our findings confirm the limited but benchmark data in the literature that long-term low-molecular-weight heparin is more effective than vitamin-K-antagonist therapy for preventing recurrent venous thromboembolism in patients with cancer and proximal venous thrombosis.

▶ This paper also failed to confirm a cancer-related death survival benefit in patients with cancer and proximal venous thrombosis treated with low-molecular-weight heparin.[1] However, the patients in this study had advanced cancer and many had advanced metastatic disease. Previous studies have suggested that survival benefit occurs only in those without metastatic disease.[2] Nevertheless, patients with advanced cancer and proximal venous thrombosis may have improved quality of life through low-molecular-weight heparin. Certainly the lack of need for laboratory monitoring, minimal bleeding risk, and decreased recurrence of venous thromboembolism would logically appear to improve quality of life. However, these patients are deteriorating for multiple reasons that may also impair quality of life, and the authors unfortunately did not include quality of life assessment as part of their protocol.

G. L. Moneta, MD

Reference

1. Kearon C, Ginsberg JS, Julian JA, et al. Comparison of fixed-dose weight-adjusted unfractionated heparin and low-molecular-weight heparin for acute treatment of venous thromboembolism. *JAMA.* 2006;296:935-942.
2. Lee AY, Rickles FR, Julian JA, et al. Randomized comparison of low molecular weight heparin and coumarin derivatives on the survival of patients with cancer and venous thromboembolism. *J Clin Oncol.* 2005;23:2123-2129.

D-Dimer Testing to Determine the Duration of Anticoagulation Therapy
Palareti G, for the PROLONG Investigators (S Orsola-Malpighi Univ, Bologna, Italy; et al)
N Engl J Med 355:1780-1789, 2006

Background.—The optimal duration of oral anticoagulation in patients with idiopathic venous thromboembolism is uncertain. Testing of D-dimer levels may play a role in the assessment of the need for prolonged anticoagulation.

Methods.—We performed D-dimer testing 1 month after the discontinuation of anticoagulation in patients with a first unprovoked proximal deep-vein thrombosis or pulmonary embolism who had received a vitamin K antagonist for at least 3 months. Patients with a normal D-dimer level did not resume anticoagulation, whereas those with an abnormal D-dimer level were randomly assigned either to resume or to discontinue treatment. The study outcome was the composite of recurrent venous thromboembolism and major bleeding during an average follow-up of 1.4 years.

Results.—The D-dimer assay was abnormal in 223 of 608 patients (36.7%). A total of 18 events occurred among the 120 patients who stopped anticoagulation (15.0%), as compared with 3 events among the 103 patients who resumed anticoagulation (2.9%), for an adjusted hazard ratio of 4.26 (95% confidence interval [CI], 1.23 to 14.6; P=0.02). Thromboembolism recurred in 24 of 385 patients with a normal D-dimer level (6.2%). Among patients who stopped anticoagulation, the adjusted hazard ratio for recurrent thromboembolism among those with an abnormal D-dimer level, as compared with those with a normal D-dimer level, was 2.27 (95% CI, 1.15 to 4.46; P=0.02).

Conclusions.—Patients with an abnormal D-dimer level 1 month after the discontinuation of anticoagulation have a significant incidence of recurrent venous thromboembolism, which is reduced by the resumption of anticoagulation. The optimal course of anticoagulation in patients with a normal D-dimer level has not been clearly established.

▶ Evidence is accumulating that D-dimer levels can be used to predict risk of recurrent venous thromboembolism (VTE) following an initial idiopathic VTE.[1,2] The 6.2% VTE recurrence rate in the patients with normal D-dimer levels after three months of anticoagulation, along with previous data, suggests that three months of anticoagulation is inadequate for patients with idiopathic VTE. A more conservative approach would be six months of anticoagulation following idiopathic VTE followed by D-dimer testing. If the D-dimer level is abnormal it may be resumption of anticoagulation is indicated.

G. L. Moneta, MD

References

1. Palareti G, Legnani C, Cosmi B, Guazzaloca G, Pancani C, Coccheri S. Risk of venous thromboembolism recurrence: high negative predictive value of D-dimer performed after oral anticoagulation is stopped. *Thromb Hemostat.* 2002;87:7-12.
2. Palareti G, Legnani C, Cosmi B, et al. Predictive value of D-dimer test for recurrent venous thromboembolism after anticoagulation withdrawal in subjects with a previous idiopathic event and in carriers of congenital thrombophilia. *Circulation.* 2003;108:313-318.

Self-management versus conventional management of oral anticoagulant therapy: A randomized, controlled trial
Christensen TD, Maegaard M, Sørensen HT, et al (Aarhus Univ, Denmark)
Eur J Intern Med 17:260-266, 2006

Background.—The efficacy of self-managed oral anticoagulant therapy has been addressed in few randomized, controlled trials, which have provided inconsistent results. The aim of this study was to compare the quality of self-managed oral anticoagulant therapy with conventional management.

Methods.—This was a pragmatic, open-label, randomized, controlled trial where 100 patients receiving long-term oral anticoagulant therapy referred to a Danish clinic for self-management was randomized to either self-management of oral anticoagulant therapy (including a teaching program of self-management followed by 6 months of self-management) or 6 months of conventional management. The primary endpoint was an intention-to-treat analysis of a composite score combining the variance (median square of the standard deviation) of the International Normalized Ratio (INR) value (using a blinded control sample analyzed monthly by a reference laboratory), death, major complications, or discontinuation from the study. Secondary endpoints — assessed in per-protocol analyses — were the variance of the INR value (using the blinded control sample) and time within therapeutic INR target range using the standard INR values from the coagulometer and laboratory measurement.

Results.—There was no significant difference in the primary endpoint between the self-management and conventional management groups (composite score 0.16 vs. 0.24, respectively, $p=0.09$). Self-management was significantly better (0.16 vs. 0.24, $p=0.003$) with regard to the variance in a per-protocol analysis. The difference in time within therapeutic INR target range was not significantly better (78.7% vs. 68.9%, $p=0.14$) using self-management.

Conclusion.—The quality of self-management of oral anticoagulant therapy is at least as good as that provided by conventional management.

▶ This study and the trial by Fitzmaurice et al[1] evaluate the ability of patients to manage their own anticoagulation. The trials took place in different countries, and had different designs and different primary endpoints. Nevertheless, the conclusions were essentially the same, in that selected patients can self manage their oral anticoagulant therapy and, in comparison to those managed conventionally, have similar INRs and similar levels of significant adverse events. It is important to keep in mind that the patients were highly selected. In the first study, the patients were referred to the clinic for self management. They were, therefore, thought to be capable of doing so. In the second study, only 25% of the patients approached for participation in the trial agreed to participate. In addition, a quarter of the patients who agreed to the trial did not complete training and self-management of anticoagulation and one out of five patients withdrew prematurely. Nevertheless, in those patients able to self manage their anticoagulation, the time within therapeutic IRN target range is remarkably similar in the two different trials (78.7% in the Danish trial and 70% in the British trial).

G. L. Moneta, MD

Reference

1. Fitzmaurice DA, Murray ET, McCahon D, et al. Self management of oral anticoagulation: randomised trial. *BMJ.* 2005;331:1057.

Catheter-direct thrombolysis versus pharmacomechanical thrombectomy for treatment of symptomatic lower extremity deep venous thrombosis

Lin PH, Zhou W, Dardik A, et al (Baylor College of Medicine; Yale Univ, New Haven, Conn)
Am J Surg 192:782-788, 2006

Background.—Rheolytic mechanical thrombectomy using the AngioJet catheter (Possis Medical, Minneapolis, MN) has been shown to be effective in the treatment of deep venous thrombosis (DVT). Additional infusion of thrombolytic agents via the device creates a novel treatment strategy of pharmacomechanical thrombectomy (PMT), which further enhances thrombectomy efficacy. The purpose of the current study was to compare the treatment outcome in patients with symptomatic DVT who underwent either catheter-directed thrombolysis (CDT) or PMT intervention.

Methods.—During a recent 8-year period, clinical records of all patients with symptomatic lower leg DVT undergoing catheter-directed interventions were evaluated. Patients were divided into 2 treatment groups: CDT or PMT. Comparisons were made with regards to the treatment outcome between the 2 groups.

Results.—A total of 93 patients who underwent 98 catheter-directed interventions for DVT were included in the study. Among them, CDT or PMT was performed in 46 (47%) and 52 (53%) procedures, respectively. In the CDT group, complete or partial thrombus removal was accomplished in 32 (70%) and 14 (30%) cases, respectively. In the PMT cohort, complete or partial thrombus removal was accomplished in 39 (75%) and 13 (25%) cases, respectively. Venous balloon angioplasty and/or stenting in the CDT or PMT groups was necessary in 36 (78%) and 43 (82%), respectively (difference not significant [NS]). Patients in the CDT groups underwent a mean of 2.5 venograms during the hospital course, in contrast to 0.4 venograms per patient in PMT cohorts ($P < .001$). Immediate (<24 hours) improvement in clinical symptoms in CDT and PMT groups was achieved in 33 (72%) and 42 (81%) cases, respectively (NS). Significant reductions in the intensive care unit (ICU) and hospital lengths of stay was noted in the PMT group (0.6 and 4.6 days) when compared to the CDT group (2.4 and 8.4 days). During follow-up visits, the primary patency rates at 1 year of CDT and PMT groups were 64% and 68%, respectively (NS). Hospital cost analysis showed significant cost reduction in the PMT group compared to the CDT group ($P < .01$).

Conclusions.—PMT with adjunctive thrombolytic therapy is an effective treatment modality in patients with significant DVT. When compared to CDT, this treatment provides similar treatment success with reduced ICU, total hospital length of stay, and hospital costs.

▶ There is a fair amount of active intervention for DVT in Houston. The data suggest that mechanical thrombolytic therapy is more efficient than catheter-directed thrombolytic therapy alone. Patient selection was odd; it appeared that individuals received pharmacomechanical therapy if they were treated by a vascular surgeon and catheter-directed therapy alone if they were treated by a radiologist. For those who are interested in study design, this is a nightmare! A proper randomized trial is suggested by the data—nothing else.

G. L. Moneta, MD

Outcomes with Retrievable Inferior Vena Cava Filters: A Multicenter Study

Ray CE Jr, Mitchell E, Zipser S, et al (Univ of Colorado, Denver; Santa Clara Valley Med Ctr, San Jose, Calif; Univ of Southern California, Los Angeles; et al)
J Vasc Interv Radiol 17:1595-1604, 2006

Purpose.—To retrospectively review the outcomes after placement and retrieval of retrievable inferior vena cava (IVC) filters at two academic medical centers.

Materials and Methods.—All patients who underwent retrievable filter placement between May 2001 and December 2005 were included. Hospital records at both institutions were reviewed, and relevant data were collected concerning the placement and retrieval of all removable filters.

Results.—A total of 197 patients underwent placement of a retrievable IVC filter. Of those, 143 patients (72.5%) had Günther Tulip filters (GTFs) placed, and 54 patients (27.5%) had Recovery filters placed. A total of 94 patients underwent attempted filter retrieval, accounting for just less than half of all retrievable filters placed during the study period (47.7%). Retrievals were successful in 80 patients (85.1%). Half the retrieval failures ($n = 7$) were the result of thrombus within the filter, and technical difficulties (eg, filter embedded in IVC wall, tilted filter) were the cause of retrieval failure in the other half. There was no significant difference in retrieval failure rates between the GTF and Recovery filter (16.4% vs 9.5%, respectively). GTFs were removed after a median implantation time of 11 days (range, 1-139 d), whereas Recovery filters were removed after a median implantation time of 28 days (range, 6–117 d).

Conclusions.—Placement and retrieval of nonpermanent IVC filters can be performed safely with a high technical success rate. In patients at high risk for venous thromboembolism and contraindication to anticoagulation, retrievable filters may be used aggressively to prevent the potentially devastating outcome of pulmonary embolism.

▶ It is interesting that less than half the patients who undergo placement of a retrievable IVC filter actually even have an attempt at removal of the filter. Retrievable filters should be placed with knowledge that they will very likely be a permanent filter.

G. L. Moneta, MD

Extended interval for retrieval of vena cava filters is safe and may maximize protection against pulmonary embolism

Stefanidis D, Paton BL, Jacobs DG, et al (F H Sammy Ross, Jr Trauma Ctr, Charlotte, NC; Carolinas Med Ctr, Charlotte, NC)
Am J Surg 192:789-794, 2006

Background.—Retrieval of optional vena cava filters (VCF) has been demonstrated to be safe and feasible in injured patients in 4 recent studies. However, 2 pulmonary emboli PE were reported in these studies with mean implant durations less than 19 days. In light of these occurrences, we changed our practice for VCF retrieval when patients had recovered from their injuries and at least 30 days after their discharge, or had been stable on therapeutic anticoagulation for deep venous thrombosis (DVT) or PE for at least 2 weeks. The aim of the current study was to assess the safety of this approach.

Methods.—A review of prospectively collected data on optional VCF over a 16-month period. The filters were inserted prophylactically per an institutional practice guideline or for the presence of DVT or PE with a contraindication and/or complication to anticoagulation. All patients underwent duplex imaging of the lower extremities and had pre- and post- retrieval cavagrams. Demographics, duration of implantation, and complications were recorded.

Results.—Eighty-three patients had optional VCF inserted since the change in our clinical practice. Indications included prophylaxis for high-risk trauma patients (n = 58), DVT or PE with acute contraindication to therapeutic anticoagulation (n = 22), or complications of anticoagulation (n = 3). Two patients developed lower extremity DVT after filter insertion and 1 patient developed a vena cava thrombosis. Retrieval was successful in 47 of 54 cases (87%) attempted. Median implantation duration was 142 days (range 17–475). A filter strut fracture occurred during retrieval without further consequences. No post-insertion or post-retrieval PE occurred in this study.

Conclusion.—Extended intervals for retrieval of VCF are safe and may maximize protection against pulmonary embolism.

▶ The study suggests there will be less permanent "temporary" inferior vena cava (IVC) filters if the period for potential filter removal is extended. It appears reasonable to consider removal of retrievable IVC filters that have been in place longer than what has been previously suggested as safe for removal. However, even with this policy, a high percentage of temporary filters will be permanent.[1] A temporary filter is not a free lunch; it very well may be a permanently implanted device.

G. L. Moneta, MD

Reference

1. Ray CE Jr, Mitchell E, Zipser S, Kao EY, Brown CF, Moneta GL. Outcomes with retrievable inferior vena cava filters: a multicenter study. *J Vasc Interv Radiol.* 2006;17:1595-1604.

Clinical Syndromes and Clinical Outcome in Patients With Pulmonary Embolism: Findings From the RIETE Registry

Lobo JL, Zorrilla V, Aizpuru F, et al (Hosp de Txagorritxu, Vitoria, Spain; Hosp de Cruces, Bilbao, Spain; Hosp de Girona, Spain; et al)
Chest 130:1817-1822, 2006

Introduction.—The influence of the clinical syndromes of pulmonary embolism (PE) on clinical outcome has not been evaluated.

Patients and methods.—The Registro Informatizado de la Enfermedad TromboEmbólica (RIETE) is an ongoing registry of consecutive patients with acute venous thromboembolism. In this study, all enrolled patients with acute PE without preexisting cardiac or pulmonary disease were classified into three clinical syndromes: pulmonary infarction, isolated dyspnea, or circulatory collapse. Their clinical characteristics, laboratory findings, and 3-month outcomes were compared.

Results.—As of January 2005, 4,145 patients with acute, symptomatic, objectively confirmed PE have been enrolled in RIETE. Of them, 3,391 patients (82%) had no chronic lung disease or heart failure: 1,709 patients (50%) had pulmonary infarction, 1,083 patients (32%) had isolated dyspnea, and 599 patients (18%) had circulatory collapse. Overall, 149 patients (4.4%) died during the first 15 days of therapy: 2.5% with pulmonary infarction, 6.2% with isolated dyspnea (odds ratio [OR], 2.6; 95% confidence interval [CI], 1.7 to 3.8), and 6.5% with circulatory collapse (OR, 2.7; 95% CI, 1.7 to 4.2). From days 16 to 90, 31 patients had recurrent PE; 5 of 14 patients (36%) with pulmonary infarction died of their new PE, compared with 5 of 10 patients (50%) with isolated dyspnea, and all 7 patients (100%) with circulatory collapse.

Conclusions.—PE patients with pulmonary infarction (50% of the whole series) had a significantly lower mortality rate both during initial therapy and after discharge.

▶ The data make sense. Patients with pulmonary infarction usually present with pleuritic chest pain or hemoptosis reflecting emboli to the lung periphery. Those with dyspnea and circulatory collapse have more central and larger emboli and, thus, have more extensive vascular occlusion. It is important to note that, no matter the initial presentation, recurrent pulmonary embolism within 90 days of the initial event is frequently fatal.

G. L. Moneta, MD

Massive Pulmonary Embolism

Kucher N, Rossi E, De Rosa M, et al (Univ Hosp Zurich, Switzerland; CINECA, Bologna, Italy; Harvard Med School)
Circulation 113:577-582, 2006

Background.—Acute massive pulmonary embolism (PE) carries an exceptionally high mortality rate. We explored how often adjunctive therapies, particularly thrombolysis and inferior vena caval (IVC) filter placement, were performed and how these therapies affected the clinical outcome of patients with massive PE.

Method and Results.—Among 2392 patients with acute PE and known systolic arterial blood pressure at presentation, from the International Cooperative Pulmonary Embolism Registry (ICOPER), 108 (4.5%) had massive PE, defined as a systolic arterial pressure <90 mm Hg, and 2284 (95.5%) had non-massive PE with a systolic arterial pressure ≥90 mm Hg. PE was first diagnosed at autopsy in 16 patients (15%) with massive PE and in 29 patients (1%) with non-massive PE ($P<0.001$). The 90-day mortality rates were 52.4% (95% CI, 43.3% to 62.1%) and 14.7% (95% CI, 13.3% to 16.2%), respectively. In-hospital bleeding complications occurred in 17.6% versus 9.7% and recurrent PE within 90 days in 12.6% and 7.6%, respectively ($P<0.001$). In patients with massive PE, thrombolysis, surgical embolectomy, or catheter embolectomy were withheld in 73 (68%). Thrombolysis was performed in 33 patients, surgical embolectomy in 3, and catheter embolectomy in 1. Thrombolytic therapy did not reduce 90-day mortality (thrombolysis, 46.3%; 95% CI, 31.0% to 64.8%; no thrombolysis, 55.1%; 95% CI, 44.3% to 66.7%; hazard ratio, 0.79; 95% CI, 0.44 to 1.43). Recurrent PE rates at 90 days were similar in patients with and without thrombolytic therapy (12% for both; $P=0.99$). None of the 11 patients who received an IVC filter developed recurrent PE within 90 days, and 10 (90.9%) survived at least 90 days. IVC filters were associated with a reduction in 90-day mortality (hazard ratio, 0.12; 95% CI, 0.02 to 0.85).

Conclusions.—In ICOPER, two thirds of the patients with massive PE did not receive thrombolysis or embolectomy. Counterintuitively, thrombolysis did not reduce mortality or recurrent PE at 90 days. The observed reduction in mortality from IVC filters requires further investigation.

▶ It is probably wrong to conclude from these data that thrombolytic therapy cannot reduce mortality in patients with massive pulmonary embolism syndrome. ICOPER is a registry. Patients receiving thrombolytic therapy may have been the worst among the worst. The apparent significant reduction in mortality associated with inferior vena cava filters deserves further investigation but may also reflect those patients who are actually well enough to receive a filter. Clearly, there is a need for improved and more standardized treatment of massive pulmonary embolism syndrome.

G. L. Moneta, MD

Effect of patient's sex on risk of recurrent venous thromboembolism: a meta-analysis

McRae S, Tran H, Schulman S, et al (Queen Elizabeth Hosp, Woodville, Australia; McMaster Univ, Hamilton, Ont, Canada; Hamilton Health Sciences, Ont, Canada)
Lancet 368:371-378, 2006

Background.—Individual risk of recurrent venous thromboembolism affects patient management and might differ between men and women. We did a meta-analysis to assess from available evidence whether men and women have the same risk of recurrent venous thromboembolism after stopping anticoagulant treatment.

Methods.—Eligible articles were identified by searches of MEDLINE (source PubMed, 1966 to February 2005), EMBase (1980 to February 2005), and the Cochrane database 2005, issue 1. Prospective cohort studies and randomised trials were eligible if they included patients with objectively diagnosed venous thromboembolism treated for a minimum of 1 month and followed up for recurrence after anticoagulant treatment was stopped. Data were extracted for study design, study quality, and the number, sex, and age of enrolled patients, risk factors for venous thromboembolism, treatment given, duration of follow-up, and the number of episodes of recurrent venous thrombosis.

Findings.—15 studies (nine randomised controlled trials and six prospective observational studies) enrolling a total of 5416 individuals (2729 men), of whom 816 (523 men) had recurrent venous thromboembolism after stopping treatment, were eligible for inclusion. The pooled estimate of the relative risk (RR) of recurrent venous thromboembolism for men compared with for women was 1.6 (95% CI 1.2–2.0). Significant heterogeneity was shown among individual study findings; however, the higher risk of recurrent venous thromboembolism in men than in women was consistent across predefined subgroups. The relative risk for recurrence in men from randomised trials (RR 1.3; 95% CI 1.0–1.8) was lower than that from observational studies (2.1; 1.5–2.9). The lower risk of recurrent venous thromboembolism in women did not seem to be accounted for by a reduced rate of recurrence after venous thromboembolism associated with oestrogen treatment or pregnancy.

Interpretation.—Men seem to have a 50% higher risk than women of recurrent venous thromboembolism after stopping anticoagulant treatment. If confirmed by further prospective studies, this difference in risk of recurrence should be considered when duration of anticoagulant treatment is determined in individual patients.

▶ This meta-analysis used strict inclusion criteria for studies and analyzed large numbers of patients with predefined subgroups. This lends strength to the authors' conclusions. There was, however, heterogeneity among studies and differences among relative risks from randomized trials versus observational studies. The trials did not have individual patient data and, therefore, a true multivariant analysis could not be done to assess individual variables on study outcome. Nevertheless, the data argue strongly for inclusion of sex as another variable in determining the length of anticoagulant therapy following venous thromboembolism.

G. L. Moneta, MD

Identification of Patients at Low Risk for Recurrent Venous Thromboembolism by Measuring Thrombin Generation
Hron G, Kollars M, Binder BR, et al (Med Univ of Vienna)
JAMA 296:397-402, 2006

Context.—Screening of patients with venous thromboembolism (VTE) for thrombophilic risk factors is common clinical practice. Because of the large number of risk factors, assessing the risk of recurrence in an individual patient is complex. A method covering multicausal thrombophilia is therefore required.

Objective.—To investigate the relationship between recurrence of VTE and a simple global coagulation assay measuring thrombin generation.

Design, Setting, and Participants.—Prospective cohort study of 914 patients with first spontaneous VTE who were followed up for an average of 47 months after discontinuation of vitamin K antagonist therapy. The study was conducted at the Department of Internal Medicine I, Medical University of Vienna, Vienna, Austria, between July 1992 and July 2005. Thrombin generation was measured by a commercially available assay system. Patients with a previous or secondary VTE; antithrombin, protein C, or protein S deficiencies; presence of lupus anticoagulant; cancer; or pregnancy were excluded.

Main Outcome Measure.—Objectively documented symptomatic recurrent VTE.

Results.—Venous thromboembolism recurred in 100 patients (11%). Patients without recurrent VTE had lower thrombin generation than patients with recurrence (mean [SD], 349.2 [108.0] nM vs 419.5 [110.5] nM, respectively; $P<.001$). Compared with patients who had thrombin generation greater than 400 nM, the relative risk (RR) of recurrence was 0.42 (95% confidence interval [CI], 0.26-0.67; $P<.001$) in patients with values between 400 nM and 300 nM; for patients with lower values, the RR was 0.37 (95% CI, 0.21-0.66; $P=.001$). After 4 years, the probability of recurrence was 6.5% (95% CI, 4.0%-8.9%) among patients with thrombin generation less than 400 nM compared with 20.0% (95% CI, 14.9%-25.1%) among patients with higher values ($P<.001$). Patients with thrombin generation less than 400 nM, representing two thirds of patients, had a 60% lower RR of recurrence than those with greater values (RR, 0.40; 95% CI, 0.27-0.60; $P<.001$).

Conclusion.—Measurement of thrombin generation identifies patients at low risk for recurrent VTE.

▶ There are data to suggest that patients with idiopathic VTE benefit from longer periods of anticoagulation than those with VTE and a recognizable risk factor such as surgery or trauma. Given the implications of long-term anticoagulant therapy, it is desirable to identify which patients with idiopathic VTE are particularly prone to recurrence. If this study can be confirmed by others, measurement of thrombin generation may prove to be a relatively simple method of stratifying patients with respect to their length of anticoagulation following a first-time episode of idiopathic VTE.

G. L. Moneta, MD

Adenoviral urokinase-type plasminogen activator (uPA) gene transfer enhances venous thrombus resolution
Gossage JA, Humphries J, Modarai B, et al (St Thomas' Hosp, London)
J Vasc Surg 44:1085-1090, 2006

Introduction.—There is an increase in the natural level of urokinase-type plasminogen activator (uPA) activity within the thrombus during venous thrombus resolution. The use of uPA as a thrombolytic agent in the treatment of acute iliofemoral deep vein thrombosis is not suitable for all patients. This study aimed to determine whether thrombus resolution could be enhanced by upregulating uPA expression using adenoviral gene transfer as an alternative method of delivery.

Methods.—The production of functional uPA by an adenoviral gene construct (ad.uPA) was confirmed by a colorimetric substrate assay and fibrin plate lysis. Thrombus was formed in the inferior vena cava of wild-type mice and injected, 48-hours after induction, with either a control virus at 10^8 plaque-forming units (pfu) or ad.uPA at 10^7 or 10^8 pfu. Thrombi were removed and weighed 7 days after treatment. Activity of metalloproteinase (MMP) 2 and 9 was measured by zymography and the release of vascular endothelial growth factor (VEGF) and D-dimer levels by enzyme-linked immunoabsorbent assay. The results were expressed as a mean ± SEM. Values were standardized for wet weight or for soluble protein content (mg/sol protein).

Results.—Treatment with ad.uPA reduced thrombus weight by twofold compared with thrombi treated by control virus (15.1 ± 1.1 mg vs 7.4 ± 1.3 mg, $P = .004$). Urokinase activity (17 ± 3 pg/mg wet weight) was detected in all treated thrombi, but there was no dose-dependent effect. D-dimer activity was increased twofold after treatment with ad.uPA (1.7 ± 0.15 ng/mg of sol protein vs 0.8 ± 0.1 ng/mg of sol protein, $P = .0015$) and was associated with a reduction in thrombus size ($P = .03$). Urokinase overexpression did not affect the activity of MMP2, MMP9, or VEGF in the thrombus.

Conclusion.—Increasing urokinase activity within the thrombus significantly enhanced natural thrombus resolution by a fibrinolytic action. Therapeutic delivery of ad.uPA in patients may provide a novel method of treating deep vein thrombosis.

Clinical Relevance.—The use of urokinase as a thrombolytic agent in the treatment of acute iliofemoral deep vein thrombosis is not suitable for all patients. This study aimed to determine whether thrombus resolution could be enhanced by upregulating urokinase expression using adenoviral gene transfer as an alternative method of therapeutic delivery. The study shows that by increasing urokinase activity within the thrombus, natural thrombus resolution can be significantly enhanced. The delivery of ad.uPA in patients may provide a novel method of treating deep vein thrombosis.

▶ This is a very interesting potential approach to treatment of venous thrombosis; inject the clot with a gene product and dramatically improve the "natural" fibrinolytic process. The adenoviral vector is a potential downside; institutional review boards hate adenoviruses as gene transfer agents! A different mechanism delivering the gene product would be nice. It also needs to be explained why reductions in thrombus weight were not dose dependent. This also suggests there may be a better method of delivering the gene product to the thrombus.

G. L. Moneta, MD

17 Chronic Venous & Lymphatic Disease

Haemodynamic and Clinical Impact of Superficial, Deep and Perforator Vein Incompetence
Ibegbuna V, Delis KT, Nicolaides AN (Imperial College, Paddington, London; Mayo Clinic, Rochester, Minn)
Eur J Vasc Endovasc Surg 31:535-541, 2006

Objective.—The purpose of this study was to assess the effect of venous incompetence of the deep, superficial and perforator veins combined (i.e. multi-system incompetence) on the venous haemodynamics and clinical condition of limbs with chronic venous disease (CVD).

Methods.—One hundred and thirty two limbs (16-C_1; 30-C_2; 20-C_3; 25-C_4; 21-C_5; 20-C_6) of 121 patients were studied. We excluded those with previous venous surgery/sclerotherapy, peripheral arterial disease, recent deep vein thrombosis ($\leq$6 months), or inability to comply with the tests. The CEAP clinical class was assessed. Duplex ultrasonography (ultrasound) enabled classification according to: the presence of superficial$_{[S]}$ ($\pm$ perforator$_{[P]}$) or deep$_{[D]}$ ($\pm$S, $\pm$P) reflux (>.5 s); the number of incompetent venous systems (single-system$_{[S/P/D]}$, dual-system$_{[S+P/S+D/P+D]}$, or triple-system$_{[S+P+D]}$), and the number of incompetent perforators$_{[0/1/2/\geq3]}$. The amount of reflux (Venous Filling Index$_{[VFI]}$); calf pump Ejection Fraction$_{[EF]}$, and Residual Volume Fraction$_{[RVF]}$ were studied with air-plethysmography.

Results.—VFI in limbs with triple-system incompetence (VFI median 6.68 [IQR: 4.7–9.7] ml/s) was higher than in limbs with dual-system incompetence (4.5 [2.1–7.4] ml/s), and VFI in the latter was higher than in limbs with single-system incompetence (1.3 [0.69–2.3] ml/s)($p<0.01$ Kruskal–Wallis). Although EF changes were small, RVF in limbs with triple-incompetence (39 [30–51] %) was higher than in single-system incompetence (26 [16–33] %) ($p<0.01$ Mann–Whitney). Limbs with superficial ($\pm P$) incompetence had a lower VFI ($p<0.01$) and RVF ($p<0.02$) than limbs with deep ($\pm$S$\pm$P) incompetence, and limbs with $\geq$2 incompetent perforator veins had a higher VFI ($p<0.04$) than those without perforators. All limbs with single-system incompetence were C_{1-3}, whereas 78% of those with triple-incompetence were C_{4-6} ($p<0.01$). The number of incompetent systems increased with clinical class ($p<0.01$).

347

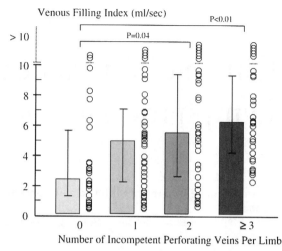

Venous Filling Index (ml/sec)

Number of Incompetent Perforating Veins Per Limb

FIGURE 3.—Venous filling index$_{\text{[VFI]}}$, presented as median and interquartile range (left) and scattergram (right), in 30 of 132 study limbs (22%) without perforator incompetence, in 40 of 132 limbs (30.3%) with one incompetent perforator, in 33 of 132 limbs (25%) with two incompetent perforators, and in 29 of 132 limbs (22%) with three or more incompetent perforators, evaluated with air-plethysmography (Mann–Whitney test adjusted with Bonferroni correction. VFI increased overall with the number of incompetent perforators ($p<0.01$, Kruskall–Wallis). (Courtesy of Ibegbuna V, Delis KT, Nicolaides AN. Haemodynamic and clinical impact of superficial, deep and perforator vein incompetence. *Eur J Vasc Endovasc Surg.* 2006;31:535-541. Reprinted by permission of the publisher.)

Conclusions.—The frequency of incompetence of more than one venous system increased with the clinical severity of venous disease and was accompanied by a 5-fold increase in the amount of reflux and a 50% rise in the RVF. The number of incompetent perforators per limb increased with the amount of reflux. The number of incompetent venous systems (superficial, deep, perforator) and perforator veins can be assessed by duplex ultrasound giving an objective indication of the functional severity of venous disease. In this way duplex ultrasound could be used to grade venous function in clinical practice as an alternative to APG measures which are less widely available (Fig 3).

▶ This carefully performed study adds to the growing literature supporting the unique strengths of the clinical, etiologic, anatomic distribution, and pathophysiologic (CEAP) classification system. CEAP was designed to identify increasing severity of chronic venous disease based on history, examination, and duplex ultrasonography. This study shows that deterioration in venous hemodynamics as measured by air-plethysmography correlates with the number of venous systems affected by valvular incompetence as identified by duplex ultrasonography. Venous filling index was increased as the number of refluxing systems increased. The incidence of venous ulcers and the CEAP score also correlated with the number of refluxing systems. Finally, residual volume fraction was higher in multisystem reflux compared with single-system reflux. Multisystem reflux, deep-system reflux, and perforator incompetence identified on ultrasonography are reliable indicators of particularly severe hemodynamic dysfunction in CVD and correlate with correspondingly high CEAP scores. Duplex ultrasonography therefore provides a good indication of hemo-dynamic dysfunction in chronic venous disease.

G. L. Moneta, MD

Development of reflux in the perforator veins in limbs with primary venous disease
Labropoulos N, Tassiopoulos AK, Bhatti AF, et al (Loyola Univ, Newark, NJ)
J Vasc Surg 43:558-562, 2006

Objective.—To determine the patterns by which perforator vein (PV) reflux develops in patients with primary chronic venous disease (CVD).

Methods.—Patients with CVD who had at least two examinations with duplex ultrasonography before any treatment were included in this study. These were patients who were offered an operation at their first visit, but for various reasons treatment was postponed. All affected limbs were classified by the CEAP classification system. A detailed map of normal and refluxing sites was drawn on an anatomic chart by using several landmarks of the skin, muscle, and bone. Reflux was induced by distal limb compression followed by sudden release by using rapid-inflation pneumatic cuffs and dorsiplantar flexion. All new reflux sites were documented. The PV reflux was divided into ascending type, descending type (re-entry flow), and those that developed in new locations, which did not have reflux in any system at that level.

Results.—The total number of patients studied was 127 (158 limbs). There were 29 limbs (18%) in 26 patients with reflux development in the PV. In total, 38 new incompetent PVs were identified. The median time for the examination was 25 months (range, 9-52 months). Reflux in a previously normal PV at a re-entry site was detected in 15, in an ascending manner from an extension of superficial vein reflux in 18, and in a new, previously intact location in 5. At the new sites, reflux in the superficial veins connected to the incompetent PVs was always present. PVs connected to the great saphenous vein system were most common (n = 27), followed by those connected to short saphenous (n = 8) and nonsaphenous (n = 3) veins. Worsening in the clinical class was observed in 11 limbs: 5 from class 2 to 3, 2 from class 2 to 4, 2 from class 3 to 4, and 2 from class 4 to 6. The worsening could not be attributed to the PV reflux alone, because other veins became incompetent as well.

Conclusions.—Reflux in PVs develops in ascending fashion through the superficial veins, at re-entry points, and at new sites. Worsening of CVD is observed with new PV reflux, but many other factors play a major role, and therefore a causative association is difficult to prove.

▶ I like this article because it supports (although falls short of proving) what most of us believe intuitively. If you wait long enough (in this case, a median of 25 months), the number of refluxing segments including perforator veins (PVs) will increase, and the severity of chronic venous disease will worsen. Although it does not prove that PV incompetence develops as a result of worsening superficial reflux, it provides compelling evidence to support this view in a rare longitudinal study. In the 29 patients that developed new PV incompetence, all had related superficial reflux. Even the 5 limbs that had deep reflux in conjunction with newly developed PV incompetence also had accompanying superficial reflux. CEAP (clinical, etiologic, anatomic distribution, and pathophysiologic) score worsened in 11 of these 29 patients. In this study, new PV incompetence developed only in the presence of superficial reflux, a compelling reason to manage superficial reflux early, and to repeat scanning in cases of delays between diagnosis and treatment to look for new sites of reflux.

G. L. Moneta, MD

Use of microcirculatory parameters to evaluate chronic venous insufficiency
Virgini-Magalhães CE, Porto CL, Fernandes FFA, et al (State Univ of Rio de Janeiro, Brazil)
J Vasc Surg 43:1037-1044, 2006

Background.—Microcirculatory impairment caused by chronic venous hypertension is usually not taken into account in chronic venous insufficiency, probably due to lack of practical means to observe it. The objective of this work was to use a new noninvasive technique to access quantitatively the cutaneous microangiopathy in female patients classified according to CEAP from C1 to C5 and matched with healthy controls.

Methods.—Forty-four patients and 13 healthy subjects (112 lower limbs), with a mean age ± SD of 48 ± 8 years, were evaluated by using orthogonal polarization spectral (OPS) imaging. Films of the internal perimaleolar region were analyzed by the CapImage software. The microcirculatory parameters evaluated were functional capillary density (number of capillaries with flowing red blood cells/mm^2), capillary morphology (percentage of abnormal capillaries), diameter (µm) of dermal papilla to quantify edema, diameter of capillary bulk (µm) to assess the degree of change, and diameter capillary limb to detect enlargement. A microcirculatory index combining these five parameters was proposed with I, II, and III stages, indicating normal microcirculation, and moderate and severe microangiopathy, respectively.

Results.—These microcirculatory parameters were significantly different ($P < .05$) from control values (C): capillary diameter and capillary morphology from C2 to C5, 8.1 ± 0.8, 3.6 ± 5.5 (C), and 9.7 ± 1.3, 27.5 ± 17.7 (C2); diameter of dermal papilla and diameter of capillary bulk from C3 to C5, 111.4 ± 13.5, 52.8 ± 8.8 (C), and 150.5 ± 31.7, 87.8 ± 26.9 (C3); and functional capillary density only from C4 to C5, 20.9 ± 6.1 (C) and 14.5 ± 4.5 (C4). The microcirculatory index showed good correlation to CEAP classification.

Conclusion.—It was possible to quantify the microangiopathy using OPS imaging and to compare the microcirculatory changes of chronic venous insufficiency patients with healthy controls. Two parameters seemed more important to identify the differences between patients and controls: capillary morphology and capillary diameter. The suggested microcirculatory index can possibly demonstrate, in future studies, a prognostic capability when combined with the CEAP classification.

▶ Chronic venous disease is ultimately a disease of the skin. The anatomic and functional changes in the dermal and subdermal microcirculation are underappreciated factors leading to chronicity of venous ulcers and their propensity to recur. Surgical treatment of the large veins is unlikely to be of benefit if the microcirculation of the skin has been destroyed. Perhaps evaluation of the microcirculation may eventually have prognostic significance in selecting patients for ablative and reconstructive procedures for the treatment of chronic venous insufficiency.

G. L. Moneta, MD

Severe Chronic Venous Insufficiency Treated by Foamed Sclerosant
Pascarella L, Bergan JJ, Mekenas LV (Vein Inst of La Jolla, Calif; Univ of California San Diego, La Jolla)
Ann Vasc Surg 20:83-91, 2006

Our objective was to chronicle our experience in using sclerosant foam to treat severe chronic venous insufficiency (CVI). Forty-four patients with 60 limbs severely affected by severe CVI were entered into the study. They had lipodermatosclerosis, CEAP 4 (seven limbs); atrophie blanche or scars of healed venous ulcerations, CEAP 5 (18 limbs); and frank, open venous ulcers, CEAP 6 (35 limbs). Patients and limbs were collected into three groups. In group I, all limbs were treated with compression without intervention. Group II consisted of crossover patients who failed compression treatment. Group III consisted of patients treated promptly with sclerosant foam therapy without a waiting period of compression. A standing Doppler duplex reflux examination was done in all cases. Compression was by Unna boot or long stretch elastic bandaging. Foam was generated from Polidocanol 1%, 2%, or 3% by the two-syringe technique and administered under ultrasound guidance. Posttreatment compression was used for 14 days. In addition to clinical and ultrasound evaluation at 2, 7, 14, and 30 days, venous severity scoring was noted at entry and discharge. In group I, 12 patients were discharged from care within 6 weeks of initiating compression. All eight of the class 6 limbs had healed. Group II consisted of four CEAP class 5 limbs and eight class 6 limbs that had failed to heal with compression. Five of eight venous ulcers healed within 2 weeks, two more healed by 4 weeks, and one required 6 weeks to heal. In group III, 7 of 11 venous ulcers healed within 2 weeks and four more within 4 weeks. Venous severity scores reflected the success of treatment, with the greatest change occurring in group III and the least in group I. Limbs treated with foam had a statistically better outcome than those without ($p = 0.041$). One patient failed foam sclerotherapy, another had pulmonary emboli 4 months after foam treatment, and a single medial gastrocnemius thrombus was discovered 24 hr after treatment. Treatment of severe CVI with compression and foam sclerotherapy causes more rapid resolution of the venous insufficiency complications and does so without an increase in morbidity.

▶ This study focuses on the potential role of foam sclerosing therapy in healing venous ulcers. Patients were informally arranged into a conservatively managed group (compression therapy), a crossover group that failed conservative management and later underwent sclerosant treatment (foamed polidocanol), and a primary sclerosant therapy group. The venous clinical severity score (VCSS) improved most in the sclerosant group but only modestly in the conservatively managed group, with intermediate scores for the crossover group. Similar results were seen for the venous segmental disease score (VSDS) and the venous disability score (VDS). However, there was no difference in the VCSS at 6 weeks of follow-up. No neurologic complications were observed. Clinical studies such as these serve to highlight the potential role that sclerosing therapy may have in the management of patients with venous disease. How does this compare with surgical or endovenous ablation? Are the results different for early versus advanced Clinical, Etiologic, Anatomic, and Pathophysiologic (CEAP) classes? What is the optimum dose? As the use of this relatively easily delivered therapy continues to expand, we need more detailed studies, with larger numbers, more defined cohorts of patients, and standardized regimens before firm decisions to change practice patterns can be made.

G. L. Moneta, MD

Ultrasound-guided foam sclerotherapy for the treatment of varicose veins
Darke SG, Baker SJA (Royal Bournemouth Hosp, England)
Br J Surg 93:969-974, 2006

Background.—The aim was to assess the early efficacy and complications of ultrasound-guided foam sclerotherapy (UGFS) in a cohort of patients with varicose veins.

Methods.—Of 192 consecutive patients referred with varicose veins over 15 months, only 11 chose surgery; the rest underwent UGFS treatment. Polidocanol was foamed 1 : 3 with air. Under ultrasound control via butterfly or Seldinger cannulation, 1 per cent foam was injected into superficial veins and 3 per cent foam into saphenous trunks, up to a total volume of 14 ml. Outcome was defined as complete when occlusion of the saphenous trunk and/or over 85 per cent of the varicosities was achieved, and partial closure when less.

Results.—In 163 legs, complete occlusion occurred after one intervention, a further 32 after a second, and one after a third (overall 91 per cent). Of the remainder, all other legs achieved partial occlusion after up to three interventions, apart from two legs with great saphenous vein (GSV) incompetence, which failed. All 23 legs with small saphenous veins had complete occlusion after one intervention compared with 64 of 97 legs with GSV incompetence ($P < 0.010$). Occlusion rates were also higher when the GSV was cannulated directly: 56 of 70 *versus* 8 of 27 ($P < 0.001$).

Conclusions.—UGFS achieved early complete occlusion safely in over 90 per cent of legs with varicose veins.

▶ Foam sclerotherapy can be safely delivered directly or indirectly (via communicating collaterals) to the great or short saphenous systems. Local and systemic complications were infrequent during the 6-week follow-up offered by the study. Given the mixed bag of etiologies and anatomy, conclusions regarding efficacy are probably premature. However, within these limitations and short follow-up, the study offers proof of concept, and allays concerns of high periprocedural complication rates. It still remains to be seen whether the anatomic results hold out over a longer period, and how clinical results stand up to a more rigorous and objective scrutiny and comparison with open and endovenous ablation.

G. L. Moneta, MD

The effect of ultrasound-guided sclerotherapy of incompetent perforator veins on venous clinical severity and disability scores

Masuda EM, Kessler DM, Lurie F, et al (Straub Clinic & Hosp, Honolulu, Hawaii; Mayo Clinic, Rochester, Minn)
J Vasc Surg 43:551-557, 2006

Purpose.—Current techniques to treat venous ulcerations and patients with severe lipodermatosclerosis include the elimination of incompetent perforator veins by open surgical ligation and division or by subfascial endoscopic perforator surgery. An alternative and less invasive means to obliterate perforator veins is ultrasound-guided sclerotherapy (UGS). We hypothesize that UGS is a clinically effective means of eliminating perforator veins and results in improvement of the clinical state (scores) without the complications associated with other more invasive methods.

Methods.—Between January 2000 and March 2004, UGS was used to treat chronic venous insufficiency in 80 limbs of 68 patients. This was a clinical series of patients who had perforator incompetence and no previous surgery for venous disease ≤2 years of their UGS procedure. Most had perforator disease without coexisting axial reflux of the saphenous or deep venous systems. Color flow duplex scanning was used to identify incompetent perforator veins in the calf, and duplex guidance was used to inject each perforator with the liquid sclerosant sodium morrhuate (5%). Patients were restudied by duplex scanning up to 5 years after treatment. Clinical results were determined by Venous Clinical Severity Score (VCSS) and Venous Disability Score (VDS) before and after treatment.

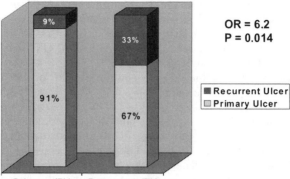

FIGURE 3.—Ulcer recurrence is associated with perforator recurrence. *IPV,* Incompetent perforator vein; *OR,* odds ratio. (Courtesy of Masuda EM, Kessler DM, Lurie F, et al. The effect of ultrasound-guided sclerotherapy of incompetent perforator veins on venous clinical severity and disability scores. *J Vasc Surg.* 2006;43:551-557. Copyright 2006 by Elsevier. Reprinted by permission.)

Results.—Of the 80 limbs treated with UGS, 98% of incompetent perforators were successfully obliterated at the time of treatment, and 75% of limbs showed persistent occlusion of perforators and remained clinically improved with a mean follow-up of 20.1 months. According to the CEAP classification, there were 46.2% with limb ulceration or C6, 1.2% C5, 28.7% C4, 17.5% C3, and 6.2% C2 with pain isolated to the site of the perforator(s). Of those who returned for follow-up, the VCSSs changed from a median of 8 before treatment (95% confidence interval [CI], 3 to 15) to a median of 2 after treatment (95% CI, 0 to 7) (P < .01). Likewise, VDSs dropped from a median of 4 before treatment (95% CI, 1 to 3) to 1 after treatment (95% CI, 0 to 2) (P < .01). There were no cases of deep vein thrombosis involving the deep vein adjacent to the perforator injected. One patient had skin complications with skin necrosis. Perforator recurrence was found more frequently in those with ulcerations than those without (Fig 3).

Conclusion.—UGS is an effective and durable method of eliminating incompetent perforator veins and results in significant reduction of symptoms and signs as determined by venous clinical scores. As an alternative to open interruption or subfascial endoscopic perforator surgery, UGS may lead to fewer skin and wound healing complications. Perforator recurrence occurs particularly in those with ulcerations, and therefore, surveillance duplex scanning after UGS and repeat injections may be needed.

▶ This report follows the rules of a well-designed study. The cohort is focused (patients with perforator incompetence), the technique standardized, and the follow-up evaluations consistent. Despite the falloff in follow-up, the authors make several pertinent points. Sclerosing agents can be safely and accurately delivered to perforators, and the complications (especially systemic) are low. Furthermore, obliteration of the perforators is associated with objective clinical improvement in CEAP (Clinical, Etiologic, Anatomic, and Pathophysiologic)

4 and 6 patients. Studies such as this beg the question, who will bell the cat and finally conduct a randomized controlled trial?

G. L. Moneta, MD

Endovenous Treatment of the Great Saphenous Vein Using a 1,320 nm Nd:YAG Laser Causes Fewer Side Effects than Using a 940 nm Diode Laser
Proebstle TM, Moehler T, Gül D, et al (Univ of Heidelberg, Germany; Univ of Mainz, Germany)
Dermatol Surg 31:1678-1684, 2005

Background.—Limited data are available about treatment-related side effects with respect to laser wavelength in endovenous laser treatment (ELT) of the great saphenous vein (GSV).

Objective.—To compare the results and side effects of a 940 nm diode and a 1,320 nm neodymium:yttium-aluminum-garnet (Nd:YAG) laser.

Methods.—Three patient cohorts (A, B, and C) received ELT of the GSV using a 940 nm diode laser at 15 W (group A) or 30 W (group B) or using a 1,320 nm laser at 8 W (group C). In all cases, energy was administered continuously with constant pullback of the laser fiber under perivenous tumescent local anesthesia.

Results.—The GSVs of group A ($n = 113$), group B ($n = 136$), and group C ($n = 33$) received ELT. An average linear endovenous energy density of 24, 63, and 62 J/cm and an average endovenous fluence equivalent of 12, 30, and 33 J/cm^2 were administered to the vein. Occlusion rates were 95% (group A), 100% (group B), and 100% (group C) at day 1 after ELT and 90.3% (group A), 100% (group B), and 97% (group C) at 3 months after ELT. With the 1,320 nm laser ELT (group C), treatment-related pain (50%) and the need for analgesics (36%) were significantly reduced ($p < .005$) in comparison with treatment-related pain (81%) and the need for analgesics (67%) after the 30 W 940 nm laser ELT (group B). Ecchymosis was also significantly reduced ($p < .05$) in group C (1,320 nm) compared with group B (30 W, 940 nm).

Conclusion.—ELT of the GSV using a 1,320 nm Nd:YAG laser causes fewer side effects compared with 940 nm diode laser ELT.

▶ Use of 810-nm ELT devices can result in temperatures up to 1200°C in animal models.[1] The goal of ELT of the GSV is to close the GSV with a minimal amount of energy so as to minimize the damage to the perivenous tissue. It may be that less than the 8 W of energy utilized in this study is also effective in achieving GSV ablation with a further reduction in postoperative pain. I strongly encourage you to read the comment accompanying the original article by Dr Robert Weiss.

G. L. Moneta, MD

Reference

1. Weiss RA. Comparison of endovenous radiofrequency versus 810 nm diode laser occlusion of large veins in an animal model. *Dermatol Surg.* 2002;28:56-61.

Reduced recanalization rates of the great saphenous vein after endovenous laser treatment with increased energy dosing: Definition of a threshold for the endovenous fluence equivalent
Proebstle TM, Moehler T, Herdemann S (Univ of Heidelberg, Germany; Univ of Mainz, Germany)
J Vasc Surg 44:834-839, 2006

Background.—Recent reports indicated a correlation between the amount of energy released during endovenous laser treatment (ELT) of the great saphenous vein (GSV) and the success and durability of the procedure. Our objective was to analyze the influence of increased energy dosing on immediate occlusion and recanalization rates after ELT of the GSV.

Methods.—GSVs were treated with either 15 or 30 W of laser power by using a 940-nm diode laser with continuous fiber pullback and tumescent local anesthesia. Patients were followed up prospectively with duplex ultrasonography at day 1 and at 1, 3, 6, and 12 months.

Results.—A total of 114 GSVs were treated with 15 W, and 149 GSVs were treated with 30 W. The average endovenous fluence equivalents were 12.8 ± 5.1 J/cm^2 and 35.1 ± 15.6 J/cm^2, respectively. GSV occlusion rates according to the method of Kaplan and Meier for the 15- and 30-W groups were 95.6% and 100%, respectively, at day 1, 90.4% and 100% at 3 months, and 82.7% and 97.0% at 12 months after ELT (log-rank; $P = .001$). An endovenous fluence equivalent exceeding 20 J/cm^2 was associated with durable GSV occlusion after 12 months' follow-up, thus suggesting a schedule for dosing of laser energy with respect to the vein diameter.

Conclusions.—Higher dosing of laser energy shows a 100% immediate success rate and a significantly reduced recanalization rate during 12 months' follow-up.

▶ Dosage of laser energy is a function of the amount of laser energy released and the surface area of the vein to be treated. Proper dosage results in 100% of the desired effect—that is, closure of the vein with minimal side effects such as skin burns or perforation of the vein. In this study, an energy dosage of 6.3 J/cm of each millimeter of vein diameter resulted in 100% closure of the vein. Dosage of laser energy should be a function of vein diameter; "one size fits all" does not apply to ELT. The minimal maximal dosage should be used for ELT, and this article gives reasonable suggestions for dosing laser energy.

G. L. Moneta, MD

Endovenous Saphenous Ablation Corrects the Hemodynamic Abnormality in Patients with CEAP Clinical Class 3–6 CVI Due to Superficial Reflux

Marston WA, Owens LV, Davies S, et al (Univ of North Carolina, Chapel Hill; Martha Jefferson Hosp, Charlottesville, Va)
Vasc Endovasc Surg 40:125-130, 2006

This investigation was designed to determine whether minimally invasive radiofrequency or laser ablation of the saphenous vein corrects the hemodynamic impact and clinical symptoms of chronic venous insufficiency (CVI) in CEAP clinical class 3–6 patients with superficial venous reflux. Patients with CEAP clinical class 3–6 CVI were evaluated with duplex ultrasound and air plethysmography (APG) to determine anatomic and hemodynamic venous abnormalities. Patients with an abnormal (>2 mL/second) venous filling index (VFI) and superficial venous reflux were included in this study. Saphenous ablation was performed utilizing radiofrequency (RF) or endovenous laser treatment (EVLT). Patients were reexamined within 3 months of ablation with duplex to determine anatomic success of the procedure, and with repeat APG to determine the degree of hemodynamic improvement. Venous clinical severity scores (VCSS) were determined before and after saphenous ablation. Eighty-nine limbs in 80 patients were treated with radiofrequency ablation (RFA) (n = 58), or EVLT (n = 31). The average age of patients was 55 years and 66% were women. There were no significant differences in preoperative characteristics between the groups treated with RFA or EVLT. Postoperatively, 86% of limbs demonstrated near total closure of the saphenous vein to within 5 cm of the saphenofemoral junction. Eight percent remained open for 5–10 cm from the junction, and 6% demonstrated minimal or no saphenous ablation. The VFI improved significantly after ablation in both the RF and EVLT groups. Postablation, 78% of the 89 limbs were normal, with a VFI <2 mL/second, and 17% were moderately abnormal, between 2 and 4 mL/second. VCSS scores (11.5 ±4.5 preablation) decreased significantly after ablation to 4.4 ±2.3. Minimally invasive saphenous ablation, using either RFA or EVLT, corrects or significantly improved the hemodynamic abnormality and clinical symptoms associated with superficial venous reflux in more than 90% of cases. These techniques are useful for treatment of patients with more severe clinical classes of superficial CVI.

▶ This article is a bit of dotting the I's and crossing the T's. We know that open surgical treatment of superficial reflux can result in improvement in some parameters of venous hemodynamic abnormality. The hemodynamic parameter chosen in this study was the VFI as determined by APG. These authors had previously shown that open surgical treatment can result in improved VFIs in patients with venous insufficiency. It is, therefore, also not surprising that similar results were achieved with endoluminal therapy as long as endoluminal therapy was successful in ablating the greater saphenous vein. It is, however, important to remember that improvement in venous hemodynamics after superficial venous surgery is not uniformly reported, and we still do not know what change in VFI is truly a real change or merely within the error parameters of the measurement.

G. L. Moneta, MD

Endovascular Radiofrequency Obliteration Using 90°C for Treatment of Great Saphenous Vein
Dunn CW, Kabnick LS, Merchant RF, et al (Ferrell Duncan Clinic Vein and Laser Ctr, Springfield, Mo; Vein Inst of New Jersey, Morristown; Reno Vein Clinic, Nev; et al)
Ann Vasc Surg 20:625-629, 2006

The recommended treatment temperature for endovascular radiofrequency obliteration (RFO) of the great saphenous vein (GSV) is 85°C. Faster catheter pullback rates are possible when the operating catheter tip temperature is increased. We studied the safety and effectiveness of RFO of the GSV using a temperature of 90°C, tumescent infiltration, and catheter pullback rates double the current standard. Sixty-eight patients (85 limbs) with ultrasound-documented saphenofemoral valve reflux underwent Closure procedure. Treatment temperature was increased to 90°C, and pullback times were increased to 5-6 cm/min. Outcome measures were occlusion of treated vein segments at 3 days and 6 months postoperatively and clinical evaluation of complications at 3 days and 6 months postoperatively. At 3 days, 96% (80/83) of GSVs were occluded and at 6 months 90% (66/73) were occluded. At 3 days and 6 months, no limbs had evidence of deep venous thrombosis or skin burns. Pullback times were shortened from 15-18 min to 8 min. Closure procedure of the GSV using 90°C and faster catheter pullback rates occluded a refluxing GSV with similar 3-day and 6-month occlusion rates as 85°C.

▶ Faster treatment times have led some clinicians to prefer laser obliteration of the GSV over radiofrequency ablation. However, it appears that both techniques can be performed with similar catheter pullback times. Given the "door to door" total time required for a catheter-based obliteration of the GSV, it does, however, seem a bit silly to be concerned about 7 or 8 minutes.

G. L. Moneta, MD

Quality of Life after Surgery for Varicose Veins and the Impact of Preoperative Duplex: Results Based on a Randomized Trial
Blomgren L, Johansson G, Bergqvist D (Capio St Göran's Hosp, Stockholm; Univ Hosp, Uppsala, Sweden)
Ann Vasc Surg 20:30-34, 2006

In a prospective randomized study, we found that the addition of a preoperative duplex scan before varicose vein (VV) surgery reduced recurrences and reoperations after 2 years. The aim of the present study was to investigate whether this correlates with an improved quality of life (QoL). We studied 293 patients scheduled for VV surgery with or without preoperative duplex. QoL was assessed preoperatively at 1 month, 1 year, and 2 years with the Short Form-36 (SF-36). Scores were compared with matched reference groups from the Swedish population. The 237 complete responders (81%) had a mean age of 47 (range 22-73) years, 169 (71%) were women, and 43 (18%) had skin changes. Both groups of VV patients scored significantly worse than the reference group in the domain Bodily Pain preoperatively ($p <$ 0.001) and better after 1 year ($p = 0.04$), with no difference found after 2 years. There was no significant difference in QoL between the duplex and control groups at any time. We conclude that preoperative duplex before VV surgery did not significantly improve QoL after 2 years in spite of improved surgical results. VV surgery per se improved QoL as measured with the SF-36.

▶ This is the first of 3 abstracts of varied results of VV surgery using endpoints likely to matter to patients. In this study, surgical treatment of uncomplicated VVs resulted in improved QoL compared with conservative management. There is not much to complain about here, except perhaps for the lack of a QoL instrument specific to patients with VVs. In general, assessment of QoL is best performed, when possible, with both generic (SF-36, Euroqual) questionnaires and disease-specific questionnaires. No disease-specific questionnaire was utilized here. The study may actually underestimate benefit in that many patients crossed over to surgical treatment, and generic QoL instruments may underestimate procedure-related benefits targeting specific disease processes.

G. L. Moneta, MD

Return to Work Following Varicose Vein Surgery: Influence of Type of Operation, Employment and Social Status
Wright AP, Berridge DC, Scott DJA (St James's Univ, Leeds, England)
Eur J Vasc Endovasc Surg 31:553-557, 2006

Objectives.—To determine factors which influence the time taken to return to work in patients undergoing varicose vein surgery.

Design.—Prospective collection of data from patients at outpatient interview.

Setting.—The Department of Vascular and Endovascular Surgery at a teaching hospital in the UK.

Participants.—Two hundred and fifteen consecutive employed or self-employed patients attending the outpatient clinic for review following varicose vein surgery.

Methods.—Data was collected from patients in the outpatient clinic approximately 6 weeks following varicose vein surgery. Type of procedure, gender, occupation status, category of occupation, the incidence of complications and the time taken to return to work (RTW) was recorded. Statistics were performed using Kruskal-Wallis H, Mann-Whitney U and chi-squared analysis.

Results.—Two hundred and fifteen patients were included, 77 (36%) men and 138 (64%) women. One hundred and ninety-two (89%) were employed and 23 (11%) self-employed. One hundred and fifty-three underwent primary saphenofemoral (SFJ) surgery, 10 bilateral procedures, 23 primary saphenopopliteal surgery (SPJ), 14 redo operations, five combined SFJ and SPJ, two mid thigh perforator ligation, six phlebectomies without groin or popliteal surgery and two bilateral surgery for recurrence. There was no relationship of gender or incidence of complications to RTW. There was a significant difference ($p < 0.0001$) between employed (median RTW 4 weeks, interquartile range 2–5 weeks) and self-employed patients (median 2 weeks, interquartile range 1–4 weeks). Occupation category did show an overall significant difference ($p < 0.0001$) on Kruskal–Wallis H-testing. Paired Mann–Whitney U-analysis showed that this difference was between occupation class I (median RTW 2 weeks, interquartile range 1–3 weeks) and IIIN (median 3.5 weeks, interquartile range 2–5 weeks), IIIM (median 5 weeks, interquartile range 2–5 weeks), IV (median 4 weeks, interquartile range 2–6 weeks) and V (median 4 weeks interquartile range 3–6 weeks), and between class II (median 3 weeks, interquartile range 2–4 weeks) and classes IIIM, IV and V.

Conclusions.—Employed patients and those involved in intensive manual labour are less likely to return to work early. There is no effect of gender or incidence of complications. On the basis of this study we would recommend that patients could return to work within 3 weeks of varicose veins surgery.

▶ This article was basically out of date before it was published. It evaluates patients treated with standard saphenous vein ligation stripping, an operation that is rapidly disappearing. The value of the article is not in telling us that patients with bilateral operations return to work more slowly, or that patients working for others or engaged in physically demanding jobs return to work more slowly than self-employed patients. What is of value here is that the median time to return to work after saphenous vein stripping is 3 weeks, which is a bit longer than I would have expected. One wonders and expects that an endovenous approach would shorten this time. Earlier return to work and normal activities is the principal advantage of the endovenous approach. Three weeks off for varicose vein surgery is just too long.

G. L. Moneta, MD

Neovalve construction in postthrombotic syndrome
Maleti O, Lugli M (Hesperia Hosp, Modena, Italy)
J Vasc Surg 43:794-799, 2006

Objective.—The purpose of this study was to evaluate a new neovalve construction technique in postthrombotic syndrome. The surgical procedure is described, and preliminary results of the first case series are given.

Methods.—From December 2000 to June 2004, neovalve construction in 18 limbs was performed on 16 patients (8 male and 8 female; median age, 55.5 years; range, 34-79 years) to treat severe chronic venous insufficiency in cases of postthrombotic syndrome. Surgical treatment was recommended in cases of nonhealing or recurrent ulcers (CEAP classification class C6). Preoperative duplex scanning, ascending/descending venography, and air plethysmography were routinely performed. Valvular cusps were created by dissecting the thickened venous wall to obtain material with which to fashion a new monocuspid or bicuspid valve. Mean follow-up was 22 months (range, 1-42 months). Postoperative duplex scanning and air plethysmography were performed in all patients. Descending venography was performed after surgery in 15 limbs.

Results.—In 16 lower extremities (89%), the ulcer healed within 4 to 25 weeks (median, 12 weeks), and no recurrences occurred. Neovalve competence was confirmed in 17 cases (95%). Postoperative duplex scan and air plethysmography showed a significant improvement in hemodynamic parameters ($P < .001$), especially in younger patients with good muscle pump function. In 17 limbs (95%), the treated segments remained primarily patent at median follow-up of 22 months. Early thrombosis below the neovalve site occurred in two patients (12%). No perioperative pulmonary embolism was observed. A late occlusion occurred in one patient (6%), 8 months after surgery. Minor postoperative complications occurred in three patients (17%).

Conclusions.—Neovalve construction seems to be effective in restoring femoral competence in postthrombotic reflux. Although these preliminary results are encouraging, long-term follow-up and a larger series are required to validate the technique.

▶ Deep venous system incompetence with ulceration is an intractable and difficult clinical problem that physicians have struggled with for decades. Opinions regarding optimal management range from compressive therapy to aggressive surgical attempts at restoring valvular competence. These include the more traditional valvuloplasty, vein transposition, and venous segment transplantation or the more recent cryopreserved valve insertion, xenografts, neovalve creation with vein imbrication, and bioprosthetic valves. The authors rightly contend that postthrombotic deep system incompetence presents a difficult scenario where most of these options may not be feasible. As we try to work through the pros and cons of currently proposed reconstructions, the authors have added another innovative technique to the list. In this interesting approach, they use the vein wall thickening associated with the postthrombotic state to their advantage and dissect out enough intima to create a neovalve. They present detailed anatomic (venographic and US) and physiologic (air plethysmography) evidence that the valves work and continue to do so over a follow-up ranging from 1 to 42 months. Since the neovalves are created from presumably primarily fibrotic tissue, why they do not continue to undergo proliferative or sclerotic processes is surprising. I am eagerly looking forward to longer follow-up reports and more of their experience. The method, if effective in the long-term, has the distinct advantage of using autogenous material without mandatory long-term anticoagulation.

G. L. Moneta, MD

Residual varicose veins below the knee after varicose knee surgery are not related to incompetent perforating veins
van Neer P, Kessels A, de Haan E, et al (Laurentius Hosp, Roermond, The Netherlands; Kemta and Horten-Zentrum Universitätsspital Zürich, Switzerland; Univ Hosp, Maastricht, The Netherlands; et al)
J Vasc Surg 44:1051-1054, 2006

Objective.—The objectives of this study were to investigate the occurrence of residual varicose veins (visible and ultrasonic) at the below-knee level after short-stripping the great saphenous vein (GSV) and to investigate the possible role of preoperative incompetent perforating veins (IPVs) on the persistence of these varicose veins.

Methods.—In this prospective study in 59 consecutive patients (74 limbs) with untreated primary varicose veins, a preoperative clinical examination and preoperative color flow duplex imaging were performed. Re-evaluation (clinical examination and color flow duplex imaging) was performed 6 months after surgery. Dissection of the saphenofemoral junction and short-stripping of the GSV from the groin to just below the knee level was performed without additional stab avulsions on the lower leg. The association between postoperative reflux in the three GSV branches below the knee level and preoperative IPV and the association between postoperative visible varicose veins in the GSV below knee level and preoperative IPV were determined with odds ratios with the help of a univariate and multivariate logistic regression analysis.

Results.—Preoperative varicosities in the GSV below the knee were visible in 62 limbs (70%) and were visible after surgery in 12 limbs (16%). The number of limbs with reflux in the 3 below-knee GSV branches was as follows: anterior branch, 34 (49%) before surgery and 31 (44%) after surgery; main stem, 59 (79%) before surgery and 62 (91%) after surgery; and posterior branch, 49 (67%) before surgery and 46 (63%) after surgery. No statistically significant association between postoperative reflux in the three GSV branches and preoperative IPV nor between postoperative visible varicose veins and preoperative IPV was found.

Conclusions.—This study shows that reflux in the GSV below knee level after the short-stripping procedure persists in all below-knee GSV branches. Approximately 20% of patients with visible varicose veins in the GSV area below the knee level will have visible varicose veins in this area 6 months after the short-strip procedure. These clinical and ultrasonic residual varicose veins are not significantly related to the presence of preoperative IPV.

▶ In summary, recurrence after varicose vein surgery depends on what "recurrence" means. The authors performed only ligation and above-knee stripping for varicose veins with GSV reflux. Below-knee varicosities were not addressed, and preoperative US was used to document perforator vein (PV) incompetence in all patients. Follow-up US (mean, 21 weeks) and clinical examinations (mean, 25 weeks) were performed early enough to enable conclusions to be made on the influence of preoperative PV incompetence on postoperative below-knee reflux in the territory of the GSV. Selecting this time frame has the advantage of reducing the confounding effects of neovascularization, remodeling, and development of new PV incompetence that occur over longer follow-up periods. It also makes for a more convenient study. None of the patients developed varicosities below the knee if they did not have them before surgery. Visible varicosities below the knee were reduced in patients who had them preoperatively (from 70% to 16%). However, US-detected reflux persisted in braches of the GSV below the knee in almost all the patients who had them preoperatively. Importantly, there was no correlation between the presence of PV incompetence before surgery and the persistence of reflux in the GSV branches after surgery—more evidence that PV incompetence does not contribute to persistent reflux in the leg at least early after GSV ligation and stripping. The number of limbs studied are low (n = 62), information on PV incompetence after surgery is notably absent, follow-up time is limited, and reflux in the absence of visible varicosities is defined as inconsequential. Therefore, the authors' strong recommendation that it is not necessary to focus on PV incompetence or perform stab avulsions during ablation of the GSV probably overstates their data. The jury is still out on this one.

G. L. Moneta, MD

Neovascularization: An "innocent bystander" in recurrent varicose veins
Egan B, Donnelly M, Bresnihan M, et al (Adelaide and Meath Hosp incorporating Natl Children's Hosp, Tallaght, Dublin)
J Vasc Surg 44:1279-1284, 2006

Objective.—Varicose vein recurrence after surgery occurs in up to 60% of patients. A variety of technical factors have been implicated, but biological factors such as neovascularization have more recently been proposed. The objective of this study was to characterize the relative contribution of technical and biological factors to recurrence in a large prospective series of recurrent varicose veins.

Methods.—Duplex and operative findings were recorded prospectively in a consecutive series of 500 limbs undergoing surgery for recurrent varicose veins between 1995 and 2005 in a university teaching hospital. Only limbs with previous saphenofemoral junction surgery were included. All limbs had preoperative duplex mapping by an accredited vascular technician who assessed the status of the great saphenous vein (GSV) in the thigh and groin, sought sonographic evidence of neovascularization, and reported on the presence of reflux in the short saphenous vein and perforator sites (typical and atypical). All operations were performed with an attending vascular surgeon as the lead operator.

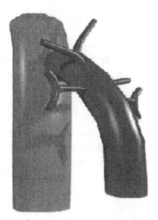

FIGURE 1.—Entirely intact long saphenous vein system. (Courtesy of Egan B, Donnelly M, Bresnihan M, et al. Neovascularization: an "innocent bystander" in recurrent varicose veins. *J Vasc Surg.* 2006;44:1279-1284. Copyright 2006 by Elsevier. Reprinted by permission.)

Results.—Primary GSV surgery was incomplete in 83.2% of limbs. A completely intact GSV system was present in 17.4% of limbs (Fig 1). An incompetent thigh saphenous vein was present in 44.2% of limbs, 37.6% had GSV stump incompetence with one or more intact tributaries, and 16% had both a residual thigh GSV and an incompetent stump with intact tributaries. Non-GSV sites of reflux were identified in 25% of limbs. Neovascularization was identified on duplex scanning in 41 (8.2%) limbs. However, in 27 of these, surgical exploration revealed a residual GSV stump with 1 or more significant tributaries. Each of the remaining 14 (2.8%) limbs had a residual incompetent thigh GSV.

Conclusions.—Despite reports to the contrary, neovascularization occurs in a relatively small proportion of patients with recurrent varicose veins. All recurrent varicose veins associated with duplex-diagnosed neovascularization are also associated with persistent reflux in the GSV stump tributaries, thigh GSV, or both. Recurrence after primary varicose vein surgery is associated with inadequate primary surgery or progression of disease, and neovascularization alone is not a cause of recurrent varicose veins.

▶ The controversy over the role of neovascularization in varicose vein recurrence is still alive and kicking! This study, however, has the power of numbers behind it. It is also thorough, including both standardized duplex US and operative findings in 500 reoperative cases, a formidable number of patients collected over a decade. At the very least, it confirms all those previous reports that recurrence after varicose vein ablation occurs more frequently than any of us would choose to admit. The authors report that incomplete GSV surgery accounted for 83.2% of recurrences. These included incomplete ablation of tributaries at the GSV–common femoral vein junction (33.4%), failure to remove/strip a ligated GSV in 44.2%, and importantly, a disheartening 17.4% had an intact GSV system (some patients had more than one problem). Only 8.2% of patients had evidence of neovascularization on preoperative US, of which 2.8% were found to have a residual incompetent GSV on operation. Only the remaining 5.4% had a GSV stump with one or more significant tributaries that could have arisen *de novo* (neovascularization) or were the result of remodeling from residual unligated tributaries. The authors did not perform histologic analyses of the groins, thereby leaving the door open for questions regarding missed neovascularization.

This study provides strong evidence against casually attributing a recurrence to neovascularization, and should energize all of us to seek complete ablation of all tributaries and of the saphenofemoral junction. It emphasizes the importance of anatomic variations of the GSV system, most important of which is a bifid system that can occur in 24% of individuals. Whether the introduction of endovenous ablation will impact recurrence rates by reducing neovascularization (due to absence of surgical dissection), or by deliberately leaving behind tributaries very close to the saphenofemoral junction (as is being recommended by many), still remains to be seen.

G. L. Moneta, MD

Combined saphenous ablation and iliac stent placement for complex severe chronic venous disease
Neglén P, Hollis KC, Raju S (River Oaks Hosp, Jackson, Miss)
J Vasc Surg 44:828-833, 2006

Background.—Severe chronic venous disease frequently has a complex pathophysiology. This study describes results after combined interventions to correct outflow obstruction and superficial reflux, even in the presence of deep venous reflux.

Methods.—Between 1997 and 2005, 99 limbs in 96 patients had percutaneous iliofemoral venous stenting combined with great saphenous vein (GSV) stripping (39 limbs), or percutaneous GSV ablation performed by radiofrequency (27 limbs) or laser (33 limbs). Clinical severity score in CEAP was C4 in 51 limbs, C5 in eight limbs, and C6 in 40 limbs; median age was 56 years (range, 27 to 87 years); left–right limb ratio, 2.3:1; female–male ratio, 1.8:1; primary–secondary etiology, 58:41. Perioperative investigations included visual analogue pain scale (VAS), degree of swelling (grade 0 to 3); quality-of-life questionnaire; venous filling index in milliliters per second (VFI_{90}), venous filling time in seconds (VFT), percentage in ambulatory venous pressure drop (AVP), duplex Doppler scanning, and radiologic studies.

Results.—Clinical follow-up was performed in 97 (98%) of 99 for up to 5.5 years. Axial deep reflux was found in 27% (27/99). At least three venous segments were refluxing in 40% of limbs. Preoperative hemodynamic parameters reflected the presence of reflux and improved significantly $(P < .01)$ after the procedure $(VFI_{90}, 3.8$ to 2.3 mL/s; VFT, 11 to 16 seconds; AVP, 55% to 65%). No patients died, and the morbidity with endovenous GSV ablation was largely limited to ecchymosis and thrombophlebitis in the thigh area. Cumulative primary, assisted primary, and secondary stent patency rates at 4 years were 83%, 97%, and 97%, respectively (Fig 1). After treat-

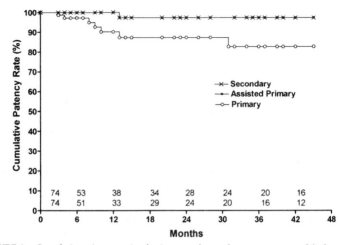

FIGURE 1.—Cumulative primary, assisted primary, and secondary patency rates of iliofemoral stents. The lower numbers represent limbs at risk for each time interval (all SEM <10%). (Courtesy of Neglén P, Hollis KC, Raju S. Combined saphenous ablation and iliac stent placement for complex severe chronic venous disease. *J Vasc Surg.* 2006;44:828-833. Copyright 2006 by Elsevier. Reprinted by permission.)

ment, limb swelling and pain substantially improved. The rate of limbs with severe pain (≥5 on VAS) fell from 44% to 3% after intervention. Gross swelling (grade 3) decreased from 30% to 6% of limbs. Cumulative analysis showed sustained complete relief of pain (VAS = 0) and swelling (grade 0) after 4 years in 73% and 47% of limbs, respectively. Ulcers healed in 26 (68%) of 38 ulcerated limbs. Cumulative ulcer-healing rate was 64% at 48 months. All quality-of-life categories significantly improved after treatment.

Conclusion.—The single-stage combination of percutaneous venous stenting and superficial ablation in patients with severe chronic venous disease is safe, gives excellent symptom relief and improvement of quality of life, and a well-maintained ulcer-healing rate. It seems logical to initially perform multiple minimally invasive interventions rather than open surgery. Any associated deep reflux can initially be ignored pending clinical response to the combined intervention.

▶ Multiple venous segment abnormalities require multiple interventions, and the availability of less invasive endovenous ablative and revascularization techniques allows several concomitant procedures to be performed successfully and effectively. With their long track record of open/endovascular ablation and revascularization procedures for venous reflux/occlusive disease, it is not surprising that the River Oaks group decided to put the two together. They have made a strong case for dealing aggressively with combined reflux and axial obstructive disease at the same time. The patency rate of stenting was excellent at 4 years (97%), while the results of GSV ablation were modest with the endovenous techniques (persistent reflux: laser, 9%; radiofrequency, 25%). However, symptomatic relief, hemodynamic improvement, quality-of-life enhancement, and ulcer healing were achieved in the majority of patients over a considerable follow-up period. Enviable results in a difficult group of patients.

G. L. Moneta, MD

Obstructive lesions of the inferior vena cava: Clinical features and endovenous treatment
Raju S, Hollis K, Neglen P (Univ of Mississippi and River Oaks Hosp, Flowood)
J Vasc Surg 44:820-827, 2006

Objective.—Chronic obstructions of the inferior vena cava (IVC) are associated with many odd features. Even total occlusions may remain entirely silent or present late with acute symptoms. Renal dysfunction is rare. Many have chronic symptoms, but often only one limb is affected. We describe the clinical features in a series of 120 patients seen over a 10-year period and the results of successful stent placement in 99 limbs.

Methods.—Patients with acute onset of symptoms due to distal thromboses underwent catheter-directed thrombolysis. Patients with significant chronic symptoms were investigated by duplex, venous function tests, transfemoral venography and finally intravascular ultrasound (IVUS). Stenotic segments were balloon dilated and occluded segments were recannalized when feasible; stents were placed under IVUS control.

Results.—In the asymptomatic group, 10 patients with total occlusions had transient or no occlusive symptoms. In the acute symptom group, four patients with chronic IVC occlusions presented with acute onset of deep venous thrombosis distal to the occlusion but became asymptomatic when the clot was lysed. In the chronic symptom group, 97 patients (99 limbs) had symptoms of chronic venous disease of variable distribution and intensity. In two-thirds, limb symptoms were unilateral. Pathology was total occlusion in 14%, and the rest were stenoses. The lesion extended above the renal vein in 18%. Common iliac obstruction was concurrent in 93%. Distal reflux was present in 66%. Modifications of the basic stent technique were required in recanalization of total occlusions (four extending up to the atrium), two bilateral stent deployments, and nine IVC filter cases. Stent deployment across the renal and hepatic veins or the contralateral iliac vein had no adverse sequelae. Stent patency (cumulative) at 2 years was 82%. Complete relief (cumulative) of pain and swelling at 3.5 years was 74% and 51%, respectively. The cumulative rate of complete ulcer healing at 2 years was 63%. Overall clinical outcome was rated as good or excellent in 70%.

Conclusions.—The unusual clinical features of IVC obstructions seem related to the rich collateralization, which has an embryonic basis. Common iliac vein patency seems to be a crucial link in collateral function, and its concurrent occlusion produces symptoms. Percutaneous stent placement has an

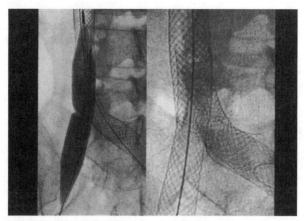

FIGURE 4.—Stent placement at the inferior vena cava (IVC) bifurcation: after the IVC stent is extended into one of the iliac veins, a fenestrum is created by balloon dilation over a guidewire. The guidewire is introduced through the opposite side and manipulated through the stent. A generous overlap of 5 cm between the stents is recommended to prevent the second stent from shrinking back through the fenestrum during postdilation. No restriction of either iliac flow has been observed when this technique has been used. (Courtesy of Raju S, Hollis K, Neglen P. Obstructive lesions of the inferior vena cava: clinical features and endovenous treatment. *J Vasc Surg.* 2006;44:820-827. Copyright 2006 by Elsevier. Reprintd by permission.)

emerging role in the treatment of IVC obstructive lesions, with good mid-term stent patency and clinical results (Fig 4).

▶ Unlike obstructive pathology in the superior vena cava, the etiology of obstruction in the IVC is almost always benign. This article details the workup, treatment, and outcome of 120 patients with IVC obstruction. It describes the tricks the authors have picked up over the decade (stenting across IVC filters, through the interstices of another stent). IVC obstruction alone is well tolerated by most patients, being compensated by abundant retroperitoneal collaterals. However, IVC obstructions in conjunction with iliac vein lesions or new distal thrombosis appear to precipitate symptoms and signs of outflow obstruction. As in the superior vena cava, endovascular maneuvers have replaced complicated open reconstructions, thereby expanding the number of patients that can be benefited. Recanalization with aggressive angioplasty and stenting can achieve 82% patency at 2 years, pain relief in 74% at 3.5 years, reduced swelling in 51% at 3.5 years, and ulcer healing in 63% at 2 years.

G. L. Moneta, MD

Successful Iliac Vein and Inferior Vena Cava Stenting Ameliorates Venous Claudication and Improves Venous Outflow, Calf Muscle Pump Function, and Clinical Status in Post-Thrombotic Syndrome

Delis KT, Bjarnason H, Wennberg PW, et al (Mayo Clinic, Rochester, Minn)
Ann Surg 245:130-139, 2007

Objectives.—Stent therapy has been proposed as an effective treatment of chronic iliofemoral (I-F) and inferior vena cava (IVC) thrombosis. The purpose of this study was to determine the effects of technically successful stenting in consecutive patients with advanced CVD ($CEAP_{3-6}$ ± venous claudication) for chronic obliteration of the I-F (±IVC) trunks, on the venous hemodynamics of the limb, the walking capacity, and the clinical status of CVD. These patients had previously failed to improve with conservative treatment entailing compression and/or wound care for at least 12 months.

Methods.—The presence of venous claudication was assessed by ≥3 independent examiners. The CEAP clinical classification was used to determine the severity of CVD. Outflow obstruction [Outflow Fraction at 1- and 4-second (OF_1 and OF_4) in %], venous reflux [Venous Filling Index (VFI) in mL/100 mL/s], calf muscle pump function [Ejection Fraction (EF) in %] and hypertension [Residual Venous Fraction (RVF) in %], were examined before and after successful venous stenting in 16 patients (23 limbs), 6 females, 10 males, median age 42 years; range, 31–77 years, left/right limbs 14/9, using strain gauge plethysmography; 7/16 of these had thrombosis extending to the IVC. Contralateral limbs to those stented without prior I-F ± IVC thrombosis, nor infrainguinal clots on duplex, were used as control limbs (n = 9). Excluded were patients with stent occlusion or stenoses, peripheral arterial disease (ABI <1.0), symptomatic cardiac disease, unrelated causes of walking impairment, and malignancy. Preinterventional data (≤30 days) were compared with those after endovascular therapy (8.4 months; interquartile range [IQR], 3–11.8 months). Nonparametric analysis was applied.

Results.—Compared with the control group, limbs with I-F ± IVC thrombosis before stenting had reduced venous outflow (OF_4) and calf muscle pump function (EF), worse CEAP clinical class, and increased RVF (all, $P <$ 0.05). At 8.4 months (IQR, 3–11.8 months) after successful I-F (±IVC) stenting, venous outflow (OF_1, OF_4) and calf muscle pump function (EF) had both improved ($P < 0.001$) and the RVF had decreased ($P < 0.001$), at the expense of venous reflux, which had increased further (increase of median VFI by 24%; $P = 0.002$); the CEAP status had also improved ($P < 0.05$) from a median class C_3 (range, C3–C6; IQR, C3–C5) [distribution, C6: 6; C4: 4; C3: 13] before intervention to C2 (range, C2–C6; IQR, C2–C4.5) [distribution, C6: 1; C5: 5; C4: 4; C2: 13] after intervention. At this follow up (8.4 months median), venous outflow (OF_1, OF_4), calf muscle pump function (EF), and RVF of the stented limbs did not differ significantly from those of the control; significantly worse ($P < 0.025$) were the amount of venous reflux (VFI), and the CEAP clinical class, despite the improvement with stenting. Incapacitating venous claudication noted in 62.5% (10 of 16, 95% CI, 35.8%–

89.1%) of patients (15 of 23 limbs; 65.2%, 95% CI, 44.2%–86.3%) before stenting was eliminated in all after stenting ($P < 0.001$).

Conclusions.—Successful I-F (±IVC) stenting in limbs with venous outflow obstruction and complicated CVD (C3–C6) ameliorates venous claudication, normalizes outflow, and enhances calf muscle pump function, compounded by a significant clinical improvement of CVD. The significant increase in the amount of venous reflux of the stented limbs indicates that elastic or inelastic compression support of the successfully stented limbs would be pivotal in preventing disease progression.

▶ The study suggests that patients with venous claudication due to an iliac venous obstruction may be improved by stenting. There are, however, several weaknesses to this study. It is essentially a retrospective analysis, the follow-up is short, there is no objective measurement of venous claudication, and only successfully treated patients are analyzed, making it impossible to determine the true efficacy of I-F IVC stenting in patients with chronic venous disease.

G. L. Moneta, MD

Conservative versus surgical treatment of venous leg ulcers: A prospective, randomized, multicenter trial
van Gent WB, Hop WC, van Praag MC, et al (Sint Franciscus Gasthuis, Rotterdam, The Netherlands; Erasmus Med Ctr, Rotterdam, The Netherlands; Meander Med Ctr, Amersfoort, The Netherlands; et al)
J Vasc Surg 44:563-571, 2006

Background.—The prevalence of venous leg ulcers is as high as 1% to 1.5%, and the total costs of this disease are 1% of the total annual health care budget in Western European countries. Treatment modalities are conservative or surgical. Subfascial endoscopic perforating vein surgery (SEPS) combined with superficial vein ligation is performed in many centers to address vein incompetence in patients with chronic venous leg ulcers. Several reports describe good healing and low recurrence rates, although a randomized trial to compare surgical treatment including SEPS and treatment of the superficial venous system to conservative modalities has never been performed. Therefore, a prospective, randomized, multicenter trial was conducted to study whether ambulatory compression therapy with venous surgery is a better treatment than just ambulatory compression therapy in venous leg ulcer patients.

Methods.—Patients with an active (open) venous leg ulcer (CEAP C6) qualified for the study. The study consisted of two treatment groups. All patients were treated by standardized ambulatory compression therapy, and half of the patients received SEPS. Concomitant superficial venous incompetence was also treated in the second group. For allocation to both treatment groups, each patient was assigned by a computer program at the randomization center. The primary goal of the study was to compare the ulcer-free pe-

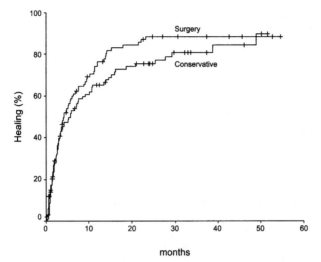

FIGURE 7.—Cumulative healing rates according to randomized treatment groups (*P* = .24). *Tickmarks* note the ends of follow-up of patients. (Courtesy of van Gent WB, Hop WC, van Praag MC, et al. Conservative versus surgical treatment of venous leg ulcers: a prospective, randomized, multicenter trial. *J Vasc Surg.* 2006;44:563-571. Copyright 2006 by Elsevier. Reprinted by permission.)

riod during follow-up in both study groups. Secondary end points were ulcer healing and recurrence rates.

Results.—From April 1997 until January 2001, 200 ulcerated legs (170 patients) were included in the study in 12 centers in The Netherlands. A total of 97 ulcers were allocated to the surgical group and 103 to the conservative group. Patient characteristics were similar in the two treatment groups at baseline, with the exception of a higher proportion in the conservative group of diabetes mellitus. Healing rates were 83% in the surgical group and 73% in the conservative group (not significant; median time to healing, 27 months) (Fig 7). Recurrence rates were the same in both treatment groups (22% surgical vs 23% conservative). During follow-up of a mean of 29 months (median, 27 months) in the surgical group and 26 months (median, 24 months) in the conservative group, we found that in the surgical group, the ulcer-free rate was 72%, whereas in the conservative group this rate was 53% (*P* = .11; Mann-Whitney test). Patients with recurrent ulceration or medially located ulcers in the surgical group had a longer ulcer-free period than those treated in the conservative group (*P* = .02 for both). A first-time ulcer and one of the centers also had a positive effect on the ulcer-free period during follow-up (*P* < .001 and *P* = .02), independent of the treatment group. Deep vein incompetence did not affect the ulcer-free period.

Conclusions.—In conclusion, we suggest that patients with medial and/or recurrent ulceration should receive surgery combined with ambulatory compression therapy. A dedicated center should provide care for those patients.

▶ This study was likely conceived to address the role of SEPS in the treatment of venous ulcers. If that was the case it failed miserably, as SEPS was combined with superficial surgery in over half of the limbs treated with SEPS. Because there was no differences in surgical and nonsurgical patients with regard to ulcer healing and recurrence, unless we believe superficial surgery action impairs ulcer healing, SEPS does not come out looking good in this study. If SEPS helps with healing and recurrence of venous ulcers, it is not proven here. All we can say from these data is that it doesn't appear to impair healing. The same evangelistic approach to perforators originally seen with SEPS is now resurfacing with laser ablation of perforators and US-guided sclerotherapy of perforators. I bet the proponents of these procedures will also find it difficult to rigorously prove the benefit of these therapies.

G. L. Moneta, MD

Chronic venous leg ulcers benefit from surgery: Long-term results from 173 legs
Obermayer A, Göstl K, Walli G, et al (Wachauklinikum Melk, Austria; Karl Landsteiner Society, Melk, Austria; Med Univ of Vienna)
J Vasc Surg 44:572-579, 2006

Objective.—The purpose of this retrospective study was to present 7 years of data from operations of currently active, chronic venous leg ulcers (CEAP: C6), focusing on the short- and long-term effects of healing and recurrence and considering concomitant risk factors.

Methods.—Between January 1997 and March 2004, 173 patients (239 legs) with a currently active, chronic venous leg ulcer were surgically treated. The surgical procedures included two main steps: (1) the surgical interruption of reflux in the superficial and perforating veins to reduce venous hypertension in the entire leg and/or the affected area and (2) the surgical procedure involving the ulcer. A total of 123 patients (173 legs) who came to the follow-up were examined. The follow-up period ranged from 3 months to 7 years. The data collection integrated a preoperative examination that included medical history and clinical diagnoses and incorporated measurements such as body mass index, ankle-brachial pressure index, and the neutral position method at the follow-up. The function of the veins was measured with duplex ultrasonography. Finally, the data were analyzed by using various statistical methods, including Kaplan-Meier analysis, Cox regression analysis, and paired t tests.

Results.—Initially, ulcer healing occurred in 87% of the cases (151 legs). A total of 13% (22 legs) of the venous ulcers never healed, and recurrent venous ulcers occurred in 5% (9 legs). The Kaplan-Meier analyses of ulcer healing showed a healing rate of 85% in 6 months for all legs. The mean time of healing was 1.5 months. Furthermore, the Kaplan-Meier analyses of ulcer recurrence showed a 1.7% rate of recurrence in 6 months for all legs. The 5-year ulcer recurrence rate was 4.6%. The mean time of recurrence was 70.4 months.

Conclusions.—On the basis of the results from the 7 years of data from functional surgery of venous leg ulcers and as a result of the outcomes of our study, we recommend surgical treatment of venous leg ulcers at any stage. We therefore conclude that surgery is indicated before an ulcer is intractable to treatment. In general, our findings are based on the understanding and identification of the causes and symptoms of venous ulceration and illustrate that standard surgical methods can be applied for the therapy of venous leg ulcers at any stage.

▶ The results of surgical treatment of ulcers that are described as ulcers failing conservative therapy are almost unbelievable. Whereas one can perhaps see an initial healing rate of 87%, a 5-year recurrence rate of 4.6% is incredible, and I am not sure if it has ever been duplicated. I will need to see comparable results from other centers before I believe this article. The authors must not be seeing the same type of patients that I see in Portland.

G. L. Moneta, MD

Excision and meshed skin grafting for leg ulcers resistant to compression therapy
Abisi S, Tan J, Burnand KG (St Thomas' Hosp, London)
Br J Surg 94:194-197, 2007

Background.—The aim of this study was to determine the success of excision and meshed skin grafting for chronic leg ulcers. The effects of different ulcer aetiology and ulcer size on outcome were also assessed.

Methods.—All patients who had excision and mesh grafting for chronic leg ulceration between January 1996 and December 2004 at St Thomas' Hospital were reviewed. Recurrence was classified as any breakdown of the ulcer during follow-up.

Results.—Sixty-two patients with 100 chronic leg ulcers underwent operation. Seventy-two of the ulcers were venous and the median ulcer size was 36 (range 1.5–192) cm². Only three patients left the hospital with their ulcers unhealed, but ulcers had recurred in 28 (28 per cent) by 2 months. A further 17 ulcers recurred later, with just over half (55 per cent) remaining healed by 5 years. There was no difference between the recurrence rates of venous ulcers and ulcers of other aetiologies ($P = 0.980$), or large (more than 10 cm²) and small ulcers ($P = 0.686$).

Conclusion.—Wide local excision and meshed skin grafting benefitted over half of these patients with refractory leg ulcers. Recurrence was most likely to occur in the first 2 months and, provided that ulcers were healed at this time, there was a low rate of further breakdown.

▶ Tangential excision and skin grafting for chronic lower extremity ulcers provides reasonable short-term results for a majority of patients and long-term ulcer healing for about half. The downside, of course, is that an outpatient disorder is transferred into an inpatient problem. The median postoperative stay for the patients in this series was 20 days, with a range of 12 to 40 days.

G. L. Moneta, MD

State-of-the-art treatment of chronic leg ulcers: a randomized controlled trial comparing vacuum-assisted closure (V.A.C.) with modern wound dressings
Vuerstaek JDD, Vainas T, Wuite J, et al (Univ Hosp Maastricht, The Netherlands; DermaClinic, Genk, Belgium; Atrium Med Centre Heerlen, The Netherlands; et al)
J Vasc Surg 44:1029-1038, 2006

Background.—Current treatment modalities for chronic leg ulcers are time consuming, expensive, and only moderately successful. Recent data suggest that creating a subatmospheric pressure by vacuum-assisted closure (V.A.C., KCI Concepts, San Antonio, Texas) therapy supports the wound healing process.

Methods.—The efficacy of vacuum-assisted closure in the treatment of chronic leg ulcers was prospectively studied in a randomized controlled trial in which 60 hospitalized patients with chronic leg ulcers were randomly assigned to either treatment by V.A.C. or therapy with conventional wound care techniques. The primary outcome measure was the time to complete healing (days). Statistical analysis was performed on the intention-to-treat basis.

Results.—The median time to complete healing was 29 days (95% confidence interval [CI], 25.5 to 32.5) in the V.A.C. group compared with 45 days (95% CI, 36.2 to 53.8) in the control group ($P = .0001$). Further, wound bed preparation during V.A.C. therapy was also significantly shorter at 7 days (95% CI 5.7 to 8.3) than during conventional wound care at 17 days (95% CI, 10 to 24, $P = .005$). The costs of conventional wound care were higher than those of V.A.C. Both groups showed a significant increase in quality of life at the end of therapy and a significant decrease in pain scores at the end of follow-up.

Conclusions.—V.A.C. therapy should be considered as the treatment of choice for chronic leg ulcers owing to its significant advantages in the time to complete healing and wound bed preparation time compared with conventional wound care. Particularly during the preparation stage, V.A.C. therapy appears to be superior to conventional wound care techniques.

▶ In this study, conventional wound care was more expensive than VAC therapy. A good proportion of the costs were from increased hospitalization times with conventional therapy. Very few chronic leg ulcers are treated with hospitalization for wound care in the United States. I doubt the cost analysis in this article, therefore, is widely applicable on this side of the pond. Nevertheless, VAC therapy appears more effective than anyone would have imagined. I suspect it is actually more expensive than more traditional compression therapy for leg ulcers, and certainly does not permit the same degree of mobility. However, if hospitalization, immobilization, or both are truly required for wound care, negative pressure therapy appears to have advantages over conventional therapy. Much to the dismay of hospital administrators, VAC therapy is used more and more as a mainstay of inpatient wound care. The results certainly seem to justify this.

G. L. Moneta, MD

Prevention of recurrence of venous ulceration: Randomized controlled trial of class 2 and class 3 elastic compression
Nelson EA, Harper DR, Prescott RJ, et al (Univ of Leeds, England)
J Vasc Surg 44:803-808, 2006

Objective.—To compare venous ulcer recurrence and compliance with two strengths of compression hosiery.

Methods.—This study was a randomized controlled trial with a 5-year follow-up. The setting was the leg ulcer clinics of a teaching and a district general hospital in Scotland, United Kingdom. Patients were 300 outpatients with recently healed venous ulcers, with no significant arterial disease, rheumatoid disease, or diabetes mellitus. Interventions were fitting and supply of class 2 or class 3 compression hosiery. Four-monthly refitting by trained orthotists and surveillance by specialist nurses were performed. The main outcome measures were recurrence of leg ulceration and compliance with treatment.

Results.—Thirty-six percent (107/300) of patients had recurrent leg ulceration by 5 years. Recurrence occurred in 59 (39%) of 151 class 2 elastic compression cases and in 48 (32%) of class 3 compression cases. One hundred six patients did not comply with their randomized compression class, 63 (42%) in class 3 and 43 (28%) in class 2. The difference in recurrence is not statistically significant, but our estimate of the effectiveness of class 3 hosiery is diluted by the lower compliance rate in this group. Restricted ankle movement and four or more previous ulcers were associated with a higher risk of recurrence.

Conclusions.—There was no evidence of a difference in recurrence rates at the classic level of significance (5%), but the lowest recurrence rates were seen in people who wore the highest degree of compression. Therefore, patients should wear the highest level of compression that is comfortable.

▶ Compliance has always been the key to preventing recurrent leg ulcers, especially venous ulcers. The authors' recommendation to go with as high a degree of compression as possible makes sense, but in many cases of elderly patients who have difficulty applying stockings or live in warm climates or who lack the funds for compression stockings, the recommendations presented here, while perhaps valid, would be frequently impractical. We also need to consider that if someone is willing to wear class 3 stockings, perhaps that person is also more compliant in other ways of treating his venous ulcers. Finally, lack of statistical significance is lack of significance, and while the authors think that class 3 stockings are better to prevent recurrence, their data do not actually prove this.

G. L. Moneta, MD

The Superior Vena Cava Syndrome: Clinical Characteristics and Evolving Etiology

Rice TW, Rodriguez RM, Light RW (Vanderbilt Univ, Nashville, Tenn; Saint Thomas Hosp, Nashville, Tenn)
Medicine 85:37-42, 2006

Malignancy is the most common cause of the superior vena cava (SVC) syndrome. With the increasing use of intravascular devices, the incidence of the SVC syndrome arising from benign etiologies is increasing. We reviewed the etiology and outcome of 78 patients with SVC syndrome over 5 years. Malignancy was the etiology in 60% of the cases, and bronchogenic carcinoma was the most common malignancy. Small cell and non-small cell lung cancer accounted for 17 (22%) and 19 (24%) cases, respectively, but a higher percentage of patients with small-cell lung cancer developed the syndrome (6% vs 1%). Lymphoma and germ cell tumors were other significant malignant causes (8% and 3% of cases, respectively). An intravascular device was the most common etiology in benign cases (22 of 31 cases; 71%), with fibrosing mediastinitis the second most common benign etiology (6 cases). The most frequent signs and symptoms were face or neck swelling (82%), upper extremity swelling (68%), dyspnea (66%), cough (50%), and dilated chest vein collaterals (38%). Dyspnea at rest, cough, and chest pain were more frequent in the patients with malignancy. Procedures performed for diagnostic or treatment purposes did not increase morbidity or mortality.

▶ The etiology of SVC obstruction has progressively evolved over the past century. In the early 20th century, the causes were equally divided between aortic aneurysms and malignancies. In the mid and late 20th century, this had shifted to almost entirely thoracic malignancies. The current experience collected from 1996 to 2001 shows yet another shift, with 60% of cases caused by thoracic malignancies and 40% by benign etiologies. Notably, 70% of benign cases were due to intravascular devices. With increasing dependence on the jugular/subclavian routes to deliver chemotherapy, antibiotics, nutrition, dialysis, pacing wires, and sundry other materials, we should anticipate this number to continue to increase. While chemoradiation is still the preferred management for malignant compression, interim relief in this situation and definitive management in benign cases can be achieved with a judicious combination of anticoagulation and endovascular revascularization.

G. L. Moneta, MD

Transfection of Human Hepatocyte Growth Factor Gene Ameliorates Secondary Lymphedema via Promotion of Lymphangiogenesis

Saito Y, Nakagami H, Morishita R, et al (Osaka Univ, Japan; Asahikawa Med Univ, Hokkaido, Japan)
Circulation 114:1177-1184, 2006

Background.—Lymphedema is a disorder of the lymphatic vascular system characterized by impaired lymphatic return and swelling of the extremities. Treatment for this disabling condition remains limited and largely ineffective. The goal of the present study was to investigate the therapeutic efficacy of hepatocyte growth factor (HGF) in animal models of lymphedema.

Method and Results.—Immunofluorescent analysis demonstrated that canine primary lymphatic endothelial cells (cLECs) were positive for lymphatic-specific markers (vascular endothelial growth factor receptor-3, LYVE-1, podoplanin, and Prox1) and the HGF receptor c-Met. Treating cLECs with human recombinant HGF resulted in a dose-dependent increase in cell growth and migration and increased activity of extracellular signal-regulated kinase and Akt. In human LECs, c-Met also was expressed, and treatment with HGF increased cell growth and migration in a dose-dependent manner. Transfection of human HGF plasmid DNA in cLECs also increased the c-*fos* promoter activity. Furthermore, weekly HGF gene transfer in a rat tail lymphedema model by disruption of lymphatic vessels resulted in a decrease in lymphedema thickness. Although expression of the endothelial cell marker PECAM-1 was increased in both HGF- and vascular endothelial growth factor 165–injected groups, expression of LEC markers (LYVE-1 and Prox1) was increased only in the HGF-injected group.

Conclusions.—These data demonstrate that expression of HGF via plasmid transfer improves lymphedema via promotion of lymphangiogenesis. Further studies to determine the clinical utility of this approach would be of benefit to patients with lymphedema.

▶ The data suggest that the phenotypic changes associated with secondary lymphedema can be attenuated with HGF gene transfer and that this occurs through local lymphangiogenesis induced by HGF. HGF is proving to be an extraordinarily interesting molecule. It appears to be a substance that allows targeted angiogenesis of both arteries and lymphatics. The huge current interest in HGF certainly seems justified.

G. L. Moneta, MD

18 Technical Notes

Is saphenofemoral junction reconstruction necessary during stripping of the saphenous vein?
Hulusi M, Ozbek C, Basaran M, et al (GATA Haydarpasa Training Hosp, Istanbul, Turkey; Camlica Hayat Hosp, Istanbul, Turkey; Sonomed Radiodiagnostic Ctr, Istanbul, Turkey)
Surgery 139:640-645, 2006

Background.—Patients who had undergone complete ankle-to-groin stripping of the greater saphenous vein were evaluated retrospectively to assess the necessity of saphenofemoral junction reconstruction during the stripping procedure. Since 1996, in addition to the conventional complete stripping operation, we routinely perform a saphenofemoral junction reconstruction in patients presenting with greater saphenous vein reflux associated with low-grade (grades I-II) saphenofemoral junctional reflux. In this method, the size of the common femoral vein was adjusted to the desired diameter by a running linear suture technique after division of the greater saphenous vein.

Methods.—Retrospective evaluation revealed that 73 limbs in 56 patients treated with this technique (group I). This group of patients was matched to another group of 65 patients (78 limbs) with similar characteristics and symptoms (group II) in whom the conventional complete ankle-to-groin stripping of greater saphenous vein was the treatment. The 2 groups were compared with respect to the incidence of complications, including recurrence of varicosities, ecchymosis, lymphocele, lymphorrhagia, wound infection, and paresthesia in the operated extremity. All patients also were evaluated by Doppler ultrasonography at 6 months, 12 months, and annually thereafter to determine the saphenofemoral junction reflux time (valve reflux time). The mean duration ± SD of follow-up was 6.7 ± 1.6 years (range, 2.1-10.8 years).

Results.—Recurrence of varicosity was noted in 14 patients, 3 in group I and 11 in group II ($P = .02$). There were no statistically significant differences between the 2 groups in terms of ecchymosis, hematoma, lymphocele, lymphorrhagia, wound infection, and paresthesia. At 6 months, a rapid decrease in valve reflux time was noted in group I ($P = .0001$). In addition, there was a significant improvement in valve reflux time at each subsequent Doppler examination in group I. Group II showed a decrease in valve reflux time, compared with the preoperative value ($P = .068$). During subsequent

Doppler examinations, a decrease in valve reflux time also was noted in group II; this difference reached statistical significance only at 24 months ($P = .04$).

Conclusions.—We believe that saphenofemoral junction reconstruction is a simple technique to perform and that addition of this method to the conventional stripping provides more durable results with a lesser incidence of recurrence. This method should be considered as a treatment modality in patients with greater saphenous vein reflux associated with low-grade (grades I-II) saphenofemoral junctional reflux.

▶ What happens to deep venous reflux following saphenous vein stripping is a bit controversial. The rate or resolution of reflux following saphenous vein stripping varies from 94%[1] to 33%[2]. Everyone agrees that it happens and that it certainly would not help long-term results. The technique described here is essentially narrowing the common femoral vein to the diameter of the femoral vein. The technique is simple to perform and may improve common femoral vein valve closure times. A bit more dissection will be required than for a simple saphenous vein ligation. However, the long-term results may be improved, and the common femoral vein has to be closed anyway, so it is reasonable to try this technique.

G. L. Moneta, MD

References

1. Sales CM, Bilof ML, Petrillo KA, Luka NL. Correction of lower extremity deep venous incompetence by ablation of superficial venous reflux. *Ann Vasc Surg.* 1996;10:186-189.
2. Puggioni A, Lurie F, Kistner RL, Eklof B. How often is deep venous reflux eliminated after saphenous vein ablation? *J Vasc Surg.* 2003;38:517-521.

Fresh Arterial Grafts as Conduits for Vascular Reconstruction in Transplanted Patients

Matia I, Adamec M, Janousek L, et al (Inst for Clinical and Medicine, Prague, Czech Republic)
Eur J Vasc Endovasc Surg 32:549-556, 2006

Objectives.—To assess the outcome of arterial allografts in patients receiving organ transplantation.

Design.—From October 1997 to June 2005, we used fresh arterial allografts as vascular conduits in 21 patients for the treatment of claudications (10), abdominal aortic aneurysm (6), complicated renal transplantation (2), acute lower extremity ischemia (2) and gangrene (1). At the time of the vascular procedure, ten of the patients (Group A) had already undergone organ transplantation. The mean follow up period was 32 months for renal and 37 months for heart recipients, respectively. In 11 patients (Group B), the vascular reconstruction was undertaken simultaneously with the renal transplantation. The mean follow up period was 49 months.

Results.—There was no arterial allograft related deaths. No signs of arterial graft infection or requirement for secondary intervention (angioplasty and/or thrombolysis) were observed during the follow up period.

Conclusions.—Our experience suggests that it is possible to use fresh arterial allografts in the treatment of arterial occlusive disease or abdominal aortic aneurysm, both in already transplanted patients and simultaneously with organ transplantation, with good results.

▶ Arterial allografts were the first arterial substitute used for arterial reconstruction. They were abandoned because of the emergence of prosthetic grafts and the patient's immune response to alloantigens. If the patient is already immune suppressed or will be because of impending transplantation, then theoretically, allografts may be useful. Indeed, the data here show they can work reasonably well under the conditions of immunosuppression. I think the use of such grafts should be very limited. Most of the patients in this series received their allografts for iliac occlusive disease, and there are, of course, other good options for treatment of occlusive iliac, such as angioplasty and endarterectomy that do not involve logistic difficulties of obtaining and implanting a fresh allograft. Nevertheless, this article reminds us that for the rare patient under unusual circumstances, fresh allografts may be appropriate. This is a technique to keep in the back of one's data bank.

G. L. Moneta, MD

Axillo-iliac Conduit for Haemodialysis Vascular Access
Hamish M, Shalhoub J, Rodd CD, et al (Charing Cross Hosp, London)
Eur J Vasc Endovasc Surg 31:530-534, 2006

Objectives.—To describe a series of venous surgical procedures performed to maintain vascular access.

Methods.—We report eight patients with end-stage renal failure (ESRF) who had complex renal access problems. Three patients had central venous occlusion and underwent veno-venous axillo-iliac bypass. In five further patients with a symptomatic central venous obstruction we performed axillo-iliac arterio-venous grafting (AVGs) in order to achieve haemodialysis access. All patients were assessed pre-operatively with duplex ultrasound and venogram of upper and lower limbs. The axillary artery or vein, and iliac vein were approached via infraclavicular and extra-peritoneal groin incisions, respectively. Non-externally-supported polytetrafluoroethylene (PTFE) was used as a conduit in all patients and anti-coagulation regimen were commenced post-operatively.

Results.—Following venous diversion surgery, there was a dramatic improvement in the facial and limb swelling experienced by the patients. There was no significant peri-operative morbidity. The veno-venous graft is still patent at 14 months in patient one, at 10 months in patient two, and 5 months in patient three. In the second group, who had arterio-venous grafts, the mean follow-up was 13.2 (7–20) months with a secondary patency rate of 80% at 6 months. Four patients had patent, usable grafts at 12 months. In two cases, graft occlusion was treated with successful thrombectomy.

Conclusion.—Axillary-iliac veno-venous diversion can overcome the symptoms and complications of superior vena cava and innominate vein obstruction. Although, axillo-iliac arterio-venous graft fistulae formation was previously described it has not been widely used. We have found the procedure to have low morbidity and advocate its use in these complex cases.

▶ The axillary vein to iliac vein conduit seems a bit of a stretch. However, they appeared to work reasonably well to both preserve an upper- extremity fistula and relieve symptoms of central venous obstruction. Six-mm nonsupported PTFE grafts were used for the venous operations. The patients received anticoagulation with warfarin postoperatively, but the target international normalized ratio was not reported.

G. L. Moneta, MD

Incidence and Management of Seroma after Arteriovenous Graft Placement
Dauria DM, Dyk P, Garvin P (St Louis Univ)
J Am Coll Surg 203:506-511, 2006

Background.—Perigraft seromas are rare complications of insertion of PTFE hemodialysis grafts. They are often difficult to treat and recurrence is common. This study evaluates the incidence, potential etiologic variables, and management strategies for seromas after prosthetic arteriovenous graft (AVG) placement.

Study Design.—A retrospective analysis of all patients undergoing AVG placement between August 2002 and December 2005 was performed to identify all patients diagnosed with seroma requiring surgical intervention. Multiple variables were analyzed to determine potential risk factors for seroma formation and outcomes of various forms of surgical management.

Results.—In this interval, 535 AVG were inserted in 427 patients. Ten patients presented with a seroma and underwent surgical treatment. Overall incidence of seroma formation was 1.7%. There was no significant difference in seroma formation based on gender, age, diabetes, lower extremity versus upper extremity placement, or loop forearm versus straight forearm grafts. A statistically significant difference was found between upper arm ($p = 0.007$) and lower arm grafts ($p = 0.04$), with upper arm grafts more prone to seroma formation. Patients undergoing bypass of the seromatous segment of graft have not had a recurrence, compared with those who were simply evacuated and have had a mean patency of 402 days.

Conclusions.—Seroma complications after AVG insertion are higher in patients with upper arm grafts. To minimize this complication, meticulous operative technique is required. If a seroma develops, the graft might still be salvageable with aggressive management, including bypass of the involved segment.

▶ The same principle of treating seromas involving extra anatomical bypass of any sort appears to apply to arteriovenous grafts. If a seroma develops, it appears the most reliable solution is to replace that segment of the graft with a new piece of polytetrafluoroethylene and tunnel this new piece through a fresh tissue plane.

G. L. Moneta, MD

Percutaneous Treatment of Dysfunctional Brescia-Cimino Fistulae Through a Radial Arterial Approach
Wang H-J, Yang Y-F (China Med Univ, Taichung, Taiwan)
Am J Kidney Dis 48:652-658, 2006

Background.—Dysfunctional Brescia-Cimino fistulae contribute to significant morbidity in hemodialysis patients. These fistulae normally are treated through a retrograde venous approach. There are no data regarding a transradial approach. Furthermore, measurement of pressure reduction in the radial artery appears to be useful.

Methods.—We retrospectively examined 50 interventions to treat 49 patients (17 men, 32 women; mean age, 61.8 ± 10.6 years) with Brescia-Cimino fistulae. Inclusion criteria were patients with palpable radial arteries and dysfunctional end-to-side Brescia-Cimino fistulae. Patients with infected fistulae, contrast allergy, upper-arm/synthetic graft/central-vein stenosis, and end-to-end Brescia-Cimino fistulae were excluded from the study. Radial arterial pressures before and after angioplasty were compared as a surrogate of stenosis relief. Anatomic and clinical success rates were calculated.

Results.—Sixty-five stenoses and 4 total occlusions were treated through radial access. All radial punctures were successful, except in 1 patient. Most lesions were located in the cephalic vein (87%). Mean length of treated lesions was 4.1 ± 2.8 cm. Mean pretreatment diameter of lesion stenoses was 76.7% ± 12.1%. Mean posttreatment diameter stenosis was 22.6% ± 8.2% ($P < 0.001$). Systolic, diastolic, and mean blood pressures recorded from the radial artery decreased from 130 ± 40, 60 ± 18, and 87 ± 27 to 88 ± 40, 43 ± 18, and 60 ± 26 mm Hg ($P < 0.001$, $P < 0.001$, and $P < 0.001$), respectively. The anatomic success rate of the transradial approach was 91.3%. The clinical success rate of the transradial approach was 96%.

Conclusion.—The transradial approach is a feasible and highly effective approach to treat dysfunctional Brescia-Cimino fistulae. Measuring blood pressure reduction through the radial artery appears promising as a hemodynamic evaluation method.

▶ The antegrade approach to a Brescia-Cimino fistula using the radial artery distal to the fistula has a number of potential advantages. First of all, 1 sheath can be used to treat any downstream lesion visualized, including occlusive lesions. The antegrade stick allows visualization of all lesions without the hassle of occluding blood pressure cuffs or tourniquets. In addition, the fistula itself does not need to be punctured or compressed at the end of the procedure. As attempts to salvage dysfunctional Brescia-Cimino fistulas with catheter-based techniques become more frequent, this seems like a good technique to remember.

G. L. Moneta, MD

Use of a Pneumatic Tourniquet Improves Outcome Following Trans-tibial Amputation

Wolthuis AM, Whitehead E, Ridler BMF, et al (Royal Devon and Exeter NHS Found Trust and Peninsula Med School, Exeter, England)
Eur J Vasc Endovasc Surg 31:642-645, 2006

Background.—It is traditionally taught that a pneumatic tourniquet is contraindicated for trans-tibial amputations in patients with peripheral arterial disease. However, tourniquets are used successfully during total knee arthroplasty in elderly patients. Vascular patients undergoing a trans-tibial amputation have a high perioperative mortality and morbidity—notably the need for wound revision or a higher amputation level. We hypothesised that a tourniquet, used during amputation, would reduce blood loss and subsequent complications without compromising healing.

Methods.—This was a prospective non-randomized study of 89 adult patients who underwent a trans-tibial amputation between January 2001 and December 2003. The endpoints were: haemoglobin levels, the need for blood transfusion, perioperative morbidity, revision rate and mortality. Patients were divided into two groups: a group with a pneumatic tourniquet ($n=42$) and a group without ($n=47$).

Results.—The haemoglobin fall was 14.8% in the non-tourniquet group and 5.6% in the tourniquet group, with a higher need for transfusion in the non-tourniquet group. The revision rate was 14.3% in the tourniquet group and significantly higher in the non-tourniquet group (38.3%). Mortality was similar in both groups: 7.1% for the tourniquet and 6.4% for the non-tourniquet group.

Conclusion.—The use of a pneumatic tourniquet is safe and significantly reduces both blood loss and transfusion requirements during trans-tibial amputation. A pneumatic tourniquet reduces revision rates by over 50%, with subsequent cost savings.

▶ This was not a randomized study. It makes sense that tourniquets could reduce blood loss, but why they appear to reduce the need for revision is not obvious and the authors do not provide a satisfactory explanation. One must conclude selection bias is the most likely reason. Nevertheless, the reduced blood loss and no real tourniquet-related complications suggest this is a reasonable adjunct to consider doing a below-the-knee amputation. There will be patients in which the technique will not work because of severe calcification of the superficial femoral artery.

G. L. Moneta, MD

Carotid Body Tumor Resection: Does the Need for Vascular Reconstruction Worsen Outcome?

Smith JJ, Passman MA, Dattilo JB, et al (Vanderbilt Univ, Nashville, Tenn)
Ann Vasc Surg 20:435-439, 2006

We evaluated outcomes after carotid body tumor resection (CBR) requiring vascular reconstruction. Patients undergoing CBR at an academic medical center between 1990 and 2005 were identified. Medical records were retrospectively reviewed for clinical data, operative details, Shamblin's classification, tumor pathology, complications, and mortality. Comparisons were performed between those undergoing CBR alone and CBR requiring vascular reconstruction (CBR-VASC). Of the 71 CBRs performed in 62 patients, 16 required vascular reconstruction (23%). Although there was no difference in mean tumor size (CBR 29.1 ± 11.9 mm, CBR-VASC 32.5 ± 9.9 mm; $p = 0.133$), carotid body tumors were more commonly Shamblin's I when CBR was performed alone (CBR 53% vs. CBR-VASC 25%, $p = 0.045$) and Shamblin's II/III when vascular reconstruction was required (CBR 47% vs. CBR-VASC 75%, $p = 0.045$). There was also a significant difference in malignant tumor pathology when vascular reconstruction was required (CBR 4.4% vs. CBR-VASC 25%, $p = 0.034$). Cranial nerve dysfunction was higher in patients requiring vascular repair (CBR 27% vs. CBR-VASC 63%, $p = 0.012$), but there was no difference in baroreflex failure (CBR 7.27% vs. CBR-VASC 0%, $p = 0.351$), Horner's syndrome (CBR 5.5% vs. CBR-VASC 6.25%, $p = 0.783$), or first bite syndrome (CBR 7.27% vs. CBR-VASC 12.5%, $p = 0.877$). There were no perioperative strokes in either group, and one death was unrelated to operation. When required, carotid artery reconstruction at the time of CBR can be performed safely. Although cranial nerve dysfunction is more common when vascular repair is required, this is more likely related to locally advanced disease and tumor pathology rather than operative techniques.

▶ Certainly one can expect more advanced tumors to require more advanced surgical techniques with a higher likelihood of local cranial nerve complications. An additional point of this article is that saphenous vein interposition grafting seems to work well in the short term. This retrospective article does not really answer the questions everybody wants to know: Is preoperative embolization ever truly necessary? Are shunts needed during vascular repair? How does the vein graft hold up over time?

G. L. Moneta, MD

19 Miscellaneous

Training with simulation improves residents' endovascular procedure skills
Dawson DL, Meyer J, Lee ES (Univ of California, Davis, Sacramento)
J Vasc Surg 45:149-154, 2007

Background.—Endovascular procedure simulators are now commercially available and in use for physician training. The purpose of this study was to evaluate the role of simulation-based training in vascular surgery residencies.

Methods.—Residents from vascular surgery programs in a five-state area were invited to participate in a series of 2-day endovascular training programs that used a high-fidelity endovascular procedure simulator (SimSuite; Medical Simulation Corporation, Denver, Colo), didactic instruction, computer-based training, and tabletop procedure demonstrations. The curriculum covered arteriography and intervention for treatment of aortoiliac, renal, and carotid artery disease. Nine residents participated, with one to three per training session. Each completed an average of 9.5 simulated endovascular cases. Performance on a standardized TransAtlantic Inter-Society Consensus B iliac angioplasty/stenting case was used to assess endovascular skills and knowledge at the beginning of the training program, and this was repeated at the completion of the training. Performance metrics were measured by the simulator, faculty observed trainees' performance of simulated cases, and trainees provided their evaluations of the usefulness of the simulation experiences.

Results.—Endovascular procedural skills on the standardized iliac intervention case improved after completion of the training program. Compared with performance early on day 1, performance improved ($P \leq .05$; paired t test): total procedure time decreased 54%, volume of contrast decreased 44%, and fluoroscopy time decreased 48% (mean change from baseline). Selection of angioplasty balloon catheters and stents was improved, and the average number of catheters used and stents deployed decreased, although this did not reach statistical significance. Faculty observation allowed identification of shortcomings of knowledge and skills, including common problems with selection of catheter, balloon, and stent sizes; correct positioning of the sheath; and intraprocedural monitoring. Postcourse evaluations indicated support for the use of simulation in vascular surgery residents' endovascular training.

Conclusions.—Training with a simulator, incorporated into an individual or small group learning session, offers a means to learn and realistically practice endovascular procedures without direct risk to patients, with measurable improvements in key performance metrics. How simulation training affects subsequent clinical performance has yet to be established.

▶ The authors apply their interest in aviation simulation to endovascular training by using a high-fidelity simulator. Simulation helped improve procedural tasks in the 9 residents with basic endovascular experience who participated in this study. Importantly, fluoroscopic time and contrast volume diminished with simulator training on straightforward iliac (TransAtlantic Inter-Society Consensus B lesions) cases and other procedures for occlusive disease. Whether this expensive training modality will have an impact on clinical performance remains unknown.

G. L. Moneta, MD

The examination assessment of technical competence in vascular surgery
Pandey VA, for the European Board of Vascular Surgery (St Mary's Hosp, London; Athens Univ, Greece; Univ Hosp, Uppsala, Sweden)
Br J Surg 93:1132-1138, 2006

Background.—The European Board of Surgery Qualification in Vascular Surgery is a pan-European examination for vascular surgeons who have attained a national certificate of completion of specialist training. A 2-year study was conducted before the introduction of a technical skills assessment in the examination.

Methods.—The study included 30 surgeons: 22 candidates and eight examiners. They were tested on dissection (on a synthetic saphenofemoral junction model), anastomosis (on to anterior tibial artery of a synthetic leg model) and dexterity (a knot-tying simulator with electromagnetic motion analysis). Validated rating scales were used by two independent examiners. Composite knot-tying scores were calculated for the computerized station. The stations were weighted 35, 45 and 20 percent, respectively.

Results.—Examiners performed better than candidates in the dissection $(P < 0.001)$, anastomosis $(P = 0.002)$ and dexterity $(P = 0.005)$ stations (Fig 1). Participants performed consistently in the examination (dissection *versus* anastomosis: $r = 0.79$, $P < 0.001$; dexterity *versus* total operative score: $r = -0.73$, $P < 0.001$). Interobserver reliability was high ($\alpha = 0.91$). No correlation was seen between a candidate's technical skill and oral examination performance or logbook-accredited scores.

Conclusion.—Current surgical examinations do not address technical competence. This model appears to be a valid assessment of technical skills in an examination setting. The standards are set at a level appropriate for a specialist vascular surgeon.

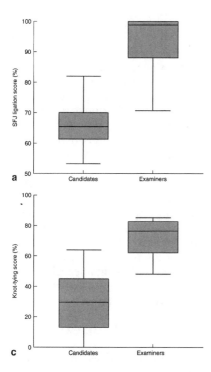

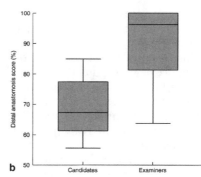

FIGURE 1.—Box plot representing performance of candidates and examiners in each station. Horizontal lines within boxes, boxes and error bars represent median, interquartile range and range of marks respectively. **a,** Saphenofemoral junction (SFJ) ligation ($P < 0.001$). **b,** Distal anastomosis ($P = 0.002$). **c,** Motion analysis on the knot-tying task ($P < 0.001$). (Courtesy of Pandey VA, for the European Board of Vascular Surgery. The examination assessment of technical competence in vascular surgery. *Br J Surg.* 2006;93:1132-1138. Reprinted by permission of Blackwell Publishing.)

▶ The authors point out that it seems silly not to assess technical skills in a certifying examination for a surgeon. Nevertheless, it is extremely unusual for technical skills to be assessed in a national certifying surgical examination. Before implementing this type of assessment, it seems prudent to correlate results of scores from this examination with established surgeons' morbidity and mortality rates, as well as rates of technical error in day-to-day practice. I know of no movement to incorporate a technical skills examination into the current North American certifying examination for vascular surgery.

G. L. Moneta, MD

Continuity of care experience of residents in an academic vascular department: Are trainees learning complete surgical care?

Gagnon J, Melck A, Kamal D, et al (Univ of British Columbia, Vancouver, Canada)
J Vasc Surg 43:999-1003, 2006

Background.—It is widely accepted that exemplary surgical care involves a surgeon's involvement in the preoperative, perioperative, and postoperative periods. In an era of ever-expanding therapeutic modalities available to the vascular surgeon, it is important that trainees gain experience in preoperative decision-making and how this affects a patient's operative and postoperative course. The purpose of this study was to define the current experience of residents on a vascular surgery service regarding the continuity of care they are able to provide for patients and the factors affecting this experience.

Methods.—This prospective cohort study was approved by the Institutional Review Board and conducted at the University of British Columbia during January 2005. All patients who underwent a vascular procedure at either of the two teaching hospitals were included. In addition to type of case (emergent, outpatient, inpatient), resident demographic data and involvement in each patient's care (preoperative assessment, postoperative daily assessment, and follow-up clinic assessment) were recorded. Categoric data were analyzed with the χ^2 test.

Results.—The study included 159 cases, of which 65% were elective same-day admission patients, 20% were elective previously admitted patients; and 15% were emergent. The overall rate of preoperative assessment was 67%, involvement in the decision to operate, 17%; postoperative assessment on the ward, 79%; and patient follow-up in clinic, 3%. The rate of complete in-hospital continuity of care (assessing patient pre-op and post-op) was 57%. Emergent cases were associated with a significantly higher rate of preoperative assessment (92% vs 63%, $P < .05$) (Fig 2). For elective cases admitted before the day of surgery compared with same-day admission patients, the rates of preoperative assessment (78% vs 58%, $P < .05$) and involvement in the decision to operate (16% vs 4%, $P < .05$) were significantly higher (Fig 3).

Conclusions.—The continuity-of-care experiences of vascular trainees are suboptimal. This is especially true for postoperative clinic assessment. Same-day admission surgery accounted for most of the cases and was associated with the poorest continuity of care. To provide complete surgical training in an era of changing therapeutic modalities and same-day admission surgery, vascular programs must be creative in structuring training to include adequate ambulatory experience.

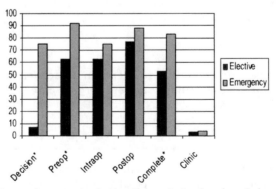

FIGURE 2.—Percent of cases associated with resident continuity of care for each phase of patient contact for emergent vs elective cases. *$P < .05$. (Courtesy of Gagnon J, Melck A, Kamal D, et al. Continuity of care experience of residents in an academic vascular department: are trainees learning complete surgical care? *J Vasc Surg.* 2006;43:999-1003. Copyright 2006 by Elsevier. Reprinted by permission.)

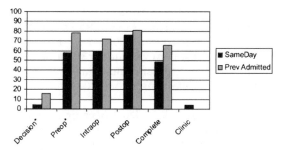

FIGURE 3.—Percent of cases associated with resident continuity of care for each phase of patient contact for elective same-day admission vs elective previously admitted patients. *$P < .05$. (Courtesy of Gagnon J, Melck A, Kamal D, et al. Continuity of care experience of residents in an academic vascular department: are trainees learning complete surgical care? *J Vasc Surg.* 2006;43:999-1003. Copyright 2006 by Elsevier. Reprinted by permission.)

▶ This study confirms what most educators suspected. Our trainees participate in aspects of patient care, but rarely have a complete continuity-of-care experience with a patient. This trend will likely worsen as more patients undergo same-day admission, and work restrictions force residents to cherry-pick parts of the surgical care of most interest (ie, the operating room). Despite the discussion of some modest residency changes, I suspect the definitive answer will be a change in training paradigms to include independent training of vascular surgeons.

G. L. Moneta, MD

Claims, Errors, and Compensation Payments in Medical Malpractice Litigation
Studdert DM, Mello MM, Gawande AA, et al (Harvard School of Public Health, Boston; Brigham and Women's Hosp, Boston; Harvard Risk Management Found, Boston)
N Engl J Med 354:2024-2033, 2006

Background.—In the current debate over tort reform, critics of the medical malpractice system charge that frivolous litigation—claims that lack evidence of injury, substandard care, or both—is common and costly.

Methods.—Trained physicians reviewed a random sample of 1452 closed malpractice claims from five liability insurers to determine whether a medical injury had occurred and, if so, whether it was due to medical error. We analyzed the prevalence, characteristics, litigation outcomes, and costs of claims that lacked evidence of error.

Results.—For 3 percent of the claims, there were no verifiable medical injuries, and 37 percent did not involve errors. Most of the claims that were not associated with errors (370 of 515 [72 percent]) or injuries (31 of 37 [84 percent]) did not result in compensation; most that involved injuries due to error did (653 of 889 [73 percent]). Payment of claims not involving errors occurred less frequently than did the converse form of inaccuracy—nonpayment of claims associated with errors. When claims not involving errors were compensated, payments were significantly lower on average than were payments for claims involving errors ($313,205 vs. $521,560, P=0.004). Overall, claims not involving errors accounted for 13 to 16 percent of the system's total monetary costs. For every dollar spent on compensation, 54 cents went to administrative expenses (including those involving lawyers, experts, and courts). Claims involving errors accounted for 78 percent of total administrative costs.

Conclusions.—Claims that lack evidence of error are not uncommon, but most are denied compensation. The vast majority of expenditures go toward litigation over errors and payment of them. The overhead costs of malpractice litigation are exorbitant.

▶ The report indicates that contrary to popular belief, the malpractice system may not be inundated with frivolous litigation. This sort of makes sense as malpractice is a business, and people tend not to pursue what is unlikely to be profitable. As the article demonstrates, frivolous claims are unlikely to result in payment. However, it also points out that 1 in 6 claims actually involving error did not result in payment. The system still seems broken. It is neither adequately sensitive nor specific, and the overhead is ridiculous. Eliminating frivolous claims may not reduce the cost of the malpractice system. However, it does seem that efforts to compensate true malpractice victims appropriately but not excessively, and limiting the overhead of the system will work to the benefit of both patients and most physicians, although perhaps not to the benefit of attorneys and so-called "experts."

G. L. Moneta, MD

Subject Index

A

Abdominal aortic aneurysm
endovascular repair
anesthesia type and outcome after, 144
AneuRx endografts for, effect of challenging neck anatomy on mid-term migration rates, 149
with branched and fenestrated endografts, 182, 183
contrast-enhanced duplex surveillance after, with continuous infusion technique, 85
CT evaluation after, elimination of arterial phase, 81
CT vs. MRI for endoleak detection and classification after, 83
duplex ultrasound scanning for endoleak detection after, 84
hypogastric artery bypass and embolization during, 146
long-term outcome
12-year experience, 139
factors affecting mortality, 142
in patients at high risk for open surgery, 141
vs. open repair
in hemodynamically stable patients after 1-year follow-up, cost analysis, 155
in VA hospitals, 143
preservation of pelvic circulation with hypogastric artery bypass during, 148
secondary interventions following, 151
treatment of type II endoleaks, 152
expansion rate, influence of sex on, 124
experimental
deletion of $p45^{phox}$ and attenuation of, 25
hypertension and upregulation of nuclear factor κB and ets in, 22
oral administration of diferuloylmethane and suppression of proinflammatory cytokines and destructive connective tissue remodeling in, 26
regression by inhibition of c-Jun N-terminal kinase, 27
temporal changes in aortic wall gene expression in, 24
ischemic colitis following repair
inferior mesentery artery replantation and incidence of, 129

intraoperative colon mucosal saturation for prevention of, 154
N-acetylcysteine for prevention of kidney injury in surgery for, 128
N-terminal pro-B-type natriuretic peptide as long-term prognostic marker following repair, 94
N-terminal pro-B-type natriuretic peptide levels and postoperative cardiac events, 96
open repair
age-stratified, perioperative, and one-year mortality after, 127
factors affecting outcomes, 130
outcome of common iliac arteries after straight aortic tube-graft placement during, 135
preoperative and intraoperative determinants of incisional bulge following, 131
wound complications and erectile dysfunction following, 132
perioperative myocardial ischemia injury in high-risk patients, incidence and clinical significance, 90
preoperative cardiac testing in intermediate-risk patients on beta-blocker therapy with tight heart rate control, 89
psychiatric morbidity after repair, 137
rupture
ACE inhibitors and, 133
matrix metalloproteinase-8 and -9 levels at site of, 21
outcomes at regional trauma centers vs. other acute care hospitals, 134
screening in women, cost-effectiveness, 123
small
continued surveillance and suitability for endovascular repair, 126
growth rate and associated factors, 125
statins and renal function after aortic cross clamping during repair, 98
Acute coronary syndrome
placental growth factor levels and adverse outcomes at four-year follow-up, 42
Acute lung injury
comparison of 2 fluid-management strategies for, 109
Aging
differential effects on limb blood flow in humans, 7

H

Hemodialysis
  access (*see also* Arteriovenous fistulae;
    Arteriovenous grafts)
    asymptomatic central venous stenosis
      in, 254
    axillo-iliac conduit for, 381
    dysfunctional, inflow stenoses in, 251
    mortality risk with change from
      catheter to arteriovenous fistula or
      graft, 253
    percutaneous treatment of
      dysfunctional Brescia-Cimino fistula
      through a radial arterial approach,
      383
    atherosclerotic renovascular disease in
      older patients starting, 249
Heparin
  fixed-dose weight-adjusted
    unfractionated vs.
    low-molecular-weight, for acute
    treatment of venous
    thromboembolism, 333
  low-molecular-weight
    long-term therapy vs. usual care in
      proximal vein thrombosis in cancer
      patients, 334
    for prevention of restenosis after
      femoropopliteal angioplasty, 216
  unfractionated, vs. enoxaparin in
    elective percutaneous coronary
    intervention, 40
Heparin immobilization
  for reduced thrombogenicity of
    small-caliber expanded
    polytetrafluoroethylene grafts, 115
Heparin-induced thrombocytopenia
  effects of argatroban therapy,
    demographic variables, and platelet
    count on thrombotic risks in, 105
Hepatocyte growth factor
  for secondary lymphedema in animal
    models, 377
Hirudin/iloprost coating
  for prevention of pseudointima and
    intimal hyperplasia in
    small-diameter expanded
    polytetrafluoroethylene grafts, 117
Homocysteine
  lowering with B vitamins, effect on
    cognitive performance in healthy
    older people, 58
  lowering with folic acid and B vitamins,
    effect on cardiovascular events in
    vascular disease, 57

Human immunodeficiency virus (HIV)
  infection
  role of combination antiretroviral
    therapy in subclinical carotid
    atherosclerosis, 298
Hyperhidrosis
  isolated axillary, T3-T4 vs. T4
    sympathectomy for, 322
  upper limb, quality of life after
    endoscopic sympathetic block for,
    323
Hypertension
  drug-resistant, implantable carotid sinus
    stimulator for, 327
  in experimental abdominal aortic
    aneurysm, effect on upregulation of
    nuclear factor κB and ets in, 22
Hypobaric hypoxia
  effect on coagulation, fibrinolysis,
    platelet function, and endothelial
    activation, 329
Hypogastric artery
  bypass and embolization during
    endovascular aneurysm repair, 146
  bypass during endovascular aneurysm
    repair, effect on pelvic circulation,
    148
Hypotension
  requiring vasopressor support after
    carotid artery angioplasty and
    stenting, factors associated with,
    276

I

Iliac artery
  aneurysm, endovascular treatment with
    a tubular stent-graft, 156
  stent placement combined with
    saphenous ablation for complex
    severe chronic venous disease, 365
  subintimal angioplasty and stenting for
    chronic total occlusion, true lumen
    re-entry devices for facilitation of,
    221
Iliac vein
  venous claudication due to obstruction
    of, inferior vena cava stenting for,
    369
Iliorenal bypass
  indications and outcomes, 161
Inferior vena cava
  leiomyosarcoma of
    prosthetic replacement for, 315
    surgery and chemotherapy for, 316
  obstructive lesions, clinical features and
    endovenous treatment, 367

Author Index